AF479165

Biological Responses in Cancer

Volume 3
Immunomodulation by
Anticancer Drugs

Biological Responses in Cancer

Series Editor
ENRICO MIHICH

Grace Cancer Drug Center
Roswell Park Memorial Institute
Buffalo, New York

Editorial Board

A Continuation Order Plan is available for this series. A continuation order will bring delivery of each new volume immediately upon publication. Volumes are billed only upon actual shipment. For further information please contact the publisher.

Biological Responses in Cancer

Volume 3
Immunomodulation by
Anticancer Drugs

Edited by
Enrico Mihich

Grace Cancer Drug Center
Roswell Park Memorial Institute
Buffalo, New York

and
Yoshio Sakurai

Cancer Chemotherapy Center
Japanese Foundation for Cancer Research
Tokyo, Japan

Advisory Board

Alexander Fefer, *Seattle, Washington*
Hiroshi Kobayashi, *Sapporo, Japan*
Federico Spreafico, *Milan, Italy*
John L. Turk, *London, England*
Takeo Wada, *Sapporo, Japan*

PLENUM PRESS • NEW YORK AND LONDON

The Library of Congress cataloged the first volume in this series as follows:

Main entry under title:

Biological responses in cancer.

  Includes bibliographical references and index.
  1. Cancer—Immunological aspects. 2. Immune response. I. Mihich, Enrico.
[DNLM: 1. Neoplasms—Physiopathology. 2. Cell transformation, Neoplastic. 3.
Neoplasm invasiveness. 4. Neoplasm metastasis. QZ 202 B6157]
RC268.3.B56 1982   616.99′4079   82-18041

ISBN 0-306-41879-7

CONTRIBUTORS

M. JANE EHRKE, Grace Cancer Drug Center, Roswell Park Memorial Institute, Buffalo, New York 14263

MASUO HOSOKAWA, Laboratory of Pathology, Cancer Institute, Hokkaido University School of Medicine, Sapporo 060, Japan

MASAAKI ISHIZUKA, Institute of Microbial Chemistry, Microbial Chemistry Research Foundation, Tokyo 141, Japan

TATESHI KATAOKA, Division of Experimental Chemotherapy, Cancer Chemotherapy Center, Japanese Foundation for Cancer Research, Tokyo 170, Japan

ALBERTO MANTOVANI, Laboratory of Human Immunology, Mario Negri Institute for Pharmacological Research, 20157 Milan, Italy

ENRICO MIHICH, Grace Cancer Drug Center, Roswell Park Memorial Institute, Buffalo, New York 14263

FRED R. MILLER, Department of Immunology, Michigan Cancer Foundation, Detroit, Michigan 48201

HOWARD OZER, Tumor Immunology Laboratory, Department of Medical Oncology, Roswell Park Memorial Institute, Buffalo, New York 14263

FEDERICO SPREAFICO, Departments of Oncology and Immunology, Mario Negri Institute for Pharmacological Research, 20157 Milan, Italy

RAINER STORB, Fred Hutchinson Cancer Research Center, and Division of Oncology, Department of Medicine, University of Washington School of Medicine, Seattle, Washington 98104

JOHN L. TURK, Department of Pathology, Royal College of Surgeons of England, London WC2A 3PN, England

ANNUNCIATA VECCHI, Departments of Oncology and Immunology, Mario Negri Institute for Pharmacological Research, 20157 Milan, Italy

PREFACE

The series of volumes entitled *Biological Responses in Cancer* provides information on approaches through which the interaction between neoplastic and normal cells may be modified. Topics to be dealt with include immunologic and host defense systems, control mechanisms of cell and population growth, cell differentiation, and cell transformation.

The regulatory mechanisms controlling the interactions between normal and tumor cells may be immunologic in nature. While the central question of tumor immunology addresses the nature and uniqueness of tumor-associated antigens in humans, the identification of the stages of differentiation and functions of the various cell types involved in immunity is advancing rapidly. The development of monoclonal antibody methodologies—together with progress in the biochemical characterization of cell markers, cell separation, and measurement of cell functions—has significantly aided in the identification and quantitation of different cell types. Establishing the role of these cells in the regulation of human immune mechanisms offers a means for evaluating the status of the immune responses in cancer patients and for assessing the effects that tumor and antitumor treatments may exert on their functionality and which, in turn, may alter the effects of antitumor treatments.

Biological responses can be modified through the administration of agents that act on cells mediating such responses. Thus, a minimal immune response may be altered by means of immunomodulating agents. The immune system and related systems such as macrophages and natural killer cells represent perhaps the most immediate targets for the development of new treatments based on biological response modification, due in large part to the recent advances that have been made in the understanding of these systems and their regulation. Among the agents that are able to exert immunomodulating effects leading to augmentation or reduction of immunologic responses to tumor are the antitumor agents, taken as a group.

In July 1983 a two-day seminar was held in Sapporo, Japan, under the auspices of the Sapporo Cancer Foundation, to discuss specifically the immunomodulating effects of anticancer agents and their potential therapeutic exploitation. In the discussions held at that meeting it became apparent that alkylating agents, antibiotics, and antimetabolites may exert different immunomodulating effects depending on the model system used and the interactions between pharmacologic and immunologic phenomena involved. It was clear that it is also possible to dissect the immune system based on responses to a drug, this approach contributing to the acquisition of new basic knowledge on the heterogeneity, cellular specifications, and control mechanisms of the system. The opportunities for selective intervention with drugs were emphasized at the seminar, as were the inherent difficulties in generalizing the potential therapeutic significance of phenomena which may be restricted to specific models and/or conditions. It became clear, however, that immunomodulation may be therapeutically exploited using drugs which are usually employed essentially for their cytotoxic action.

The undersigned were of the opinion that it would be timely to discuss immunomodulation by anticancer agents in a volume which would be inspired by the topics discussed at the Sapporo Cancer Seminar without, however, representing the proceedings of that meeting. An *ad hoc* advisory board was formed which included Drs. A. Fefer, H. Kobayashi, F. Spreafico, J. L. Turk, T. Wada, E. Mihich, and Y. Sakurai under the chairmanship of Dr. Sakurai, and in view of the obvious appropriateness of the subject discussed the decision was made to publish the volume within this series.

In this volume current knowledge on the regulation of the immune response is briefly outlined only to provide a background on which to visualize the specific effects induced by drugs. The immunomodulating effects of antimetabolites are reviewed based on the examples provided by the thiopurines, DTIC, pyrimidine analogues, antifolates, and Ara C. The selective effects of Adriamycin and the augmenting or permissive effects of several antibiotics, most of them developed in Japan, are discussed. The effects of alkylating agents, particularly those of cyclophosphamide, on the regulation of the immune systems are reviewed. Immunomodulation by *Vinca* alkaloids, platinum complexes, nitrosoureas, dicarbazine, adenosine deaminase inhibitors, and glucocorticoids is reviewed. The use of anticancer drugs in bone marrow transplantation is also briefly discussed. In conclusion, in this volume the evidence that anticancer drugs have immunomodulating activity is discussed with emphasis on the large number of questions that still need to be answered to understand the action of the individual agents considered as well as the generality of the phenomena observed. It is the objective of this volume to contribute to progress in the area discussed through stimulation of further research and productive interactions among readers with diversified expertise.

ACKNOWLEDGMENT. The editors wish to express their appreciation for the excellent support provided by Ms. Jessie Crowe in editorial matters related to the preparation of this volume.

Buffalo, New York, USA   E. Mihich
Tokyo, Japan   Y. Sakurai
Sapporo, Japan   H. Kobayashi

CONTENTS

CHAPTER 2

INTERACTIONS OF ANTIMETABOLITES WITH TUMORS AND THE IMMUNE SYSTEM

FRED R. MILLER AND TATESHI KATAOKA

CHAPTER 3

IMMUNOMODULATION BY ANTIBIOTICS

ENRICO MIHICH, M. JANE EHRKE, AND MASAAKI ISHIZUKA

CHAPTER 4

EFFECTS OF ALKYLATING AGENTS ON IMMUNOREGULATORY MECHANISMS

HOWARD OZER

CHAPTER 5

THE IMMUNOMODULATORY ACTIVITY OF CERTAIN CANCER CHEMOTHERAPEUTIC AGENTS

FEDERICO SPREAFICO AND ANNUNCIATA VECCHI

CHAPTER 6

EFFECT OF GLUCOCORTICOID HORMONES ON THE IMMUNE SYSTEM

ALBERTO MANTOVANI

CHAPTER 7

ANTICANCER AGENTS IN BONE MARROW TRANSPLANTATION

RAINER STORB

CHAPTER 1

REGULATION OF THE IMMUNE RESPONSE

JOHN L. TURK and MASUO HOSOKAWA

1. GENERAL ASPECTS

1.1. Introduction

Immune responses are ultimately controlled by genes, most of which are found in the major histocompatability complex (MHC). Both control and regulation of immune responses are a function of the I region of the MHC and are mainly under *Ir* (immune response) gene control. Regulation results from the interaction of T lymphocytes, B lymphocytes, and macrophages, by both cell surface interaction and the secretion of soluble products.

This chapter outlines the mechanisms of regulation. The first half gives a general description of regulatory mechanisms as they affect the immune response as a whole. The second part is concerned with the regulation of the immune response as it occurs, particularly in experimental and human models of cancer. Many regulatory systems have only been identified as a result of their abrogation by immunosuppressive agents. There is therefore some degree of overlap with what is said in other chapters. However, this may help to emphasize the close interaction between data obtained from the search for therapeutic agents and fundamental biological research.

Regulation of the immune response is known to involve idiotypic determinants through the idiotypic network, T-cell receptors through helper and suppressor factors, and immunoglobulins that may reduce a cell-mediated immune response by the process known as "immunological enhancement." In addition we consider the phenomenon of immunological tolerance

---

JOHN L. TURK ● Department of Pathology, Royal College of Surgeons of England, London, WC2A 3PN, England.   MASUO HOSOKAWA ● Laboratory of Pathology, Cancer Institute, Hokkaido University School of Medicine, Sapporo 060, Japan.

in the absence of demonstrable suppressor cells, which could result from specific inhibition of clonal proliferation that might be induced directly by antigen. Another subject considered is the role of macrophages in regulating the immune response. Macrophages are important in handling and presenting antigen. However, they have also been found to play a supporting role in the regulation of lymphocyte proliferation, as well as in controlling cellular infiltration in the periphery. Subpopulations of mononuclear phagocytes involved in immunoregulation appear to carry surface-membrane-associated Ia antigens similar to those carried by lymphocytes involved in the immune response (Table I).

1.2. The Role of the Major Histocompatibility Complex in the Regulation of the Immune Response

The MHC is situated on chromosome 6 in man and chromosome 17 in the mouse. In man it is referred to as the human leukocyte A (HLA) system and in the mouse as the H2 system. The HLA controls three major characteristics: (1) alloantigens, (2) thymus-dependent immune responses, and (3) some components of the complement cascade. The thymus-dependent immune responses are controlled by genes that lie in the I region of the MHC. This region also codes for Ia antigens, which are specific glycoproteins that play an integral part in the regulation of the immune response. These are identified in man as DR antigens. In the mouse the I region has two genetic subregions coding for Ia molecules. There are two sets of Ia antigens, the I–A and the I–E in the mouse, and correspondingly it is likely that there are two sets of DR antigens in man (Morling *et al.*, 1982). Ia antigens are present on the surface of macrophages as well as lymphocytes and thus also play an important role in antigen presentation. The surface membrane expression of Ia antigens of these cell types is particularly important in the mechanism of action of the associated *Ir* genes in the genetic control of the immune response. The ability of macrophages to process antigen for presentation to

TABLE I
Mechanisms of Regulation of the Immune Response

Genetic control by major histocompatibility complex
Network formed by autoantiidiotypic antibodies
Helper T lymphocytes
Suppressor T lymphocytes
Suppressor B lymphocytes
Immunological enhancement by blocking antibody
Inhibition of clonal proliferation by antigen (immunological tolerance)
Lymphokines
Prostaglandins
Thymic hormones
Macrophages

T cells is also under genetic control and shows marked restriction at the I region (Rosenthal and Shevach, 1973). The interaction between the T cell on the one hand and foreign antigen and MHC (Ia) antigen could take place in a number of ways involving separate receptors on the T cell or a single composite receptor. The foreign antigen on the surface of the macrophage may be separate from the Ia antigen or combined with the Ia antigen.

Another example of genetic restriction of the immune response is the demonstration that cytotoxic T cells will lyse only virus-infected cells with which they share a major transplantation antigen (Zinkernagel and Doherty, 1974). It has therefore been suggested that the MHC could form part of the antigen specificity in T-cell-mediated reactions with target cells. This gave rise to the *altered self* concept: it was suggested that virus-immune T cells are sensitized to altered self cell surface antigens, whose expression might be controlled by genes at or near the H2-K or H2-D loci in the mouse. A similar genetic restriction has been found for the specificity of mouse splenic lymphocytes cytotoxic for trinitrophenyl (TNP)-modified target cells, which must share antigens whose expression is controlled at the K and I region to obtain maximum effect (Forman, 1975). This finding, together with the observations of Miller and his colleagues (Vadas *et al.*, 1977) that identity at the MHC was essential for successful transfer of delayed hypersensitivity in mice, could be interpreted as support for the altered self concept in delayed hypersensitivity. The mechanisms through which antigen associates with MHC-coded gene products to form a new altered self or altered antigen is far from clear. Thus in the case of a soluble antigen such as fowl gamma globulin, absolute identity at the I region is necessary, whereas with contact sensitivity identity at either K, I, or D is sufficient.

Two hypotheses exist to explain genetic restriction of the immune response (Zinkernagel and Doherty, 1977). In the first the requirement is for dual recognition. In this hypothesis T cells interact with specific antigen and then subsequently interact with "self." In the second or altered self hypothesis, the individual is sensitized to altered cell surface structures. Such a hypothesis is easy to envisage in a virus or contact sensitivity model. However, it is more difficult to imagine with antigens such as fowl gamma globulin.

HLA restriction of immune reaction has also been demonstrated in a number of *in vitro* human systems involving the lysis by cytotoxic T cells of influenza-virus-infected or haptenated (DNP) target cells (McMichael *et al.*, 1977; Dickmeiss *et al.*, 1977). These findings together with the well-known association between HLA and disease confirm the importance of the MHC in the control and regulation of the immune system in man.

1.3. Antiidiotypic Antibody: The Network Theory

The antigen-combining site of an antibody not only combines with antigen but is antigenic in its own right. The antigenicity of the site is dependent on its specific amino acid sequence in the variable region. This also provides it with its unique antigenicity, which thus reflects its antigen-combining ability and is referred to as its idiotypic determinant (Id). The Id can thus induce an anti-Id antibody. According to the network theory (Jerne, 1974), the idiotypic determinants of the antibody molecules elicit an anti-Id auto-antibody response during a normal immune response. The antigen-combining sites of T cells show a similar idiotype to the antigen-combining site of immunoglobulins directed against the same epitope (antigenic determinant). Thus naturally occurring idiotype suppressor T cells may also be observed.

The network theory considers the immune system as a web of idiotype–antiidiotype interactions. Antiidiotypic antibodies can stimulate or depress the immune response, thus providing positive and negative immunoregulatory control. Specific antiidiotypic antibodies given immediately before or just after immunization have been found to decrease significantly delayed hypersensitivity responses to pneumococcal vaccine (Julius et al., 1977). Small doses stimulated the development of delayed hypersensitivity to the same determinant. Similar results were found by Sy et al. (1980) using the response to the azobenzene arsonate hapten. In studies on contact sensitivity to dinitrofluorobenzene, which is a transient phenomenon in the mouse occurring on day 5 after sensitization and declining on day 8, Sy et al. (1979) found an inhibitory factor in the serum that behaved as an anti-idiotype autoantibody. This factor was removed by antimouse Ig immuno-sorbent and immune lymphoid cells but not by dinitrophenylated keyhole limpet hemocyanin or anti-DNP antibody immunoadsorbent. It has been suggested that suppressor B cells, which are found to regulate T-cell function in certain delayed hypersensitivity reactions (Katz et al., 1974), might also be producing similar antiidiotype autoantibodies.

1.4. Regulatory T Lymphocytes and B Lymphocytes

Another major advance in our understanding of the immune response has been the realization that T lymphocytes are not just involved directly in cell-mediated immune reactions but are important in the regulation of almost all immune responses. The action of these cells is usually antigen specific. However, many of the factors produced once the cells have interacted with antigen act nonspecifically on cells involved in the immune reaction, whether T cells, B cells, or macrophages. The regulatory activity of T cells may play a positive or negative role. Thus we talk about *helper T* (T_H) *cells* or *suppressor T* (T_S) *cells.* Helper T cells and suppressor T cells in the mouse belong to distinct subpopulations of T cells (Cantor and Boyse, 1975) that can be recognized by specific antigenic determinants. Helper T cells in the mouse are Lyt 1^+23^-, while T_S cells are Lyt 1^-23^+. Helper T cells are cyclophosphamide insensitive, whereas T_S cells are a cyclophosphamide-sensitive population. In man helper cells have also been shown to carry distinct antigens recognizable by specific monoclonal antibodies. Helper T cells carry OKT_4 or Leu_3 antigens, whereas T_S cells are OKT_8 or Leu_2

positive. In a number of acquired immunodeficiency states in man, there is a reversal of the normal T_H/T_S ratio, related directly to the immunosuppressed state.

The first observation leading to an identification of T_H cells was the demonstration that normal thymus function was important for the full manifestation of a B-cell response. Identification of a specific population of T_H cells has led to the demonstration in a number of experiments of the release of soluble T helper factors. Progress in this field was slow until the use of T-cell cloning techniques (Fischer *et al.*, 1981). A number of reports on the soluble products of T_H-cell clones indicate that these products may be a heterogeneous mixture of antigen-specific and MHC-restricted factors with molecular weight varying between 10,000 and 70,000. Helper-T-cell function does not appear to play a role in the immune response to polysaccharide antigens, although it seems to be important in the response to antigens containing a protein moiety. Much of the work on T-helper factors has been with influenza virus, as well as sheep erythrocytes as antigens in the mouse.

There is some controversy as to whether T_H cells always act through soluble T helper factor. This is particularly important with reference to cell surface antigens, which matter most in various models of cancer. Mitchison (1980) has suggested that there may be direct cell-to-cell instruction by means of a bridge between the T and B cell consisting of antigen together with the Ia molecule, and believes that this perhaps plays an important role in the response to the MHC. There appears to be evidence also that the T_H cells show marked genetic restriction, which cannot be abrogated by the addition of appropriate macrophages.

The demonstration that the state of immunological tolerance could be transferred from one animal to another by lymphocytes (Gershon and Kondo, 1971) opened up the whole field of suppressor cells that can suppress or regulate the immune response. Initially most of the models studied were those of *immunological tolerance*, in which an animal was made unresponsive by a large dose of antigen generally given by the intravenous route. These suppressor cells were mainly T lymphocytes (Zembala and Asherson, 1973). Suppressor T cells in initial animal studies were found to be mainly antigen specific. Suppressor T cells in human and mouse lymphocyte cultures can be stimulated nonspecifically by the plant mitogen concanavalin A (Con A). In mouse models a soluble immune response suppressor (SIRS) can be released from Con-A-activated Lyt 2^+ T cells that nonspecifically suppresses the immune response of B cells to sheep erythrocytes *in vitro* (Rich and Pierce, 1973). The target of SIRS is the macrophage suppressor factor, which acts not only on normal proliferating B cells but also on proliferating neoplastic cells *in vitro* (Aune and Pierce, 1983). SIRS has been produced by a T-cell hybridoma and has been shown to be a single polypeptide chain of molecular weight 21,500.

Antigen specific T_S have now been demonstrated in a wide range of immune responses, both T cell mediated and involving antibody production. These include many tumor models as well as chemical contact sensitivity

(Glaser, 1979a,b; Schwartz *et al.*, 1978). In a number of these studies the precursors of these cells have been shown to be sensitive to cyclophosphamide. Treatment of animals with cyclophosphamide results, therefore, in an increase in the immune response and in the case of tumor-bearing animals, in an increase in the mean time to death.

Studies in the laboratory of one of us (JLT) over the past 12 years have indicated a population of B lymphocytes that regulates delayed hypersensitivity reactions in the guinea pig (Turk and Parker, 1982). These suppressor cells are not destroyed by anti-T-cell serum that destroys the T cells that transfer delayed hypersensitivity in the guinea pig (Ota *et al.*, 1979). At the same time the suppressor cells may be removed by passage through a degalan bead column coated with specific anti-guinea-pig immunoglobulin antibody prepared in the rabbit, indicating that they have surface Fc receptors (Katz *et al.*, 1974). These cells will specifically suppress the delayed hypersensitivity reactions in guinea pigs whose own suppressor cells have temporarily been destroyed by cyclophosphamide pretreatment. Other evidence for suppressor B lymphocytes has been provided during normal sensitization of the mouse with picryl chloride by Zembala *et al.* (1976) using similar transfer studies.

The specificity of reaction of such B cells in the guinea pig (Katz *et al.*, 1974) and the failure of transfer with serum from the same animals, indicate a membrane-bound receptor that is probably an immunoglobulin. A recent suggestion is that this may turn out to be an autoantiidiotypic antibody. Another possibility is that this is an enhancing antibody with affinity for antigen stronger than the T-cell receptor that mediates the delayed hypersensitivity reaction.

1.5. Regulation of the Immune Response by Antibodies against the Immunogen

Suppression of the immune response by "blocking antibody" has been termed *immunological enhancement* (Kaliss, 1958) or *immunological facilitation* (Voisin, 1971). Immunological enhancement refers particularly to "enhancement of tumor growth" in those models where suppression of the immune response leads to increased tumor growth. Feldman (1972) preferred the term *immunological blockade*, defining this as the inhibition or delay by antibodies of an immune response to specific antigens. Although originally described in relation to tumor growth, antibody has been shown to block delayed hypersensitivity, experimental autoimmune disease, and renal graft rejection. Blocking antibody has mainly been found to be IgG, often associated with cytotoxic or hemagglutinating activity. However, Fabre and Batchelor (1975), working on passive enhancement of renal allografts, found no link whatsoever between enhancing and cytotoxic antibodies. Voisin (1980) found strong anaphylactic but no complement-fixing activity in enhancing sera. Chemical characterization suggested IgG1, rather than IgG2. Other laboratories found enhancing activity in both IgG1 and IgG2, while occasionally it was found in the IgG2 fraction only. In other experiments Voisin (1980) found enhancing antibody in the IgA fraction. In addition, it was found that progressive dilution of sera caused a loss of IgG1-enhancing activity and an increase in IgG2-enhancing activity. Moreover, after forming an immune complex with H-2 antigens, IgG2 acquired enhancing properties.

There have been a number of studies that have demonstrated the enhancing activity of immune complexes. These have been found to be effective in the regulation of the immune response to protein as well as allograft antigens. In some situations immune complexes are enhancing in antigen excess, in others in antibody excess, depending on the specificity of the antigenic determinant and immunoglobulin class (Voisin, 1980). Antibodies are thought to exert a regulatory action on antigenic determinants by masking the determinants. The formation of immune complexes could also signal the formation of suppressor rather than effector cells, or the induction of anti-idiotypic antibodies. Anaphylaxis could be an immunoregulatory mechanism in its own right.

Finally, the question arises whether enhancing antibodies or immune complexes act on the efferent as well as the afferent limb of the immunization arc. Can they act by preventing antigen from interacting with T-cell receptors peripherally as well as centrally? Another possibility is that they might form immune complexes with soluble antigen and the complex could block the T-cell receptor in an irreversible manner by causing cross-linkages of antigenic determinants attached to specific receptors on the T-cell surface.

The theory of afferent blockade implies that antibodies with enhancing activity bind to target cellular antigens and block them from reaching the immunocompetent cells of the host. These may either be in the periphery or residing in central lymphoid tissue. The concept of afferent blockade rests on two findings:

1. Target tissues, either tumor cells or normal tissue grafts, bind the antibody as shown by fluorescent or isotope techiques. These tissues when grafted onto allogeneic recipients then show increased graft survival.
2. There is specific uptake of enhancing antibody by the graft.

The main argument against blockade is that specific immune cells may develop at the same time in the enhanced as in the normal host. It has, however, been considered that afferent blockade may occur at the level of macrophage recognition rather than at the T cell.

Efferent blockade occurs after immunity has been established. The block occurs at the periphery of the graft that is to be rejected, where blocking antibodies cover the antigens and prevent effector elements from seeing their targets. There are a number of experiments in the tumor field where coating tumors with blocking antibody has resulted in their increased survival in the immunized host, indicating that they prevent or diminish target destruction by effector cells. A major argument against efferent blockade as the mechanism of immunological enhancement has been that blocking antisera given repeatedly to recipients with enhanced neoplastic or normal tissue grafts do not prolong graft survival indefinitely. Moreover, computation of the number of blocking antibodies in an experiment indicates that these are insufficient to cover all antigenic sites (Haughton and Nash, 1969).

Finally, there is the theory of central blockade which suggests that antibodies regulate or inhibit the production of antibodies or sensitized lymphocytes that might react specifically with target antigens. The block is presumably at the level of efferent lymphocytes in the lymph nodes and spleen. Feedback inhibition of T-lymphocyte proliferation by antibody and a reduced production of effector T cells would appear to be a plausible mechanism for immunological enhancement. However, the distinction between these three mechanisms, which may occur together in parallel, may be extremely difficult.

1.6. Immunological Tolerance

The term immunological tolerance was at one time used synonymously with all forms of antigen-specific immunological unresponsiveness. It had been shown by Billingham *et al.* (1953) that mice injected with allogenic lymphocytes either *in utero* or neonatally would accept skin grafts from donors of the same allogeneic strain. At that time Burnet (1957) had put forward his clonal selection theory for the immune response. It was then considered that many forms of tolerance resulted from clonal elimination. Clones of immunologically active cells were particularly susceptible to elimination during the period of immunological immaturity in mice. Moreover, even in adult life, extremely high levels of antigen could also induce a state of tolerance. The theory of clonal elimination was particularly important to explain the normal absence of clones of cells that carry reactive sites corresponding to the body's determinants.

At that time blocking antibody and immunological enhancement was considered an idiosyncrasy of cancer immunology. However, in 1971 Hellström, Hellström, and Allison suggested that neonatally induced allograft tolerance might be mediated by serum-borne factors similar to those involved in immunological enhancement. This was based on a study using a cytotoxic test to show that mice, made tolerant neonatally, had lymphocyte-mediated immunity detectable *in vitro* against target cells of the strain to which they were tolerant (Hellström *et al.*, 1971). They also showed that serum from the tolerant animals could inhibit this reactivity. Although in this model it has been difficult to show that serum can actually transfer a state of tolerance from animal to animal, the demonstration of T suppressor cells in tolerance to sheep erythrocytes (Gershon and Kondo, 1971) and to the picryl hapten (Zembala and Asherson, 1973) seriously reduced the number of models in which the theory of clonal elimination could be invoked.

Clonal elimination by high levels of antigen is still the hypothesis of choice where T suppressor cells or blocking antibody cannot be demonstrated as able to transfer antigen specific immunological unresponsiveness *in vivo*. The term *immunological tolerance* usually implies specific clonal elimination. However, this mechanism is generally hypothetical and as it is difficult to prove with a positive experiment, it is a term used when all other positive mechanisms have been excluded. However, it must be emphasized that exclusion may be by *in vivo* demonstration of positive factors and not just by the demonstration of *in vitro* blocking factors as in the experiments of Hellström *et al.* (1971). Immunological tolerance caused by clonal elimination is still considered the hypothesis of choice for explaining the classical experiments of Billingham *et al.* (1953).

1.7. Lymphokines and Monokines

1.7.1. Interleukins

Among the most important regulatory molecules produced by lymphocytes and monocytes are the interleukins. The role of these molecules has been defined in mainly *in vitro* experiments using lymphocyte proliferation. Interleukin 1 (IL 1) was originally described as a lymphocyte-activating factor present in macrophage culture supernatants that would replace macrophages in the proliferative response of lymphocytes to alloantigens. This was followed by the demonstration that a factor present in the culture fluids of lipopolysaccharide-stimulated human and murine macrophages could enhance the response of murine thymus cells and peripheral T cells to mitogens such as phytohemagglutinin (PHA). It is now known that IL 1 is a peptide molecule of molecular weight between 10,000 and 20,000. The molecule has a number of properties and one of the most interesting is that it is also the endogenous pyrogen that has been known for some time. It will, among other activities, (1) induce interleukin 2 (IL 2) release from T cells, (2) enhance antibody responses *in vitro* by an action on both T_H and B cells, (3) enhance cytotoxicity of lymphocytes, (4) induce Lyt markers, (5) enhance stable E-rosette formation, (6) induce collagenase and prostglandin synthesis in synovial cells, (7) induce fibroblast proliferation, and even cause (8) the production of serum amyloid. It may also be involved in T-cell suppression (Simon and Willoughby, 1982; de Weck *et al.*, 1983).

The discovery of IL 2 (T-cell growth factor) was the result of the observation that the supernatant from mitogen (Con-A)-stimulated human peripheral blood leukocytes contained a factor that resulted in the proliferation of cells *in vitro*. The availability of IL 2 has allowed the long-term cultures of cloned T-cell populations. Purified IL 2 has been shown to (1) trigger the proliferative expansion of activated T-cell clones, (2) enhance thymocyte mitogenesis, (3) provide T-cell help for the generation of plaque-forming cells from nude (T-cell deficient) mice to sheep erythocytes, and (4) induce alloantigen-specific thymocyte and nude mouse cytolytic T-cell reactivity (Watson *et al.*, 1982). IL 2 is a glycoprotein that appears to elute from gel filtration columns with molecules in the range of 25,000–40,000 daltons. Other studies indicate a molecular weight of nearer 20,000.

It is thought that IL 2 production is both stimulated and regulated by IL 1. However, some workers feel that IL 1 is not mandatory for IL 2 production, only for the regulation of its production (Stadler and Oppenheim, 1982). These authors consider that IL 2 serves as the ultimate extracellular mitogenic signal for both antigenically and polyclonally activated T cells. The mitogenic property of IL 2 leads to the clonal expansion of immature thymocytes and lymphocytes which then differentiate into mature cytotoxic, suppressor or helper cells.

In addition to the interleukins, lymphokines that activate macrophages can have a profound effect on the regulation of the immune response. Lymphokines were first discovered by Bloom and Bennet (1966) and David (1966) as soluble factors derived from lymphocytes activated *in vitro* that would inhibit the migration of macrophages from capillary tubes. They are now known to affect profoundly the metabolic activity of macrophages. Their effects include raised levels of glucose-6-phosphate dehydrogenase, NADPH oxidation activity, succinic dehydrogenase activity and β glucuronidase activity (Poulter and Turk, 1975). Other studies showed raised levels of intracellular cyclic GMP but not cyclic AMP (Pick *et al.*, 1979; Rouveix *et al.*, 1980.

1.7.2. Interferon

Interferon (IFN) is another macromolecule that may play a role in the regulation of the immune response. This may also be lymphocyte derived. IFN has been shown to have a number of immunomodulatory activities. These include both suppression and enhancement of antibody responses, suppression of delayed hypersensitivity and graft rejection, suppression of lymphocyte mitogenesis, macrophage activation, and enhancement of lymphocyte surface antigen expression and of histamine release by basophils. In addition, interferon can increase T-cell cytotoxicity, antibody-dependent cell cytotoxicity and natural killer cell activity (Sonnennfeld, 1980). These activities have mainly been shown with type I interferon (IFN-α) that can be derived from both B and T lymphocytes as well as macrophages. Some of these functions have also been demonstrated with type II interferon (IFN-γ) derived from activated T lymphocytes.

1.8. Prostaglandins

Prostaglandins (PGs) are a widely distributed family of compounds derived from the polyunsaturated fatty acid arachidonic acid by cyclo-oxygenase activity. PGE_2, $PGF_{2\alpha}$, PGI_2 (prostacyclin), and TXA_2 (thromboxane), have been shown to be synthesized by macrophages from a number of species. Macrophages have an active cyclo-oxygenase system. Lymphocytes have not been shown to synthesize PGs. Thus it was logical to look for an effect of PGs on T cells. PGE_1 and PGE_2 but not $PGF_{1\alpha}$ or $PGF_{2\alpha}$ can induce a rapid two- to fourfold increase in thymocyte cyclic AMP, which results 2 to 4 hr later in thymocyte proliferation (Franks *et al.*, 1971). PGE_1 can also induce more rapid expression of the Thy-1 antigen in mouse embryo thymus cultures (Singh and Owen, 1975). Most studies on the immunoregulatory effect of PGs on T-cell function have been on their effect on mitogen- or antigen-induced T-cell blastogenesis. There have been a large number of reports of the suppression of mitogen-induced blastogenesis by PGE_1 and PGE_2 (Goldyne and Stobo, 1980), and this has been reversed by treatment with indomethacin. Another approach has been that of Bray, Gordon, and Morley (Gordon *et al.*, 1976) who showed that PGE significantly inhibited the production of the lymphokine migration inhibitory factor by T cells. PGEs can also inhibit the ability of sensitized T cells specifically to lyse tumor target cells. However, this needs high concentrations of PGs (Henney *et al.*, 1972).

It is thought that PGEs have their inhibitory effect on lymphocyte proliferation through activation of adenylate cyclase and elevation of intracellular levels of cyclic AMP. PGEs, which increase intracellular cyclic AMP, augment blastogenesis in thymocytes, whereas they inhibit blastogenesis in unfractionated circulating T cells. Thus it has been postulated that the major action is through suppressor cells in the peripheral blood. Prostaglandin synthesis inhibitors such as indomethacin have been shown to inhibit the development of T_S cell function in Con A lymphocyte cultures (Orme and Shand, 1981). PGs can also have a modulating role in B-cell function. Indomethacin, a prostaglandin synthesis inhibitor, causes an enhancement of formation of antibody-producing cells to sheep erythrocytes (Webb and Nowowiejski, 1977). It is likely that the action of PGs is on T_H as well as B cells.

1.9. Thymic Hormones

A number of preparations of the thymus have been produced since the role of the thymus in regulating the immune response was first discovered by Miller (Miller, 1961). A number of these have been chemically characterized. There are four main preparations: (1) thymosin, (2) thymopoietin, (3) thymic humoral factor, and (4) *facteur thymique sérique* (FTS).

1.9.1. Thymosin

This preparation is a crude extract of calf serum used mainly by A. L. Goldstein and associates (Thurman *et al.*, 1980), and the active preparation that is studied is usually referred to as *Thymosin fraction 5*. Thymosin fraction 5 consists of a number of polypeptides, some of which are derived from the thymic epithelium. Other are of thymocyte origin. The amino acid sequence of a number of these with biological activity has been determined; one, $thymosin_{\alpha 1}$, contains 28 amino acid residues. Thymosin fraction 5 and certain biologically active peptides derived from it have been used in a number of experimental models. In addition, they have been used in immunodepressed patients with cancer or severe viral infections. Most T-cell functions have been shown to be induced or enhanced by this and other factors. However, it is of importance to note that as well as increasing T-effector-cell function, thymosin fraction 5, and particularly thymosin$_{\alpha 7}$, have been shown to induce suppressor cell formation in mice (Asherson *et al.*, 1976). A similar effect has been demonstrated in man (Wolf, 1979). Thus the rational use of this type of preparation will have to await the purification of the individual peptides and an accurate definition of their particular target cells.

1.9.2. Thymopoietin

Thymopoietin was originally isolated in studies on experimental models of myasthenia gravis and was characterized according to its effect on neuromuscular transmission by G. Goldstein (1974). It has also been shown to act on early T-cell differentiation. Thymopoietin has been chemically characterized and shown to have a 49-amino-acid polypeptide chain. Subsequently, Goldstein and colleagues isolated a pentapeptide with similar biological activity, which they named TP5. TP5 has been investigated in a number of experimental models in mice. For example, it can facilitate recovery from experimentally induced autoimmune disease in mice (Lau and Goldstein, 1980).

1.9.3. Thymic Humoral Factor

This is a 3000-molecular-weight peptide derived from a dialysate of a crude thymic extract prepared initially by Trainin and associates (Trainin *et al.*, 1980). It is assayed by an *in vitro* graft-versus-host assay and, as with other similar preparations, it is capable of restoring immunological activity to neonatally thymectomized mice and has been used in the treatment of immunodepressed patients.

1.9.4. *Facteur Thymique Serique*

This is the only "thymic hormone" that is not prepared from an extract of calf thymus. It is a 900-molecular-weight nonpeptide derived originally from serum, but now synthesized. It was first demonstrated through its ability to induce T-cell markers (Thy-1 membrane antigen) in T-cell precursors. It is absent from the serum of thymectomized mice (Bach and Dardenne, 1973). FTS is thought to act similarly, but not identically, to thymopoietin in a number of assay systems.

Another approach to the study of thymic factors has been ageing. Both thymopoietin and FTS levels in the serum decline with age. Immune deficiencies of old mice can be reversed by an injection of TP5. FTS in high concentration can be shown to have a stimulatory effect on T suppressor cells similar to that described for thymosin, in that it can cause the suppression of dinitrofluorobenzene sensitivity and skin graft rejection. In man, FTS has been shown under certain circumstances to depress the generation of T suppressor cells *in vitro*.

1.10. Summary of the Role of Macrophages in Regulating the Immune Response

Throughout this survey emphasis has been placed on the role of macrophages in regulating the immune response (Table II). There is no doubt that these cells are as important in regulation as in antigen presentation. Allison (1978) indicated a number of soluble products of activated macrophage origin that would act directly on T- or B-cell function to inhibit the response of these cells. These include thymidine, arginase, and polyamine oxidase. The role of complement has been emphasized in the studies of Klaus and Humphrey (1977), who depleted thymectomized mice of circulating C3 by treatment with cobra venom factor after primary immunization with dinitrophenylated keyhole limpet hemocyanin. This treatment abrogated the development of B-cell memory and appeared to involve impaired precursor proliferation following primary immunization. Lack of C3 also prevents uptake of antigen by dendritic cells.

The role of PGs, cyclic AMP, INF, and IL 1 have been discussed previously. Other factors such as B-cell and thymic differentiating factors and the T-cell activating molecule (Unanue, 1978) await further chemical characterization.

There are very few reports of the direct suppression of immunobiological reactivity by macrophages *in vivo*. However, recent studies in the laboratory of one of us (JLT) have demonstrated that purified peritoneal exudate macrophages injected intravenously into guinea pigs sensitized with DNP-bovine gamma globulin, nonspecifically suppressed delayed hypersensitivity reactions to this antigen (Katayama *et al.*, 1982).

2. TUMOR IMMUNITY

2.1. Introduction

The regulation of immunological responses against cancer has become a central matter in tumor immunity, as it is particularly difficult to evoke

TABLE II
Products of Activated Macrophages Regulating
Lymphocyte Responses[a]

Thymidine
Arginase
Polyamine oxidase
Complement cleavage products (C3, C4, C2, Factor B)
Prostaglandins
Cyclic AMP
Interferon
Interleukin 1
B-cell-differentiating factor
T-cell-activating molecule
Thymic differentiating factor

[a]From Addison (1978) and Unanue (1978).

immune resistance against tumors in cancer patients. Although there is much evidence indicating that animals can respond to autochthonous or syngeneic tumor cells, there have been no satisfactory reports of successful immunotherapy in man. Regulation of immune response in tumor immunity is not considered to differ basically from that to a foreign antigen, since tumors express antigenic molecules on their cell surface. However, tumor antigens are rather weak and the immunosuppressed status of cancer patients with large tumors may contribute to the difficulty in evoking an antitumor response. Furthermore, it has been observed that tumor cells grow successfully even in individuals who can respond immunologically to their own tumor cells. The mechanisms by which tumors may escape or evade immunological destruction are considered.

Both cell-mediated and humoral immune responses have been observed against human and animal tumor cells. Protection against tumors, however, is mainly cell-mediated depending on T lymphocytes, with other cells such as macrophages, granulocytes, and natural killer cells also involved in the effector phase of tumor rejection. The interaction between the different groups of immunocompetent cells is of paramount importance in tumor immunity. An antibody directed against a particular cell antigen may participate in the tumor escape mechanism whereas it may also kill the tumor cell with the cooperation of complement or K cells in an antibody-dependent cell-mediated cytotoxicity (ADCC) reaction.

One of the most important goals in tumor immunology is to augment the activity of effector cells that protect the body against tumor growth *in vivo* and to overcome the escape mechanisms by which tumor cells evade the host's immunological reactions.

2.2. Induction of Antitumor Resistances

A central issue in studies of tumor immunology is the concept that tumor cells express antigens not present on normal cells. It has been observed that many experimental tumor cells express antigens that induce a certain degree of transplantation-type resistance against tumor challenge in syngeneic animals or even in the same individual (Foley, 1953; Prehn and Main, 1957; Klein *et al.*, 1960; Takeda *et al.*, 1968) (see Table III). It is accepted that tumor cells express antigens called tumor-associated transplantation antigen (TATA), and the degree of antigenicity of TATA varies with the cause of the tumor and the stage of the tumor growth, as well as with host factors.

It has been noted that the immunizing activity of TATAs may be affected by the manner of antigenic presentation. It is particularly important for the induction of resistance against experimental cancer that the immunizing tumor cells retain their viability. Viable but nonreplicating cells, therefore, are used as tumor vaccines in most cases. X-irradiated tumor cells may have a comparatively effective immunizing activity, and this technique was used in original demonstrations of transplantation resistance against autochtho-

TABLE III

Methods Used for Induction of Specific Antitumor Resistance

Viable tumor cells
   Smaller dose of tumor cells than minimum take dose
   Surgical removal after tumor growth
   Ligation and release after tumor growth
   Xenogeneic tumor cells
   Allogeneic tumor cells
Attentuated tumor cells
X-ray (γ-ray)-irradiated cells
   Ultraviolet-irradiated cells
   Mitomycin-C-treated cells
   Iodoacetamide-treated cells
Killed tumor cells
   Formaldehyde-treated cells
   Glutaraldehyde-treated cells
   Frozen–thawed cells
   Homogenate of tumor cells
Extracted tumor-associated antigen
   Crude membrane
   3 M KCl-extract
   Hypotonic and sonicated extract
   Enzymatic digestion (papain, etc.)
   Non-ionic detergent extract (deoxycholate, NP-40, etc.)

nous tumors (Klein *et al.*, 1960). The use of irradiated tumor cells has become a standard against which other antigen-modifying treatments are compared. The antitumor drug, mitomycin C may be used for this purpose, as well as irradiation with ultraviolet or γ-rays. The effectiveness of attenuated tumor cells may be related to the degree of retention of viability. Indeed, when animals are immunized with viable tumor cells modified by a virus infection and rejected by syngeneic hosts, strong resistance develops against the original unmodified tumor cells (Kobayashi *et al.*, 1970).

Tumor cells killed with chemicals may also be used for the immunization. Formaldehyde (Lin *et al.*, 1969; Oikawa *et al.*, 1979) and glutaraldehyde (Sanderson and Frost, 1974; Frost and Sanderson, 1975) have been used to obtain safe and stable tumor vaccines. Tumor cells treated with iodoacetate or iodoacetamide have also produced resistance to tumors (Apffel *et al.*, 1966; Prager *et al.*, 1974). Other methods for the attenuation of tumor-replicating activity such as freezing and thawing or homogenation cause a loss of immunizing activity. However, heated homogenates of Sarcoma 180 cells induce an enhanced growth of tumor in allogeneic mice (Hosokawa *et al.*, 1975). Deoxycholate-solubilized tumor antigens of a fibrosarcoma in rats were found to induce enhancement of tumor growth, despite producing specific antitumor responses detected by delayed type hypersensitivity reaction and the tumor-neutralizing assay (Winn's assay) (Minami *et al.*, 1979). The enhanced tumor growth in rats immunized with the solubilized antigen was related to the generation of suppressor T cells (Minami et al., 1980). In their attempts to get immunogenic TATA solubilized, Kahan and co-workers separated tumor-protective antigen and tumor-facilitating antigen from 3 M KCl-solubilized tumor extracts of a mouse 3-methylcholanthrene-induced sarcoma (Yamagishi et al., 1979; Pellis et al., 1980). Natori et al. (1978) reported that highly purified TATA of 3-methylcholanthrene tumors still retained some specific tumor rejection property.

The immunizing activity of TATAs seems to be generally weak and unstable. The procedures mentioned previously for the attenuation of the replicating activity of tumor vaccine seem to cause a loss of TATA immunogenicity. There have been many attempts to increase TATA immunizing activity by modifying tumor cells (Kobayashi, 1982). One of the methods used is to attach tumor cells to antigenic molecules, which are more easily recognized by the host and thus elicit a stronger immune response against the weakly antigenic TATA. This concept was supported by the suggestion that T–T cell interaction increased antigenic help (Hamaoka et al., 1979). Viable rat tumor cells modified by infection with murine leukemia viruses, which cannot grow in normal syngeneic rats, induce strong responses to both the virus-associated antigen (VAA) and to TATA. It was suggested that the increased immunogenicity of TATA was not only due to viable cell-immunization but also to antigenic help by VAA in the recognition of tumor cells. This suggestion was supported by evidence that virus-infected tumor cells produced stronger resistance against noninfected tumors even after they had been attenuated by irradiation, if the right amount of VAA was used (Yamaguchi et al., 1982). However, too strong a response to the modifying dose of VAA reduced the response to the original TATA because of antigenic competition (Hosokawa et al., 1983). The use of antigen modification in the conversion of the original TATA to an immunogen suitable for increasing tumor resistance has been clearly supported by the observation that purified protein derivatives (PPD) bound to tumor cells (Lachmann and Sikora, 1978; Takatsu et al., 1978) or TNP-coupled tumor cells (Hamaoka et al., 1979) produced definite transplantation resistance in mice. Helper T lymphocytes were found to react to the modifying antigen (PPD or TNP). Moreover, no anti-TATA response was produced by the unmodified tumor cells.

With regard to the route of immunization, intradermal injection of TATA is most effective for the induction of a cell-mediated immune response. Intravenous injection of antigen may induce enhancement of tumor growth caused by the generation of T_S cells or stimulation of antibody-producing B cells. Despite this, it is difficult to make generalizations in the absence of sufficient information on which of the mechanisms of the regulation of the immune response might be more favorable to the induction of antitumor resistance. Much of the information acquired to date has been obtained using transplantable tumor models under conditions that may not directly reflect the physiopathology of autochthonous tumors. The role of different effector cells implicated in antitumor resistance will be very briefly mentioned in the following sections.

2.3. Positive Effectors of Antitumor Resistance

Protection against tumors involves both specific immune responses to TATA and nonspecific antitumor mechanisms. Table IV lists the positive effectors of antitumor resistance.

2.3.1. Cytotoxic T Lymphocytes

The TATA-specific resistance against tumors is thought to be mediated by T cells sensitized against TATA. This is suggested by experiments in which specific resistance to tumors can be transferred to normal animals by spleen or lymph node cells but not if they are depleted of T cells. The tumor-neutralizing test (Winn's assay) also indicates that antigen specific antitumor effector cells are T cells, while nonspecific effector cells are found mainly in the non-T-cell populations. Cytotoxic T lymphocytes (CTL) have been found in TATA-immune or tumor-bearing mice and have been shown to be Lyt $1^-2^+3^+$ lymphocytes by *in vitro* cytotoxicity tests such as the chromium release assay. Antitumor CTL are generated *in vitro* in mixed lymphocyte tumor cultures with the collaboration of T_H cells or amplifier T (T_A) cells, or one of the soluble factors such as IL 2 produced by T_H cells. Since CTL have been found to kill target tumor cells effectively after a short incubation period in *in vitro* cytotoxicity assay, it is thought that CTL could participate in the specific resistance against tumor cells *in vivo*. However, recently evidence has accumulated in adoptive lymphocyte transfer experiments that the participation of Lyt $1^+2^-3^-$ T lymphocytes (a marker of T_H or T_A cells) is also likely in protection against tumor growth (Greenberg *et al.*, 1981). It is possible that there is continuous generation of CTL in tumor-bearing hosts with the assistance of transfered T_H cells. It is also possible that lymphokines produced by T_H cells activate nonspecific effector cells, macrophages or natural killer cells. The possibility that Lyt 1^+2^- lymphocytes may act as direct effectors in the destruction of tumor cells remains to be established.

2.3.2. Macrophages

Macrophages are believed to be important effector cells in the destruction of tumors. Macrophages armed with products of specifically sensitized lymphocytes have been shown to kill tumor cells (Evans and Alexander,

TABLE IV
Positive Effectors of Antitumor Resistance

Cytotoxic T lymphocytes (CTL)
Armed macrophages
Killer (K) cells
Activated macrophages
Natural killer (NK) cells
Lymphokine-activated killer (LAK) cells

1972). Antibody-dependent macrophage-mediated cytotoxicity has been found in situations where macrophages are activated and express Fc receptor (Yamazaki *et al.*, 1975). Nonspecific cytolysis of tumor cells by activated macrophages *in vitro* has been well investigated. The *in vivo* role of macrophages is likely to be more complex. It has been reported that the growth of subcutaneously implanted tumors may be enhanced in mice treated with carrageenan, which is toxic to macrophages (Wu and Kearney, 1979). The artificial metastasis of a melanoma was inhibited by the addition of activated macrophages to the injection mixture or injection of the macrophage-activating agent muramyldipeptide (Fidler *et al.*, 1981; Sone and Fidler, 1980). In *in vitro* cytotoxicity experiments activation of macrophages to kill tumor cells has been achieved by the addition of antitumor drugs such as Adriamycin® (Tomazic *et al.*, 1980; Mantovani *et al.*, 1980; Martin *et al.*, 1982) and mitomycin C (Ogura *et al.*, 1982). Recently it has been found that bleomycin also activated macrophages to be cytotoxic to tumor cells (Morikawa *et al.*, 1985). The explanation for this action of antitumor drugs remains to be investigated. Regarding macrophage participation in tumor immunity, interaction of macrophages with other cell types is also important. Macrophages process TATA and present it to T cells to recognize and also produce IL 1, which assists T-cell maturation when precursor cells are stimulated by TATA or other antigen. Macrophages are activated by macrophage-activating factors produced primarily by stimulated T cells or other cells. Moreover, granulocytes can also be activated by products of T cells and exert nonspecific cytotoxicity to tumor cells (Sendo *et al.*, 1981; Inoue and Sendo, 1983).

2.3.3. K Cells, Natural Killer Cells, and Lymphokine-Activated Killer Cells

In addition to macrophages, granulocytes, and T cells, "null" lymphocytes can have cytotoxic effects against tumor cells. K cells are effector cells in ADCC and kill target tumor cells coated with small amounts of specific antibody *in vitro*. It is not yet clear whether or not in vivo ADCC has a role in protection against tumor cells. The specific antibody binds to the Fc receptor of lymphoid cells. K cells include monocytes and other lymphocytes that also express Fc receptors but do not express T- and B-cell marker, and do not have phagocytic activity. K-cell activity is regulated by factors that stimulate the expression of Fc receptors. Natural killer (NK) cells have been characterized as large granular lymphocytes in both animals and humans (Herberman and Holden, 1978; Timonen *et al.*, 1979). They are antigen-nonspecific effector cells that are thought to protect against small numbers of tumor cells and to inhibit metastasizing tumor cells (Hanna and Burton, 1981). The *in vivo* activity of NK cells in tumorigenesis has been suggested based on evidence that the incidence of tumors is not high in athymic nude mice in which NK cells are particularly active (Riesenfeld *et al.*, 1980) and that growth and metastasis of tumor cells are enhanced in beige mice in which NK activity is genetically low (Talmadge *et al.*, 1980). Moreover, it has been reported that xenografted human tumors grow better in nude mice depleted of NK activity by treatment with anti-asialo GM1 serum (Kasai *et al.*, 1981; Habu *et al.*, 1981). NK activity is augmented by IFN *in vitro* and by IFN inducers and other lymphokines (Minato *et al.*, 1980).

Recently, it has been reported that peripheral blood leukocytes from cancer patients could be activated in culture by preparations of IL 2. This resulted in the development of effector cells cytotoxic for autologous fresh solid tumor cells in the chromium release assay (Lotze *et al.*, 1981). Lymphokine-activated killer cells, distinct from CTL and NK cells, have also been suggested to play a role in immune protection against NK-resistant solid tumors and to have a possible role in adoptive immunotherapy of tumors (Grimm *et al.*, 1982, 1983).

2.4. Negative Regulation of Antitumor Resistance

If the host's immunological system were fully capable of recognizing tumor cells as foreign, then the tumor would be unable to grow successfully. It is evident that an antitumor response is detectable in most individuals in which a tumor is growing unless the immune system is suppressed. Immune responses to tumor cells, however, are not necessarily protective against tumors. Negative regulation of antitumor resistance (see Table V) is observed in tumor-bearing hosts and in individuals immunized with TATA.

2.4.1. Antibody and Shed Antigens

Blocking factors inhibiting the cytotoxic action of lymphocytes are found in sera of tumor-bearing individuals. Specific antibodies directing against tumor antigens can abrogate the cytotoxic activity of lymphocytes by binding to the tumor cell surface (Hellström and Hellström, 1974). The observation that blocking activity in serum disappeared within 72 hr of surgical removal of the tumor, however, suggests that blocking might not be purely because

TABLE V
Negative Responses for Antitumor Resistance

Specific to tumor antigens
  Suppressor T cells
  Blocking antibody
  Shedding antigen
  Immune complex
Nonspecific to tumor antigens
  Suppressor macrophages
  Other suppressor cells
  Immunoregulatory alphaglobulin (IRA)
  Alpha-1-antitrypsin
  C-reactive protein (CRP)
  Alpha-1-acidic glycoprotein (AAG)
  Immunosuppressive acidic protein (IAP)

of specific antibodies (Baldwin *et al.*, 1973). Soluble tumor antigens can bind to antigen receptors and block the effector cells. The presence of circulating soluble antigens has been demonstrated in the sera of tumor-bearing animals as well as humans (Alexander, 1974). It has been suggested, furthermore, that antigen–antibody complexes in the sera of an animal with a large tumor might paralyze the effector response to tumor cells (Baldwin *et al.*, 1973; Robins and Baldwin, 1974). It is now known that blocking activity is not demonstrated in sera from animals bearing regressing tumors and these sera may even delay the influence of blocking antibody (Sjögren *et al.*, 1971). The most likely explanation, therefore, is that the blocking activity in the sera of tumor-bearers is caused by soluble tumor antigens shed into the circulation and/or antigen–antibody complexes and that "unblocking regressor sera" represent a shift on the binding curve from antigen to antibody excess as a consequence of tumor decline (see review by Ozer, 1982).

Another possible mechanism of antibody-mediated escape from cytotoxic effector cells may involve the complete or partial loss of tumor antigens or their suppressed expression *in vivo* as a result of antigenic modulation (Stackpole and Jacobson, 1978). Antigenic modulation was originally demonstrated in the TL-antigen system of mice by the observation that TL-antigen expression on leukemia cells in C57BL/6 mice was inhibited *in vivo* and *in vitro* by the presence of anti-TL antibody (Old *et al.*, 1968). Loss of antigen from the cell surface by antigenic modulation or by immunological selection in immunocompetent hosts is a possible cause for the escape of tumor cells from the effect of cytotoxic T lymphocytes.

It is possible that the humoral response to tumor antigen delays the development of immunological protection against tumors, although the question remains whether ADCC has a role in the destruction of tumor cells *in vivo*. Some observations indicate that the selective inhibition of the humoral response by antitumor drugs is favoring tumor rejection. Heppner and Calabresi (1972) reported that a low dose of cytosine arabinoside (10 mg/kg) was effective in the treatment of mammary tumors in C3H/He mice through a selective inhibition of antibody production against the tumor cells. A large dose of the drug (20–40 mg/kg) also suppressed cell-mediated immunity and was less effective in inducing antitumor effects (Heppner *et al.*, 1974). A similar role for chemotherapy in experimental tumor models has been suggested by other investigators. Blocking factors detectable in sera of rats bearing polyoma-virus-induced tumors (Steele *et al.*, 1974) and in sera of chickens with Marek's disease (Lu *et al.*, 1976) are markedly decreased after treatment with cyclophosphamide.

2.4.2. Suppressor Cells

As mentioned earlier, many experimental tumors are able to grow in normal syngeneic animals, whereas they can be rejected in animals immunized with TATA. These tumors have been found to induce suppressor cells which negatively regulate the immune response to the tumor during their initial growth in normal hosts (Berendt and North, 1980).

The role of suppressor cells in neoplastic diseases has been reviewed by Naor (1979). Tumor-antigen-specific suppressor cells were first found in A/J mice bearing methylcholanthrene-induced Sarcoma 1509a and were characterized to be cortisone-resistant T cells found in the thymus, spleen, draining lymph node, and bone marrow cells but not in peripheral lymphocytes of tumor-bearing mice (Fujimoto et al., 1976a,b). These T_S cells were detected by adoptive transfer into mice immunized by surgical removal of the tumor followed by further injections of tumor cells, which had developed antitumor resistance. The T_S cells were also found in animals immunized with TATA. For example, spleen cells of WKA rats immunized with deoxycholate-solubilized antigens of a syngeneic fibrosarcoma, and in which the tumor growth was enhanced, abrogate the tumor-neutralizing activity of immune spleen cells detected by Winn's assay (Minami et al., 1979). The suppressor activity found in vitro in cytotoxic assays was mediated by T cells (Minami et al., 1980). These suppressor cells appear to act on the effector arm of the immune response. Other suppressor cells act on the induction of cytotoxic effector cells. It has also been found that T_S cells in the thymus and spleen from syngeneic P815 mastocytoma-bearing DBA/2 mice inhibit the in vitro generation of specific cytotoxic lymphocytes (Takei et al., 1977). Naor and his co-workers (Galili et al., 1976, 1978; Devens et al., 1978) demonstrated the interesting finding that Moloney-leukemia-virus-induced lymphoma YAC cells growing in vivo induced suppressor cells. The A/J mice immunized with mitomycin-C-treated YAC cells could not reject low doses of viable tumor cells. On the other hand, mice immunized with mitomycin-C-treated cells of a culture line of the tumor termed YAC-1 could reject viable YAC cells (Devens et al., 1978, 1979). Furthermore, spleen cells generated cytotoxic effector cells after sensitization with YAC-1 cells in vitro. The effector cytotoxic cells after cocultivation with YAC-1 cells could kill both the in vivo grown YAC cell line and the in vitro YAC-1 cells. They concluded, therefore, that in vivo grown YAC cells stimulated suppressor cells and that these suppressor cells recognized and inactivated memory cells. However, in vitro grown YAC-1 cells induced memory cells that reacted also with YAC cells. In addition they observed that YAC cells conjugated with the TNP group as well as allogeneic tumor cells that cross-reacted with YAC antigen induced significant resistance against a low dose of viable YAC cells (Galili et al., 1976, 1978).

Another interesting example of suppressor cells is that of specific suppressor cells to the UV-irradiation-induced sarcoma that develops in UV-irradiated mice. It was found that UV-irradiation of C3H mice induced fibrosarcomas that grow progressively. The tumor could not be transplanted into normal syngeneic mice unless they had been UV-irradiated (Kripke, 1980). When inoculated into X-irradiated mice, lymphoid cells from the UV-irradiated mice prevented the recipients from rejecting the UV-induced tumors. In contrast, most of the recipients that had been injected with normal lymphoid cells were able to reject the tumors. It was suggested, therefore, that UV irradiation induced specific suppressor cells which inhibited the cytotoxic cells directed against UV-induced tumors. These suppressor cells were shown to be T cells, as they were sensitive to anti-T-cell serum and complement (Spellman and Daynes, 1977; Fisher and Kripke, 1978). It was suggested that UV-irradiation caused a modification of skin antigens and these UV-modified antigens induced the development of the T_S cells.

Immunosuppressive macrophages, B cells, and null cells have also been found in tumor-bearing hosts (see review by Naor, 1979). It has been found that spleen cells from tumor-bearing mice generated significantly lower proliferative responses after stimulation with the T-cell mitogens, PHA and Con A, than spleen cells from normal mice (Kirchner et al., 1974a). The removal of cells that adhered to rayon columns or that had a phagocytosing activity completely restored the ability of the spleen cells from tumor-bearing mice to proliferate in response to PHA (Kirchner et al., 1974b). Similarly, removal of phagocytosing cells with carrageenan restored the ability of spleen cells to respond to allogeneic spleen cells in the mixed lymphocyte reaction (Fernbach et al., 1976). In addition, these cells were insensitive to anti-T-cell serum and irradiation with 2500 rad (Kirchner et al., 1975a,b). The above-mentioned evidence concerning the suppressive activity of the spleen cells of tumor-bearing animals suggests that these suppressor cells are macrophages. Suppressor macrophages inhibit the proliferative response of T lymphocytes in vitro after stimulation with mitogens, alloantigens, or tumor antigens. Similar suppressor macrophages have been found in animals immunized with Bacillus Calmette–Guerin (BCG) (Baldwin and Pimm, 1973; Wepsic et al., 1976; Bennett et al., 1978; Bennett and Mitchell, 1979; Drucker et al., 1981). Although BCG is known for its effects against tumors (Mitchell and Murakata, 1979), these reports indicate the BCG induces suppressor cells that may be detected by in vitro lymphocyte-proliferating tests and enhance tumor growth in vivo. The suppressive activity of macrophages in tumor-bearing animals or in animals immunized with BCG could be mediated through the production of PGE_2. Suppressor macrophages have been shown to produce PGE_2 (Pelus and Bockman, 1979) and their activity is reduced after treatment with indomethacin (Shibata et al., 1983). It is possible that these suppressor macrophages may also regulate the immune response directed against specific tumor antigens, although suppression mediated by macrophages is usually antigen nonspecific.

Suppressive activity mediated by T cells or macrophages in tumor-bearing animals has been found to disappear after tumor removal (Fujimoto et al., 1976b; Shibata et al., 1983). It is suggested, therefore, that suppressor cells are generated during the course of tumor growth. Some investigations have shown that suppressor cell activity is eliminated in vivo by certain types of antitumor drugs. Preferential diminution of suppressor cell precursor activity has been observed by pretreatment of tumor recipients or tumor-immune animals with cyclophosphamide (Glaser, 1979a,b; Terashima et al.,

1980; Minami *et al.*, 1980; Greene *et al.*, 1979). It has been reported, moreover, that a low dose of cyclophosphamide in the treatment of tumor-bearing animals inhibits the activity of suppressor cells and augments the host effector potentials against tumors (Jun and Johnson, 1979; Ray and Raychaudhuri, 1981; Hengst *et al.*, 1980, 1981; Nakajima *et al.*, 1981). A similar effect of cyclophosphamide has been suggested during carcinogenesis by methylcholanthrene treatment in BALB/c mice (Hellström and Hellström, 1978). Recently it has been found that tumor-specific suppressor T cells are eliminated and the induction of antitumor resistance is augmented by the antileukemia drugs busulfan (Mizushima *et al.*, 1981) and bleomycin (Hosokawa *et al.*, 1985) in rats immunized with irradiated tumor cells. Kataoka *et al.* (1980, 1981) reported that suppressor macrophages in L1210-bearing mice receiving a Con-A-bound tumor vaccine were diminished by antitumor drugs such as 6-mercaptopurine and mitomycin C.

2.4.3. Serum Factors

In addition, to the regulation of positive antitumor responses by suppressor cells, serum factors capable of suppressing the immune response appear to provide one of the more important tumor escape mechanisms. There have been many reports of serum immunosuppressive factors in cancer patients and tumor-bearing animals, other than the serum blocking factors described earlier that are tumor antigen specific and act by inhibiting the action of cytotoxic effector cells on tumor cells. Although the nature and significance of these serum factors has not yet been established, studies have been made on their inhibitory action on lymphocyte-proliferating responses to mitogens *in vitro*. Among these factors are the immunoregulatory alpha-globulin (IRA) (Cooperband *et al.*, 1972), alpha-1-antitrypsin (Arora *et al.*, 1978), C-reactive protein (Mortensen and Gewurz, 1976), and alpha-1-acid glycoprotein (Chiu *et al.*, 1977; Tamura *et al.*, 1981). These are known to exist in normal serum and to increase in sera from tumor-bearing individuals, although little is known about their role in cancer patients. There have been some reports of specific mechanisms. For example, IRA acts at the earliest stage of antigen uptake by a steric effect such as masking or coating and inhibiting directly or indirectly antigen receptors on T lymphocytes (Cooperband *et al.*, 1972). Alpha-2-macroglobulin, which was observed to increase in the sera of gastric cancer (Urushizaki *et al.*, 1977). Similarly, Ishida and his co-workers reported that immunosuppressive acidic protein increases in tumor-bearing individuals and induces suppressor macrophages after its transfer into normal mice (Tamura *et al.*, 1981; Shibata *et al.*, 1978). The source of these immunosuppressive factors still remains to be investigated. They may be produced by host cells, tumor cells, or both.

2.5. Conclusion

It is apparent that the immune system can respond to tumor cells, which exist as variants of self in the host. These responses are not necessarily positive in that they protect from unlimited growth of tumor cells. They may also be negative, representing immunological escape mechanisms. In this situation, the stimulus of tumor-associated antigen generates a negative response rather than a positive response resulting in host resistance against the tumor. It should be noted that tumors that have grown to a size that is detectable in the host already have shown the ability to escape from host defense effector mechanisms. Weak antigenicity or lack of immunogenicity of tumor cells, perhaps in part resulting from immunoselection, may be one of the reasons why such tumor cells can escape host defense responses. Modification of tumor cells may be one way to overcome a poor antitumor immune response. The pharmacological and/or immunological procedures that may be developed to effectively inhibit the development of a negative response or to eliminate suppressive activity may provide one of the more important opportunities to augment antitumor immunity.

REFERENCES

Alexander, P., 1974, Escape from immune destruction by the host through shedding of surface antigens: Is this a characteristic shared by malignant and embryonic cells? *Cancer Res.* **34:**2077–2082.

Allison, A. C., 1978, Mechanisms by which activated macrophages inhibit lymphocyte responses, *Immunol. Rev.* **40:**3–27.

Apffel, C. A., Arnason, B. G., and Peters, J. H., 1966, Induction of tumour immunity with tumour cells treated with iodoacetate, *Nature* **209:**694–696.

Arora, P. K., Miller, H. C., and Aronson, L. D., 1978, Alpha-1-antitrypsin is an effector of immunological stasis, *Nature* **274:**589–590.

Asherson, G. L., Zembala, M., Mayhew, B., and Goldstein, A. L., 1976, Adult thymectomy prevention of the appearance of suppressor T cells which depress contact sensitivity to picryl chloride and reversal of adult thymectomy effect by thymus extract, *Eur. J. Immunol.* **6:**699–703.

Aune, T. M., and Pierce, C. W., 1983, Mechanism of action of soluble immune response suppressor (SIRS), in : *Advances in Immunopharmacology*, Volume 2 (J. W. Hadden, L. Chedid, P. Dukor, F. Spreafico, and D. Willoughby, eds.), Pergamon Press, Oxford, pp. 597–602.

Bach, J. F., and Dardenne, M., 1973, Studies on thymus products II. Demonstration and characterization of a circulating thymus hormone, *Immunology* **25:**353–366.

Baldwin, R. W., and Pimm, M. V., 1973, Immunotherapy of pulmonary growths from intravenously transferred rat tumour cells, *Br. J. Cancer* **27:**48–54.

Baldwin, R. W., Embleton, M. J., and Robins, R. A., 1973, Cellular and humoral immunity to rat hepatoma-specific antigens correlated with tumour status, *Int. J. Cancer* **11:**1–10.

Bennett, J. A., and Mitchell, M. S., 1979, Induction of suppressor cells by intravenous administration of Bacillus Calmette-Guerin and its modulation by cyclophosphamide, *Biochem. Pharmacol.* **28:**1947–1952.

Bennett, J. A., Rao, V. S., and Mitchell, M. S., 1978, Systemic Bacillus Calmette-Guerin (BCG) activates natural suppressor cells, *Proc. Natl. Acad. Sci. USA* **75:**5142–5144.

Berendt, M. S., and North, R. S., 1980, T cell-mediated suppression of antitumor immunity. An explanation for progressive growth of an immunogenic tumor, *J. Exp. Med.* **151:**69–76.

Billingham, R. C., Brent, L., and Medawar, P. B., 1953, "Actively acquired tolerance" of foreign cells, *Nature* **172:**603–606.

Bloom, B., and Bennett, B., 1966, Mechanism of a reaction *in vitro* associated with delayed-type hypersensitivity, *Science* **153:**80–82.

Burnet, F. M., 1957, A modification of Jerne's theory of antibody production using the concept of clonal selection, *Aust. J. Sci.* **20:**67–69.

Cantor, H., and Boyse, E. A., 1975, Functional subclasses of T-lymphocytes bearing different Ly antigens. II. Cooperation between subclasses of Ly$^+$ cells in the generation of killer activity, *J. Exp. Med.* **141:**1376–1389.

Chiu, K. M., Mortensen, R. P., Osmand, A. P., and Gewurz, H., 1977, Interactions of alpha-1-acid glycoprotein with the immune system. I. Purification and effects upon lymphocyte responsiveness, *Immunology* **32:**997–1005.

Cooperband, S. R., Badger, A. M., and Davis, R. C., 1972, The effect of immunoregulatory globulin upon lymphocytes *in vitro*, *J. Immunol.* **109:**154–163.

David, J. R., 1966, Delayed hypersensitivity *in vitro*: Its mediation by cell-free substances formed by lymphoid cell-antigen reaction, *Proc. Natl. Acad. Sci. USA* **56:**72–77.

Devens, B., Galili, N., Deutsh, O., Naor, D., and Klein, E., 1978, Immune responses to weakly immunogenic virally induced tumors. II. Suppressive effects of the *in vivo* carried tumor YAC, *Eur. J. Immunol.* **8:**573–578.

Devens, B., Schochot, L., and Naor, D., 1979, Immune responses to weakly immunogenic virally induced tumors. IV. Short *in vitro* cultivation of YAC changes its antigenic properties, *Cell. Immunol.* **44:**442–453.

de Weck, A. L., Kristensen, F., Bettens, F., and Joncourt, F., 1983, The biology of the interleukins, in: *Advances in Immunopharmacology*, Volume 2 (J. W. Hadden, L. Chedid, P. Dukor, F. Spreafico, and D. Willoughby, eds.), Pergamon Press, Oxford, pp. 593–596.

Dickmeiss, E., Soeberg, B., and Svejgaard, A., 1977, Humoral cell-mediated cytotoxicity against modified target cells is restricted by HLA, *Nature* **270:**526–528.

Drucker, B. J., Wepsic, H. T., Alaimo, J. C., and Murray, N., 1981, The negative systemic effect of BCGcw inoculated intraperitoneally. II. *In vitro* demonstration of the presence of suppressor cells in BCGcw-immunized rats, *Cancer Immunol. Immunother.* **10:**227–237.

Evans, R., and Alexander, P., 1972, Mechanism of immunologically specific killing of tumour cells by macrophages, *Nature (London)* **236:**168–170.

Fabre, J. W., and Batchelor, J. R., 1975, Passive enhancement of renal allografts: Specificity of the enhancing antisera, *Transplantation* **20:**269–271.

Feldman, J. D., 1972, Immunological enhancement: A study of blocking antibodies, *Adv. Immunol.* **15:**167–214.

Fernbach, B. R., Kirchner, H., Bonnard, G. D., and Herberman, R. B., 1976, Suppression of mixed lymphocyte response in mice bearing primary tumors induced by murine sarcoma virus, *Transplantation* **21:**381–386.

Fidler, I. J., Raz, A., Fogler, W. E., Hoyer, L. C., and Poste, G., 1981, The role of plasma membrane receptors and the kinetics of macrophage activation by lymphokines encapsulated in liposomes, *Cancer Res.* **41:**495–504.

Fischer, A., Beverley, P. C. L., and Feldmann, M., 1981, Long-term human T-helper lines producing specific helper factor reactive to influenza virus, *Nature* **294:**166–168.

Fisher M. S., and Kripke, M. L., 1978, Further studies on the tumor-specific suppressor cells induced by ultraviolet radiation, *J. Immunol.* **121:**1139–1144.

Foley, E. J., 1953, Antigenic properties of methylcholanthrene-induced tumors in mice of strain of origin, *Cancer Res.* **13:**835–837.

Forman, J., 1975, On the role of the H-2 histocompatibility complex in determining the specificity of cytotoxic effector cells sensitized against syngeneic trinitrophenyl-modified targets, *J. Exp. Med.* **142:**403–418.

Franks, D. J., McManus, J. P., and Whitfield, J. F., 1971, The effects of prostaglandins on cyclic AMP production and cell proliferation in thymic lymphocytes, *Biochem. Biophys. Res. Commun.* **44:**1177–1183.

Frost, P., and Sanderson, C. J., 1975, Tumor immunoprophylaxis in mice using glutaraldehyde-treated syngeneic tumor cells, *Cancer Res.* **35:**2646–2650.

Fujimoto, S., Greene, M. I., and Sehon, A. H., 1976a, Regulation of the immune response to tumor antigens. I. Immunosuppressor cells in tumor-bearing hosts, *J. Immunol.* **116:**791–799.

Fujimoto, S., Greene, M. I., and Sehon, A. H., 1976b, Regulation of the immune response to tumor antigens. II. The nature of immunosuppressor cells in tumor-bearing hosts, *J. Immunol.* **116**:800–806.

Galili, N., Naor, D., Åsjö, B., and Klein, G., 1976, Induction of immune responsiveness in a genetically low-responsive tumor-host combination by chemical modification of the immunogen, *Eur. J. Immunol.* **6**:473–476.

Galili, N., Devens, Naor, D., Bocker, S., and Klein, E., 1978, Immune responses to weakly immunogenic virally induced tumors. I. Overcoming low responsiveness by priming mice with a syngeneic *in vitro* tumor line or allogeneic cross-reactive tumor, *Eur. J. Immunol.* **8**:17–22.

Gershon, R. K., and Kondo, K., 1971, Infectious immunological tolerance, *Immunology* **21**:903–914.

Glaser, M., 1979a, Augmentation of specific immune response against a syngeneic SV40-induced sarcoma in mice by depletion of suppressor T cells with cyclophosphamide, *Cell. Immunol.* **48**:339–345.

Glaser, M., 1979b, Regulation of specific cell-mediated cytotoxic response against SV40-induced tumor associated antigens by depletion of suppressor T cells with cyclophosphamide in mice, *J. Exp. Med.* **149**:774–779.

Goldstein, G., 1974, Isolation of bovine thymin: A polypeptide hormone of the thymus, *Nature* **247**:11–14.

Goldyne, M., and Stobo, J., 1980, Prostaglandin E2 as a modulator of macrophage–T lymphocyte interactions, *J. Invest. Dermatol.* **74**:297–300.

Gordon, D., Bray, M. A., and Morley, J., 1976, Control of lymphokine secretion by prostaglandins, *Nature* **262**:401.

Greenberg, P. D., Cheever, A. B., and Fefer, A., 1981, Eradication of disseminated murine leukemia by chemoimmunotherapy with cyclophosphamide and adoptively transferred immune syngeneic Lyt-1$^+$2-lymphocytes, *J. Exp. Med.* **154**:952–963.

Greene, M. I., Perry, L. L., and Benacerraf, B., 1979, Regulation of the immune response to tumor antigen, *Am. J. Pathol.* **95**:159–169.

Grimm, E. A., Mazunder, A., Zhang, H. E., and Rosenberg, S. A., 1982, Lymphokine-activated killer cell phenomenon. Lysis of natural killer-resistant fresh solid tumor cells by interleukin 2-activated autologous human peripheral blood, *J. Exp. Med.* **155**:1823–1841.

Grimm, E. A., Ramsey, K. M., Mazunder, A., Wilson, D. J., Djeu, J. Y., and Rosenberg, S. A., 1983, Lymphokine-activated killer cell phenomenon. II. Precursor phenotype is serologically distinct from peripheral T lymphocytes, memory cytotoxic thymus-derived lymphocytes and natural killer cells, *J. Exp. Med.* **157**:884–897.

Habu, S., Fukui, H., Shimamura, K., Kassai, M., Nagai, Y., Okumura, K., and Tamaoki, N., 1981, *In vivo* effects of anti-asialo GMI. I. Reduction of NK activity and enhancement of transplanted tumor growth in nude mice, *J. Immunol.* **127**:34–38.

Hamaoka, T., Fukiwara, H., Tsuchida, T., Kinoushi, T., and Aoki, H., 1979, Induction of immune resistance against tumor by immunization with hapten-modified tumor cells in the presence of hapten-reactive helper T cells, in: *Gann Monograph on Cancer Research 23* (H. Kobayashi, ed.), Japan Science Society Press, Tokyo, pp. 123–141.

Hanna, N., and Burton, R. C., 1981, Definitive evidence that natural killer (NK) cells inhibit experimental tumor metastases *in vivo*, *J. Immunol.* **127**:1754–1758.

Haughton, G., and Nash, D. R., 1969, Specific immunosuppression by minute doses of passive antibody, *Transplant. Proc.* **1**:616–618.

Hellström, K. E., and Hellström, I., 1974, Lymphocyte-mediated cytotoxicity and blocking serum activity to tumor antigens, *Adv. Immunol.* **18**:209–277.

Hellström, I., and Hellström, K. E., 1978, Cyclophosphamide delays 3-methylcholanthrene serum induction in mice, *Nature* **275**:129–130.

Hellström, I., Hellström, K. E., and Allison, A. C., 1971, Nenoatally induced allograft tolerance may be mediated by serum-borne factors, *Nature* **230**:49–50.

Hengst, J. C. D., Mokyr, M. B., and Dray, S., 1980, Importance of timing in cyclophosphamide therapy of MOPC-315 tumor-bearing mice, *Cancer Res.* **40**:2135–2141.

Hengst, J. C. D., Mokyr, M. B., and Dray, S., 1981, Cooperation between cyclophosphamide tumoricidal activity and host antitumor immunity in the cure of mice bearing large MOPC-315 tumors, *Cancer Res.* **41**:2163–2167.

Henney, C. S., Bourne, H. R., and Lichtenstein, L. M., 1972, The role of cyclic 3′,5′-adenosine monophosphate in the specific cytolytic activity of lymphocytes, *J. Immunol.* **108:**1526–1534.

Heppner, G. H., and Calabresi, P., 1972, Suppression by cytosine arabinoside of serum-blocking factors of cell-mediated immunity to syngeneic transplants of mouse mammary tumors, *J. Natl. Cancer Inst.* **48:**1161–1167.

Heppner, G. H., Griswold, D. E., DiLoorenzo, J., Polin, E. A., and Calabresi, P., 1974, Selective immunosuppression by drugs in balanced immune responses, *Fed. Proc.* **33:**1882–1885.

Herberman, R. B., and Holden, H. R., 1978, Natural cell-mediated immunity, *Adv. Cancer Res.* **27:**305–377.

Hosokawa, M., Mihich, E., Watanabe, T., and Pressman, D., 1975, Effect of antimyeloma cell antiserum on immunological enhancement, *Cancer Res.* **25:**591–595.

Hosokawa, M., Okayasu, T., Ikeda, K., Katoh, H., Suzuki, Y., and Kobayashi, H., 1983, Alteration of immunogenicity of xenogenized tumor cells in syngeneic rats by the immune responses to virus-associated antigens produced on immunizing cells, *Cancer Res.* **43:**2301–2305.

Hosokawa, M., Suzuki, Y., Takimoto, M., Morikawa, K., Mizushima, Y., and Kobayashi, H., 1985, Elimination of suppressor cells by bleomycin for augmentation of antitumor resistance in WKA rats immunized with irradiated tumor cells (submitted).

Inoue, T., and Sendo, F., 1983, *In vitro* induction of cytotoxic polymorphonuclear leukocytes by supernatant from a concanavalin A-stimulated spleen cell culture, *J. Immunol.* **131:**2508–2514.

Jerne, N. K., 1974, Towards a network therapy of the immune system, *Ann. Immunol. (Paris)* **125c:**373–389.

Julius, M. H., Augustin, A. A., and Cosenza, H., 1977, Recognition of a naturally occurring idiotype by autologous T cells, *Nature* **265:**251–253.

Jun, M. H., and Johnson, R. H., 1979, Effect of cyclophosphamide on tumour growth and cell-mediated immunity in sheep with ovine squamous cell carcinoma, *Res. Vet. Sci.* **27:**155–160.

Kaliss, N., 1958, Immunological enhancement of tumor homografts in mice: A review, *Cancer Res.* **18:**992–1003.

Kasai, M., Yoneda, T., Habu, S., Maruyama, Y., Okumura, K., and Tokunaga, T., 1981, *In vivo* effect of anti-asialo GM1 antibody on natural killer activity, *Nature* **291:**334–335.

Kataoka, T., Ogihara, K., and Sakurai, Y., 1980, Immunoprophylactic and immunotherapeutic response by concanavalian A-bound tumor vaccine enhanced by chemotherapeutic agents eliminating possible suppressors, *Cancer Res.* **40:**3839–3845.

Kataoka, T., Oh-Hashi, F., Sakurai, Y., and Ogihara, K., 1981, Effect of antineoplastic agents on the induction of suppressor macrophages by concanavalin A-bound tumor vaccine, *Cancer Res.* **41:**5151–5157.

Katayama, I., Parker, D., and Turk, J. L., 1982, In vivo macrophage suppression of delayed hypersensitivity in the guinea pig, *Immunology* **47:**709–716.

Katz, S. I., Parker, D., and Turk, J. L., 1974, B-cell suppression of delayed hypersensitivity reactions, *Nature* **251:**550–551.

Katz, S. I., Parker, D., Sommer, G., and Turk, J. L., 1974, Suppressor cells in normal immunisation as a basic homeostatic phenomenon, *Nature* **248:**612–614.

Kirchner, H., Chused, T. M., Herberman, R. B., Holden, H. T., and Lavrin, D. H., 1974a, Evidence of suppressor cell activity in spleens of mice bearing primary tumors induced by Moloney sarcoma virus, *J. Exp. Med.* **139:**1473–1487.

Kirchner, H., Herberman, R. B., Glaser, M., and Larvin, D. H., 1974b, Suppression of in vitro lymphocyte stimulation in mice bearing primary Moloney sarcoma virus-induced tumors, *Cell. Immunol.* **13:**32–40.

Kirchner, H., Holden, H. T., and Herberman, R. B., 1975a, Inhibition of *in vitro* growth of lymphoma cells by macrophages from tumor-bearing mice, *J. Natl. Cancer Inst.* **55:**971–975.

Kirchner, H., Muchmore, A. V., Chused, T. M., Holden, H. T., and Herberman, R. B., 1975b, Inhibition of proliferation of lymphoma cells and T lymphocytes by suppressor cells from spleens of tumor-bearing mice, *J. Immunol.* **114:**206–210.

Klaus, G. B., and Humphrey, J. H., 1977, The generation of memory cells. I. The role of C3 in the generation of B memory cells, *Immunology* **33:**31–40.

Klein, G., Sjögren, H. O., Klein, E., and Hellström, K. E., 1960, Demonstration of resistance against methylcholanthrene-induced sarcoma in the primary autochthonous host, *Cancer Res.* **20:**1561–1572.

Kobayashi, H., 1982, Modification of tumor antigenicity in therapeutics: Increase in immunologic foreignness of tumor cells in experimental model systems, in: *Immunological Approaches to Cancer Therapeutics* (E. Mihich, ed.), John Wiley and Sons, New York, pp. 405–440.

Kobayashi, H., Sendo, F., Kaji, H., Shirai, T., Saito, H., Takeichi, N., Hozokawa, M., and Kodama, T., 1970, Inhibition of transplanted rat tumors by immunization with identical tumor cells infected with Friend virus, *J. Natl. Cancer Inst.* **44:**11–19.

Kripke, M. L., 1980, Immune reactivity to autochthonous tumors in ultraviolet carcinogenesis, in: *Cancer Biol. Review 1* (J. J. Marchalonis, M. G. Hanna, and I. J. Fidler, eds.), Marcel Dekker, New York, pp. 221–250.

Lachmann, P. J., and Sikora, K., 1978, Coupling PPD to tumour cells enhances their antigenicity in BCG-primed mice, *Nature* **271:**463–464.

Lau, C., and Goldstein, G., 1980, Functional effects of thymopoietin$_{32\text{-}36}$ (TP5) on cytotoxic lymphocyte precursor units (CLP-U). I. Enhancement of splenic CLP-U *in vitro* and *in vivo* after suboptimal antigenic stimulation, *J. Immunol.* **124:**1861–1865.

Lin, J. S. L., Huber, N., and Murphy, W. H., 1969, Immunization of C58 mice to line Ib leukemia, *Cancer Res.* **29:**2157–2162.

Lotze, M. T., Grimm, E. A., Mazunder, A., Stransser, J. L., and Rosenberg, S. A., 1981, Lysis of fresh and cultured autologous tumor by human lymphocytes cultured in T-cell growth factor, *Cancer Res.* **41:**4420–4425.

Lu, Y-S, Kermani, V., and Moll, T., 1976, Cyclophosphamide-induced amelioration of Marek's disease-susceptible chickens, *Am. J. Vet. Res.* **37:**687–692.

Mantovani, A., Luini, W., Candiani, G. P., and Spreafico, F., 1980, Effect of chemotherapeutic agents on natural and BCG-stimulated macrophage cytotoxicity in mice, *Int. J. Immunopharmacol.* **2:**333–339.

Martin, F., Caignard, A., Olsson, O., Jeannin, J. F., and Leclerc, A., 1982, Tumoricidal effect of macrophages exposed to Adriamycin *in vivo* or *in vitro*, *Cancer Res.* **42:**3851–3857.

McMichael, A. J., Ting, A., Zweerink, H. J., and Askonas, B. A., 1977, HLA restriction of cell-mediated lysis of influenza virus-infected human cells, *Nature* **270:**524–526.

Miller, J. F. A. P., 1961, Immunological function of the thymus, *Lancet* **2:**748–749.

Minami, A., Mizushima, Y., Takeichi, N., Hosokawa, M., and Kobayashi, H., 1979, Dissociation of anti-tumor immune responses in rats immunized with solubilized tumor-associated antigens from a methylcholanthrene-induced fibrosarcoma, *Int. J. Cancer* **23:**358–365.

Minami, A., Kasai, M., Mizushima, Y., Takeichi, N., Hosokawa, M., and Kobayashi, H., 1980, Characterization of immunosuppressor cells in rats immunized with solubilized tumor-associated antigens prepared from a methylcholanthrene-induced fibrosarcoma, *Cancer Res.* **40:**2129–2134.

Minato, N., Reid, L., Cantor, H., Lengyel, P., and Bloom, B. R., 1980, Mode of regulation of natural killer cell activity by interferon, *J. Exp. Med.* **152:**124–137.

Mitchell, M. S., and Murakata, R. I., 1979, Modulation of immunity by bacillus Calmetti-Guerin (BCG), *Pharmacol. Ther.* **4:**329–353.

Mitchison, N. A., 1980, Regulation of the immune response to cell surface antigens, in: *Regulatory T-Lymphocytes* (B. Pernis and H. J. Vogel, eds.), Academic Press, New York, pp. 147–158.

Mizushima, Y., Sendo, F., Takeichi, N., Hosokawa, M., and Kobayashi, H., 1981, Enhancement of antitumor transplantation resistance in rats by appropriately timed administration of busulfan, *Cancer Res.* **41:**2917–2921.

Morikawa, K., Hosokawa, M., Hamada, J., and Kobayashi, H., 1985, Activation of macrophage-mediated cytotoxicity against tumor cells in rats treated with bleomycin (in preparation).

Morling, N., Jakobsen, B. K., Platz, P., Ryder, L. P., Svejgaard, A., and Thomsen, M., 1982, Typing for human alloantigens with the primed lymphocyte typing technique, *Adv. Immunol.* **32:**65–156.

Mortensen, R. F. and Gewurz, H., 1976, Effects of C-reactive protein on the lymphoid system.

II. Inhibition of mixed lymphocyte reactivity and generation of cytotoxic lymphocytes, *J. Immunol.* **116**:1244–1250.

Nakajima, H., Abe, S., Masuko, Y., Yamazaki, M., and Mizuno, D., 1981, Elimination of tumor-enhancing cells by cyclophosphamide and its relevance to cyclophosphamide therapy of mammary tumor, *Gann* **72**:723–731.

Naor, D., 1979, Suppressor cells: Permitters and promoters of malignancy? *Adv. Cancer Res.* **29**:45–125.

Natori, T., Law, L. W., and Appella, E., 1978, Immunochemical evidence of a tumor-specific surface antigen obtained by detergent solubilization of the membranes of a chemically induced sarcoma, Meth A, *Cancer Res.* **38**:359–364.

Ogura, T., Shindo, H., Shinzato, O., Namba, M., Masuno, T., Inoue, T., Kishimoto, S., and Yamamura, Y., 1982, In vitro tumor cell killing by peritoneal macrophages from mitomycin C-treated rats, *Cancer Immunol. Immunother.* **13**:112–117.

Oikawa, T., Gotohda, E., Austin, F. C., Takeichi, N., and Boone, C. W., 1979, Temperature-dependent alteration in immunogenicity of tumor-associated transplantation antigen monitored via paraformaldehyde fixation, *Cancer Res.* **39**:3519–3523.

Old, L. J., Stockert, E., Boyse, E. A., and Kim, J. H., 1968, Antigenic modulation: Loss of TL antigen from cells exposed to TL antibody. Study of the phenomenon *in vitro*, *J. Exp. Med.* **127**:523–539.

Orme, I. M., and Shand, F. L., 1981, Inhibitors of prostaglandin synthetase block the generation of suppressor T cells induced by Concanavalin A, *Int. J. Immunopharmacol.* **3**:15–19.

Ota, F., Parker, D., and Turk, J. L., 1979, Further evidence for non-T-cell regulation of delayed hypersensitivity in the guinea pig, *Cell. Immunol.* **43**:263–270.

Ozer H., 1982, Tumor immunity and escape mechanisms in humans, in: *Immunological Approaches to Cancer Therapeutics* (E. Mihich, ed.), John Wiley and Sons, New York, pp. 39–73.

Pellis, N. R., Yamagishi, H., Macek, C. M., and Kahan, B. D., 1980, Specificity and biological activity of extracted murine tumor-specific transplantation antigens, *Int. J. Cancer* **26**:443–449.

Pelus, L. M., and Bockman, R. S., 1979, Increased prostaglandin synthesis by macrophages from tumor-bearing mice, *J. Immunol.* **123**:2118–2125.

Pick, E., Honig, S., and Griffel, B., 1979, The mechanism of action of soluble lymphocyte mediators. VI. Effect of migration inhibitory factor (MIF) on macrophage microtubules, *Int. Arch. Allergy Appl. Immunol.* **58**:149–159.

Poulter, L. W., and Turk, J. L., 1975, Studies on the effect of soluble lymphocyte products (lymphokines) on macrophage physiology. II. Cytochemical changes associated with activation, *Cell. Immunol.* **20**:25–32.

Prager, M. D., Baechtel, F. S., Ribble, R. J., Ludden, C. M., and Mahta, J. M., 1974, Immunological stimulation with modified lymphoma cells in a minimally responsive tumor host system, *Cancer Res.* **34**:3203–3209.

Prehn, R. T., and Main, J. M., 1957, Immunity to methylcholanthrene-induced sarcomas, *J. Natl. Cancer Inst.* **18**:769–778.

Ray, P. K., and Raychaudhuri, S., 1981, Low-dose cyclophosphamide inhibition of transplantable fibrosarcoma growth by augmentation of the host immune response, *J. Natl. Cancer Inst.* **67**:1341–1345.

Rich, R. R., and Pierce, C. W., 1973, Biological expressions of lymphocyte activation. II. Generation of a population of thymus-derived suppressor lymphocytes, *J. Exp. Med.* **137**:649–659.

Riesenfeld, I., Örn, A., Gidlund, M., Axberg, I., Alm, G. V., and Wigzell, H., 1980, Positive correlation between *in vitro* NK activity and *in vivo* resistance towards AKR lymphoma cells, *Int. J. Cancer* **25**:399–403.

Robins, R. A., and Baldwin, R. W., 1974, Tumour-specific antibody neutralization of factors in rat hepatoma-bearer serum which abrogate lymph-node-cell cytotoxicity, *Int. J. Cancer* **14**:589–597.

Rosenthal, A. S., and Shevach, E. M., 1973, Function of macrophages in antigen recognition by guinea pig T lymphocytes. I. Requirement for histocompatible macrophages and lymphocytes, *J. Exp. Med.* **138**:1194–1212.

Rouveix, B., Badenoch-Jones, P., Larno, S., and Turk, J. L., 1980, Lymphokine-induced macrophage aggregation: The possible role of cyclic nucleotides, Immunopharmacology 2:319–326.

Sanderson, C. J., and Frost, P., 1974, The induction of tumour immunity in mice using glutaraldehyde-treated tumour cells, Nature 284:690–691.

Schwartz, A., Askenase, P. W., and Gershon, R. K., 1978, Regulation of delayed-type hypersensitivity reactions by cyclophosphamide-sensitive T cells, J. Immunol. 121:1573–1577.

Sendo, F., Seiji, K., Watabe, S., Fuyama, S., and Arai, S., 1981, Collaboration of polymorphonuclear leukocytes (PMN) with con-A-stimulated lymphocytes in the inhibition of tumor growth, Transplant. Proc. 13:1927–1928.

Shibata, Y., Tamura, K., and Ishida, N., 1983, In vivo analysis of the suppressive effects of immunosuppressive acidic protein, a type of α_1-acid glycoprotein, in connection with its high level in tumor-bearing mice, Cancer Res. 43:2889–2896.

Simon, P. L., and Willoughby, W. F., 1982, Biochemical and biological characterization of rabbit interleukin-1 (IL-1), in: Lymphokines 6: Lymphokines in Antibody and Cytotoxic Responses (S. B. Mizel, ed.), Academic Press, New York, pp. 47–64.

Singh, V., and Owen, J. J. T., 1975, Studies on the effect of various agents on the maturation of thymus stem cells, Eur. J. Immunol. 5:286–288.

Sjögren, H. O., Hellström, I., Bansal, S. C., and Hellström, K. E., 1971, Suggestive evidence that the "blocking antibodies" of tumor-bearing individuals may be antigen-antibody complexes, Proc. Natl. Acad. Sci. USA 68:1372–1375.

Sone, S., and Fidler, I. J., 1980, Synergistic activation by lymphokines and muramyl dipeptide of tumoricidal properties in rat alveolar macrophages, J. Immunol. 125:2454–2460.

Sonnenfeld, G., 1980, Modulation of immunity by interferon, in: Lymphokine Reports I (E. Pick, ed.), Academic Press, New York, pp. 113–132.

Spellman, L. W., and Daynes, R. A., 1977, Modification of immunological potential by ultraviolet radiation. II. Generation of suppressor cells in short-term UV-irradiated mice, Transplantation 24:120–126.

Stackpole, C. W., and Jacobson, J. B., 1978, Antigenic modulation, in: The Handbook of Cancer Immunology 2 (H. Waters, ed.), Garland STPM Press, New York, pp. 55–160.

Stadler, B. M., and Oppenheim, J. J., 1982, Human interleukin-2: Biological studies using purified IL-2 and monoclonal anti-IL-2 antibodies, in: Lympokines 6: Lymphokines in Antibody and Cytotoxic Responses (S. B. Mizel, ed.), Academic Press, New York, pp. 117–136.

Steele, J. G., Sjögren, H. O., and Ankerst J., 1974, The effects of cyclophosphamide on in vitro correlates of tumor immunity, Int. J. Cancer 14:743–752.

Sy, M. S., Bach, B. A., Dohi, Y., Nisonoff, A., Benacerraf, B., and Greene, M. I., 1979, Antigen- and receptor-driven regulatory mechanisms. I. Induction of suppressor T-cells with anti-idiotypic antibodies, J. Exp. Med. 150:1216–1228.

Sy, M. S., Brown, A. R., Benacerraf, G., and Greene, M. I., 1980, Antigen- and receptor-driven regulatory mechanisms. III. Induction of delayed-type hypersensitivity to azobenzenearsonate with anti-cross-reactive idiotypic antibodies, J. Exp. Med. 151:896–909.

Takatsu, K., Tominaga, A., and Kitagawa, M., 1978, Induction of antitumor activity in mice presensitized with mycobacterium by immunization with tuberculin-coated tumor, Gann 69:597–598.

Takeda, K., Kikuchi, Y., Yamawaki, S., Ueda, T., and Yoshiki, T., 1968, Treatment of artifical metastases of methylcholanthrene-induced rat sarcomas by autoimmunization of the autochthonous hosts, Cancer Res. 28:2149–2154.

Takei, F., Levy, J. G., and Kilburn, D. G., 1977, Characterization of suppressor cells in mice bearing syngeneic mastocytoma, J. Immunol. 118:412–417.

Talmadge, J. E., Meyers, K. M., Prieur, D. J., and Starkey, J. L., 1980, Role of NK cells in tumour growth in metastasis in beige mice, Nature 284:622–624.

Tamura, K., Shibata, Y., Matsuda, Y., and Ishida, N., 1981, Isolation and characterization of an immunosuppressive acidic protein from ascitic fluids of cancer patients, Cancer Res. 41:3244–3252.

Terashima, M., Takeichi, N., Suzuki, K., Itaya, T., Gotohda, E., and Kobayashi, H., 1980, Enhanced immunogenicity of xenogenized tumor cells in rats pretreated with cyclophospha-mide, *Tohoku J. Exp. Med.* **132:**355–361.

Thurman, G. B., Marshall, G. D., Low, T. L. K., and Goldstein, A. L., 1980, Thymosin: Structural studies and immunoregulatory role in host immunity, in: *Thymus, Thymic Hormones, and T-Lymphocytes* (F. Aiuti and H. Wigzell, eds.), Academic Press, New York, pp. 175–185.

Timonen, T., Saksela, E., Ranki, A., and Hayry, P., 1979, Fractionation, morphological, and functional characterization of effector cells responsible for human natural killer activity against cell-line targets, *Cell. Immunol.* **48:**133–148.

Tomazic, V., Ehrke, M. J., and Mihich, E., 1980, Modulation of the cytoxic response against allogeneic tumor cells in culture by Adriamycin, *Cancer Res.* **40:**2748–2755.

Trainin, N., Umiel, T., and Yakir, Y., 1980, Biological effects of THF on thymus cell subpo-pulations in mice, in: *Thymus, Thymic Hormones, and T-lymphocytes* (F. Aiuti and H. Wigzell, eds.), Academic Press, New York, pp. 201–211.

Turk, J. L., and Parker, D., 1982, Effect of cyclophosphamide on immunological control mech-anisms, *Immunol. Rev.* **65:**99–113.

Unanue, E. R., 1978, The regulation of lymphocyte functions by the macrophage, *Immunol. Rev.* **40:**227–255.

Urushizaki, I., Ishitani, K., Nagai, T., Gocho, Y., and Koyama, R., 1977, Immunosuppressive factors in serum of patients with gastric carcinoma, *Gann* **68:**413–421.

Vadas, M. A., Miller, J. F. A. P., Whitelaw, A. M., and Gamble, J. R., 1977, Regulation by the H-2 gene complex of delayed type hypersensitivity, *Immunogenetics* **4:**137–153.

Voisin, G. A., 1971, Immunological facilitation: A broadening of the concept of the enhancement phenomenon, *Prog. Allergy* **15:**328–485.

Voisin, G. A., 1980, Role of antibody classes in the regulatory facilitation reaction, *Immunol. Rev.* **49:**3–59.

Watson, J., Frank, M. B., Mochizuki, D., and Gillis, S., 1982, The biochemistry and biology of interleukin-2, in: *Lymphokines 6: Lymphokines in Antibody and Cytotoxic Responses* (S. B. Mizel, ed.), Academic Press, New York, pp. 95–116.

Webb, D. R., and Nowowiejski, I., 1977, The role of prostaglandins in the control of the primary 19s immune response to sRBC, *Cell. Immunol.* **33:**1–10.

Wepsic, H. T., Harris, S., Sander, J., Alaimo, J., and Morris, H., 1976, Enhancement of tumor growth following immunization with *Bacillus Calmette-Guerin* cell walls, *Cancer Res.* **36:**1950–1953.

Wolf, R. E., 1979, Thymosin-induced suppression of proliferative response of human lympho-cytes to mitogens, *J. Clin. Invest.* **63:**677–683.

Wu, R. L., and Kearney, R., 1979, Effect of carrageenan on the non-specific resistance of mice to injected syngeneic tumour cells, alone or in mixtures, *Br. J. Cancer* **39:**241–246.

Yamagishi, H., Pellis, N. P., and Kahan, B. D., 1979, Tumor-protective and -facilitating antigens from 3M KCl-solubilized tumor extracts, *J. Surg. Res.* **26:**392–399.

Yamaguchi, H., Moriuchi, T., Hosokawa, M., and Kobayashi, H., 1982, Increased or decreased immunogenicity of tumor-associated antigen according to the amount of virus-associated antigen in rat tumor cells infected with Friend virus, *Cancer Immunol. Immunother.* **12:**119–123.

Yamazaki, M., Shinoda, H., and Mizuno D., 1975, Cooperation between macrophages and a factor from lymphocytes in tumor lysis *in vitro*, *Gann* **66:**489–497.

Zembala, M., and Asherson, G. L., 1973, Depression of the T cell phenomenon of contact sensitivity by T cells from unresponsive mice, *Nature* **244:**227–228.

Zembala, M., Asherson, G. L., Nowowlski, T., and Mayhew, B., 1976, Contact sensitivity to picryl chloride: The occurrence of B suppressor cells in the lymph nodes and spleen of immunized mice, *Cell. Immunol.* **25:**266–278.

Zinkernagel, R. M., and Doherty, P. C., 1974, Restriction of *in vitro* cell-mediated cytotoxicity in lymphocytic choriomeningitis within a syngeneic or semi-allogeneic system, *Nature* **248:**701–702.

Zinkernagel, R. M., and Doherty, P. C., 1977, Major transplantation antigens, viruses, and specificity of surveillance T cells, in: *Contemporary Topics in Immunobiology*, Volume 7 (O. Stutman, ed.), Plenum Press, New York, pp. 179–220.

CHAPTER 2

INTERACTIONS OF ANTIMETABOLITES WITH TUMORS AND THE IMMUNE SYSTEM

FRED R. MILLER and TATESHI KATAOKA

1. INTRODUCTION

The evidence that antimetabolites have immunosuppressive activity, accumulated for over a quarter of a century, is overwhelming. Some, such as azathioprine, are used primarily as immunosuppressive agents rather than as anticancer drugs. Our aim is not simply to review the evidence that antimetabolites are immunosuppressive but to address the interplay of these agents with both tumor and host.

It is widely recognized that different tumors have different levels of resistance to individual drugs so that there is a need to identify drugs that are active against cancer cells from individual patients. Subpopulations of individual tumors can, likewise, have different levels of resistance (Barranco *et al.*, 1972; Hakansson and Trope, 1974; Heppner *et al.*, 1978; Tsuruo and Fidler, 1981). Subpopulations of heterogeneous tumors are not autonomous but are intercommunicative such that one tumor subpopulation can influence the drug resistance of a second one (Miller *et al.*, 1981; Miller *et al.*, 1983). Furthermore, the sensitivity of host cells can be altered by the presence of tumor cells in that the severity and duration of drug-induced immunosuppression may be influenced by the presence of a tumor. (DeWys and Mansky, 1973; Harrison *et al.*, 1980). Of course, drug-induced immunosuppression may be superimposed on an already depressed state of immunity in the tumor bearer.

FRED R. MILLER ● Department of Immunology, Michigan Cancer Foundation, Detroit, Michigan 48201.   TATESHI KATAOKA ● Division of Experimental Chemotherapy, Cancer Chemotherapy Center, Japanese Foundation for Cancer Research, Tokyo 170, Japan.

Drug treatment can alter the antigenic stimulus as well as the response. Treatment of mice bearing tumors may result in the growth of genetically stable drug-resistant variants that are more immunogenic than the parental tumor line. This was first demonstrated by Mihich (1969b) and Bonmassar *et al.* (1970) with L1210 cells; it may occur after treatment with a spectrum of drugs (Nicolin *et al.*, 1972). Susceptibility of tumor cells to host defense mechanisms can be transiently increased by metabolic inhibitors *in vitro* (Segerling *et al.*, 1975; Hunyadi *et al.*, 1981).

A desirable antineoplastic agent does the cancer patient more good than harm, i.e., it has a favorable therapeutic index. To this end, experimental pharmacologists have sought drugs that selectively kill tumor cells rather than host cells or, alternatively, drugs that selectively rescue host cells from the toxic effects of another drug. Because the immune response to a tumor is a very complex network of cell interactions, various drugs and regimens suppress different parts of the host response. Thus it may be possible to selectively suppress immune components, such as suppressor cells (Rollinghoff *et al.*, 1977; Tarnowski *et al.*, 1978; Orbach-Arbouys and Castes, 1979) or "blocking serum" (Heppner and Calabresi, 1972; Buchman *et al.*, 1979), so that tumor growth is ultimately inhibited. Combination chemoimmunotherapy may not be markedly different from other toxic drug/rescue drug regimens; an adjuvant, such as Bacillus Calmette–Guérin (BCG) may be considered by some to be operationally comparable to a rescuing agent. Although many studies have attempted to induce tumor-specific immunity with various vaccine preparations, these attempts have not been highly successful. However, the value of nonspecific immune stimulation should not be discounted since "70% of patients with acute leukemia and about 50% of patients with solid tumors and lymphoma die of infection" (Ketchel and Rodriguez, 1978), and prevention of opportunistic infections may be an achievable goal of chemoimmunotherapy regimens.

2. THIOPURINES

A number of purine analogues have been synthesized and examined for antitumor activity in animal models. Among them, 6-mercaptopurine (6-MP) and 6-thioguanine (6-TG) are currently in clinical use in cancer therapy.

6-MP has long been known as a potent immunosuppressant. Azathioprine, a nitromidazole derivative of 6-MP, is a well-known immunosuppressant used in experimental and clinical transplantation studies. Many experimental studies have described 6-MP- and 6-TG-induced immunosuppression. It was assumed that the antitumor mechanisms of these agents are confined to anticellular effects by which these agents would inhibit purine metabolism in tumor cells.

Advances in immunopharmacology, however, urged us to reconsider whether these drugs suppress immune responses of tumor-bearing hosts in the protocols in which they are therapeutically beneficial. In fact, very early studies pointed to the augmentation of host immunity by 6-MP under certain conditions (Chanmougan and Schwartz, 1966). It is now known that, among the differentiated cells involved in host defenses, i.e., T cells, B cells, and macrophages, and among T-lymphocyte subpopulations, i.e., helper, cytotoxic, and suppressor cells, a clear difference can be seen in the *in vitro* and *in vivo* susceptibility to drugs, especially to purine analogues. These observations suggest that, under appropriate conditions, thiopurines may preferentially eliminate some immunocyte populations, resulting in the eventual potentiation of antitumor immunity. Furthermore, thiopurines are known to be potent differentiation inducers and may act on selected immunocyte subpopulations, thus favoring the induction of host antitumor immunity.

2.1. Immunosuppression

Thiopurine-induced suppression of antibody production is dependent on the dose of 6-TG. When mice given formalin-treated sheep red blood cells intraperitoneally (i.p.) on day 0 were administered 6-TG i.p. on day 2, the number of plaque-forming cells per spleen of these mice on day 5 was 0.1–10% of the control, dependent on the 6-TG dose which ranged from 1 to 100 mg/kg (Berenbaum, 1969).

The suppression of the primary antibody production was dependent on the timing of drug administration as well, the suppression being evident when the drug was administered soon after the sensitization, within 48 hr in most cases (Frish and Davies, 1962; Winkelstein *et al.*, 1971). The same total dose was more efficient when given in several fractions than in a single dose (Nathan *et al.*, 1960). In contrast to the suppression of the primary response, that of the secondary response was observed less frequently (Winkelstein *et al.*, 1971).

A difference has been noted in the sensitivity of the response of various immunoglobulin classes to thiopurines. Depending on dose and time of administration, 6-MP suppressed IgG production more readily than IgM production (Borel *et al.*, 1965, Sahiar and Schwartz, 1964). When primed mice were given 6-MP and a second antigenic challenge, they produced antibody of the IgM type, whereas they normally produced antiboody of the IgG type.

Furthermore, 6-MP was found to discriminate between IgG subclasses. In guinea pigs, IgG1 and IgG2 antibodies reactive to bovine gamma globulin (BGG) were produced by the primary sensitization with dinitrophenylated BGG. When 6-MP was administered on days 1–7 after the priming, the BGG-carrier-specific IgG1 response was completely suppressed, whereas the carrier-specific IgG2 response was not affected at all for the 28-day observation period. The suppression was limited to the primary response; the secondary carrier-specific IgG1 antibody production after boosting with BGG was not influenced under the experimental conditions tested (Drossler *et al.*, 1983).

Some of the phenomena described previously could be elicited by other drugs. The suppression of the induction of hemolysin-forming cells in mouse spleen was achieved both by 6-MP and by cyclophosphamide in a dose-dependent fashion. However, further analysis showed that the dose–response curve of cyclophosphamide was exponential whereas that of 6-MP was hyperbolic (Berenbaum, 1969). Furthermore, in inducing the primary anti-BGG antibody in guinea pigs, 6-MP suppressed IgG1 but not IgG2 response, whereas cyclophosphamide suppressed both IgG1 and IgG2 antibody production without selectivity (Drossler et al., 1983). These results indicate that 6-MP could more readily interact with one immunocyte population than with others.

The 6-MP-dependent suppression of delayed hypersensitivity (DH) seems somewhat complex. 6-MP suppressed DH to purified protein derivative (PPD) of BCG in guinea pigs and, in these animals, in vitro lymphocyte response to PPD was decreased (Winkelstein, 1973). Another study also showed that guinea pigs primarily sensitized with Mycobacterium tuberculosis and then treated with 6-MP (days 3–12) had suppressed DH while their lymphocytes responded in vitro to PPD quite well (Phillips and Zweiman, 1973). Phillips et al. (1979) later determined that the defect was caused by qualitative changes in cells of the monocyte–macrophage series so that those cells were poorly responsive to lymphokines. These results may reflect not only the complexity of DH but, also, the differential effects of 6-MP in inducing immunocyte modulation.

Thiopurines may selectively suppress cellular immunity. Arabinosyl 6-MP, but not 6-MP itself, suppressed homograft reaction, whereas it did not suppress antibody production against sheep red blood cells (sRBC) (Kimball et al., 1965). Furthermore, 6-MP prevented the DH to thyroid antigens in allergic experimental thyroiditis in guinea pigs, whereas it did not change the production of the corresponding humoral antibodies (Spiegelberg and Miescher, 1963).

2.2. Immunopotentiation

During the course of a very early study of immune suppression by thiopurines, it was found that, under specified conditions, 6-MP enhanced antibody synthesis. Test rabbits were given 6-MP of 10 mg/kg per day for 7 days. Two, five, or twenty days after the last injection of the drug, they received a single intravenous (i.v.) injection of either 0.02, 2.0, or 200 mg of BGG, and serum antibody activity was measured. A markedly enhanced antibody production was found for a 16-day period in animals receiving 6-MP and 0.02 mg BGG. At higher doses of BGG the enhancement was less evident. Furthermore, IgM and IgG production responded differently. When BGG was given 2 days after the last dose of a 1-week course of 6-MP, the enhancement was found in antibody of IgM type but not of IgG type. At longer intervals (5 or 20 days) after 6-MP injections, BGG induced an enhanced production of both IgM and IgG antibody (Chanmougan and Schwartz, 1966).

6-MP-dependent enhancement of humoral immunity was also found in antihapten antibody production (Drossler et al., 1983). The injection of dinitrophenylated BGG induced both hapten-reactive and carrier-reactive antibodies. 6-MP enhanced the hapten-reactive antibody production selectively. The production of IgG1 was enhanced; that of IgG2 was suppressed.

The enhancement was not restricted to humoral immunity. 6-MP enhanced the chronic allogeneic disease (graft-versus-host reaction) occurring in B6D2F$_1$ mice injected with C57BL/6 spleen cells (Schwartz and Beldotti, 1965). 6-MP enhanced the activity of effector cells in antibody-dependent cellular cytotoxicity (Medzihradsky et al., 1982). When mice given 6-TG at 30 mg/kg i.v. on day 0 were given sRBC i.p. on day 1, antibody production and DH to sRBC were suppressed as determined after an eliciting injection of sRBC subcutaneously. However, when the interval between 6-TG administration and immunization with sRBC was prolonged from 1 day to 5–9 days, DH was enhanced by up to 50%. The enhancement was dependent on dose of immunogen (Van Dijk and Voermans, 1978).

The mechanism of thiopurine-induced enhancement is not known. Cyclophosphamide, which also is able to potentiate DH, may affect a regulatory T-cell subpopulation or subpopulations leading to the enhancement (Mitsuoka et al., 1976; Schwartz et al., 1978). Such also may be the case with thiopurine-induced enhancement (Medzihradsky et al., 1981). Although some analogy was indicated between 6-TG- and cyclophosphamide-induced enhancement in terms of the inducing conditions (Van Dijk and Voermans, 1978), the difference between 6-MP and cyclophosphamide in their effect on antihapten antibody production should be noted (Drossler et al., 1983).

2.3. Antitumor Immunity

The potency of thiopurines as antitumor agents has been attributed to their cytostatic inhibition of tumor cells. In addition, thiopurines may modulate host antitumor immunity to help the host eliminate the tumor. Sarcoma 180 grows initially in 100% of Swiss HaICR female mice but is eventually rejected in 0–25% of them. The incidence of regression is greatly increased by therapeutic treatments with 6-MP. Mice transplanted subcutaneously with Sarcoma 180 were given 6-MP at a dose of 25 mg/kg per day once daily i.p. for 7 days starting the day after tumor implantation. Half of these mice were completely cured, whereas 20% of nontreated mice were cured. In neonatally thymectomized mice, 6-MP-induced regression incidence was reduced to less than 10% indicating that the regressions of Sarcoma 180 in 6-MP-treated mice were dependent upon immunologic responses of the host. In mice splenectomized about 2 weeks prior to tumor implantation, 6-MP-induced regression incidence was increased to about 80%. These results do not tell us whether 6-MP actively modulated the host antitumor immunity. However, it is clear that host antitumor immunity was involved in the 6-MP-induced therapeutic response (Mihich, 1969a).

A recent study of therapeutic effects of thiopurines in L1210-leukemia-bearing mice indicated the immunomodulating potency of 6-MP in antitumor immunity (Kataoka et al., 1984). The survival of L1210-bearing mice treated with tumor cell vaccine and antineoplastic agents was examined. Combination of the vaccine with 6-MP, but not with cyclophosphamide, cytosine arabinoside (Ara-C), or 5-fluorouracil (5FU) produced an augmented therapeutic response, although, as single agents, the three other agents were therapeutically equivalent to or better than 6-MP. The augmented therapeutic response was induced by the combination of the vaccine and 6-TG, azathioprine, or 6-MP indicating that, in this experimental model, thiopurines were distinguished from other antineoplastic agents. 6-MP injected on day 5 after L1210 implantation was more protective than 6-MP injected on day 3, although as a single agent, 6-MP on day 3 induced a better therapeutic response than 6-MP on day 5 (Kataoka *et al.*, 1984). In this study, the therapeutic response was tumor-specific since the combination of tumor vaccine and 6-MP was not effective in mice bearing P388 leukemia. In mice successfully treated with tumor vaccine and 6-MP, antitumor T cells were detected, whereas in untreated mice and in mice treated with either agent alone, antitumor immunocytes were not detected (Kataoka *et al.*, 1983). At this moment, it is not clear how 6-MP augments antitumor T-cell production.

2.4. Induction of Hematological Differentiation

Some antineoplastic agents, including thiopurines (Prasad, 1973) have long been known to be potent inducers of cell differentiation. Animal and human tumor cells, including those of myelogeneous leukemia, neuroblastoma, mammary carcinoma, and melanoma, can be induced by antineoplastic agents to differentiate *in vitro*. Some therapeutic success with such agents has been reported in animal models using myelogeneous leukemia and in cancer patients with leukemia or neuroblastoma (Hozumi, 1983).

The effectiveness of thiopurines as inducers of erythroid differentiation in cultured murine erythroleukemia has been tested (Gusella and Housman, 1976). 6-MP and 6-TG, as well as the naturally occurring purine, hypoxanthine, were shown to be extremely potent inducers. 6-TG was effective at a concentration of 60 μM, 750-fold lower than the concentration of dimethyl sulfoxide, the most widely used inducer. All three compounds were potent inducers of hypoxanthine-guanine phosphoribosyltransferase-negative cell lines; hence incorporation of purines into DNA and inhibition of cell growth were not required for induction of differentiation (Gusella and Housman, 1976).

Granulocyte differentiation was inducible by 6-TG. HL60 human leukemia cells were differentiated in the presence of 0.5 μM 6-TG after 7 days' cultivation. Maturation of HL60 cells was attainable without significant cytotoxicity, and differentiated cells had granulocyte morphology and were capable of generating superoxide anion during the respiratory burst typical of mature phagocytic cells (Papac, 1980).

Under the proper conditions, 6-MP induced the production of host hematological cells, possibly through differentiation (Kataoka *et al.*, 1981). When mice were sensitized with tumor cell vaccine and treated with four other antineoplastic agents, host cells recovered from the peritoneal cavity were decreased in number as compared with those from mice only sensitized with tumor cell vaccine. However, under the same conditions, 6-MP increased the number of peritoneal cells recovered.

In tumor-bearing hosts, 6-MP could increase the number of peritoneal macrophages. Peritoneal macrophages of L1210 leukemia-bearing mice were potent suppressors in *in vitro* polyclonal spleen cell blastogenesis. When 6-MP at 100 mg/kg was administered to these mice at day 5 after tumor implantation, the number of peritoneal macrophages at day 7 were tripled as compared with that in nontreated mice. Nevertheless, their suppressor activity was decreased by more than 50% (Kataoka *et al.*, 1983).

2.5. Anticellular Effect on Immunocytes

As previously discussed, thiopurines have been shown to suppress humoral and cellular immunity. It was noted, however, that under appropriate conditions the induced suppression was not uniform. In animals sensitized with dinitrophenylated BGG, 6-MP affected antihapten- and anticarrier-reactive antibody production differently. Furthermore, the suppressive effect detected was dependent on IgG subclasses measured. It was also noted that induction of humoral and of cellular immunity was affected by 6-MP differently. 6-MP prevented DH to thyroid antigens whereas it did not change the production of corresponding humoral antibody (Spiegelberg and Miescher, 1963). These findings indicate the possibility that 6-MP may preferentially interact with some of the immunocyte populations and interfere with their immunological function or kill them.

The effects of 6-MP (7.5 mg/kg) and cyclophosphamide (15 or 30 mg/kg) on peripheral blood cells have been compared in mice. Injections were given daily for 5–8 weeks. 6-MP decreased the levels of circulating polymorphonuclear leukocytes, monocytes, and large lymphocytes; small and medium lymphocyte counts remained unchanged. In contrast, cyclophosphamide decreased mainly the small and medium lymphocytes, leaving the other cell types unchanged. From these results, it was suggested that 6-MP exerted an antiproliferative action on the bone marrow as shown by a decrease of short-lived cells in the blood. Cyclophosphamide, on the other hand, appeared to have mainly a cytotoxic effect on circulating cells, resulting in depletion of the long-lived small lymphocytes (Lemmel *et al.*, 1971).

T and B cells may be preferentially affected by thiopurines. This can be inferred from experimental evidence that thiopurines suppressed T-cell-dependent responses more than humoral antibody production as noted in the comparative study in the response to thyroid antigens (Speigelberg and Miescher, 1963).

The cellular basis of T-cell-preferential immunosuppression by thiopurines is not clear. T and B cells differ in purine metabolism. In cultured human lymphoblasts, a clear difference in levels of ecto-5′-nucleotidase was found. T lymphoblasts contained 1.3 nmol/hr 5′-nucleotidase per 10^6 cells, assayed using deoxyadenosine monophosphate as a substrate, whereas B lymphoblasts contained 9.15 nmol/hr 5′-nucleotidase per 10^6 cells, although the apparent Michaelis constant was the same in both cells (Wortmann *et al.*, 1979). In the peripheral blood lymphocytes of healthy volunteers, adenosine deaminase activity and purine nucleotide phosphorylase activity were enriched in T cells, whereas etco-5′-nucleotidase was enriched in B cells. No difference was found in kinases of deoxycytidine, deoxyguanosine, deoxyadenosine, and adenosine (Massaia *et al.*, 1982). A recent study points to the potential importance of soluble deoxyguanosine activity as compared with the corresponding ectoenzyme (Carson *et al.*, 1981). In rats, it was reported that terminal deoxynucleotidyl transferase as well as 5′-nucleotidase and adenosine deaminase were higher in T cells than B cells (Barton and Goldschneider, 1978). These differences between T and B cells in enzymes involved in purine metabolism suggest that these enzymes could be the target of thiopurines in preferentially inhibiting T cells. At the moment, this has not been well substantiated by the experimental findings, but the feasibility of such an approach may be suggested by the following studies.

Deoxyguanosine inhibited human T and B lymphoblasts differently. At 10 μM, deoxyguanosine completely inhibited cell growth and killed 50% of T lymphoblasts, whereas it did not affect B lymphoblasts at all (Ochs *et al.*, 1979). In a separate experiment, deoxyguanosine markedly inhibited T-lymphoblast growth and phytohemagglutinin- (PHA) induced T-cell proliferation but did not affect the differentiation of B cells to an antibody-secreting stage. Deoxyadenosine was much less inhibitory to these T-cell responses, but in the presence of an inhibitor of adenosine deaminase, its effects on T-lymphoblast growth and PHA-induced T-cell proliferation were markedly potentiated (Gelfand *et al.*, 1979).

The preferential inhibition of T cells by deoxyguanosine or deoxyadenosine plus an inhibitor of adenosine deaminase was biochemically analyzed further. It was found that elevation of the corresponding deoxyribonucleoside triphosphates occurred in T cells but not in B cells. The addition of deoxycytidine resulted in lower intracellular concentrations of the corresponding deoxyribonucleoside triphosphates and prevented deoxyribonucleoside toxicity (Mitchell *et al.*, 1978).

Although T and B cells originate from common progenitor cells, they have clear differences in purine nucleotide metabolism, suggesting that the differentiation is associated with this factor. This may extend to T-cell subpopulations of different maturation stages and/or having different immunologic activity, in which case they may be expected to be differentially susceptible to purine analogues. This hypothesis is supported by experimental findings. As compared to more mature T cells of peripheral blood, proliferation of T cells from the thymus was more sensitive to inhibition by deoxyguanosine. This was related to a higher level of deoxynucleoside kinase and a lower level of 5′-nucleotidase, suggesting that these enzymes could serve as differentiation markers of T-cell maturation (Cohen *et al.*, 1980).

Adenosine deaminase may also be associated with T-cell maturation. The specific activity of this enzyme was 3- to 10-fold higher in thymocytes than in lymphocytes from thoracic duct, lymph node, spleen, and bone marrow. This high adenosine deaminase activity in thymocytes appeared to be preferentially associated with cortical thymocytes. "Immature" cortical thymocytes and thymocyte progenitors appeared to have low adenosine deaminase activity; low enzyme levels were found in fetal thymus at 16 days of embryonic life, in the early phases of thymus regeneration, and in a "null" cell population isolated from bone marrow (Barton et al., 1979). This finding may be related to another finding that the less matured cortical thymocytes agglutinable by peanut lectin were more susceptible to adenosine deaminase inhibition by 2′-deoxycoformycin than the more mature medullary thymocytes not agglutinable by peanut lectin (Ballow and Pantschenko, 1981).

Among the functionally distinct T-cell subpopulations, suppressor T cells seem more sensitive to deoxyguanosine than the other functional T cells. The effect of deoxyguanosine on the *in vitro* generation of concanavalin-A-induced suppressor T cells was tested on the secondary anti-sRBC response *in vitro*. It was found that deoxyguanosine administered *in vivo* (1 mg per mouse, i.p. daily for 4 days) strongly inhibited the *in vitro* production of suppressor T cells in the spleen, whereas cytotoxic T-cell production was not inhibited. It was also shown that production of natural killer cells of mice injected with deoxyguanosine was not affected, indicating the preferential inhibition of suppressor T cells by deoxyguanosine (Varely et al., 1983). Another study disclosed that deoxyguanosine *in vitro* inhibited the action of suppressor T cells but not of helper T cells on the response to ovalbumin (Gelfand et al., 1979). *In vivo* deoxyguanosine administration resulted in a similar result, i.e., inhibition of production of suppressor T cells but not of helper T cells (Dosch et al., 1980).

3. DTIC

5-(3,3′-Dimethyl-1-triazeno)-imidazole-4-carboxamide (DTIC) is both an antipurine and alkylating antineoplastic agent; it has been shown to be therapeutically effective against a limited number of tumors including melanoma. Not much information is available on its activity in modulating the host immune status. Nevertheless, this drug has received much attention as an immunomodulating agent because of its potency in enhancing the immunogenicity of tumor cells. Although the effects of this drug are discussed extensively in Chapter 5, a brief summary of these effects is outlined in this section because of the antimetabolite nature of the agent.

3.1. Immunosuppression

In one study, DTIC exhibited limited immunosuppressive activity in melanoma patients. It was concluded that DTIC possessed little immunosuppressive activity in man and that this property would make the combined modality of DTIC with antigenic melanoma cell vaccine more beneficial

(Bruckner *et al.*, 1974). Berkelhammer *et al.* (1977) also found no evidence that DTIC treatment of melanoma patients altered lymphocyte number or *in vitro* cytoxic activity for tumor cells.

In mice, however, DTIC has been shown to suppress both cellular and humoral immunity. DTIC was suppressive when given before antigen, whereas cyclophosphamide was suppressive when given after antigen. DTIC was less suppressive than cyclophosphamide on a mg/kg basis, but DTIC-induced suppression was more prolonged than cyclophosphamide-induced suppression, although both agents displayed a qualitatively equal activity in reducing bone marrow stem cells (Vecchi *et al.*, 1976; Puccetti *et al.*, 1978).

It has also been reported that DTIC suppresses macrophage-mediated tumor cell killing but not natural killer activity in mice (Mantovani *et al.*, 1978; Spreafico, 1980). Tumoricidal activity of both normal macrophages and BCG-stimulated macrophages was suppressed by DTIC (Mantovani *et al.*, 1980).

3.2. Enhancement of Tumor Cell Antigenicity

Several variants of L1210 lines have acquired strong antigenicity (Bonmassar *et al.*, 1970). This variation appeared stable. For a detailed discussion of this phenomenon, see Chapter 5.

The strong antigenicity may have been acquired through a somatic mutation induced by DTIC because the antimutagenic compound quinacrine prevented the formation of these L1210 lines; quinacrine did not inhibit the DTIC-induced immunosuppression (Giampietri *et al.*, 1980). DTIC-dependent enhancement of antigenicity was found in L5178Y lymphoma, LSTRA and RBL5 leukemia, and Sarcoma 51033 and in different mouse strains as well (Bonmassar *et al.*, 1975; Houchens *et al.*, 1976).

Other drugs may also enhance the antigenicity of tumor cells. It was found that L1210 sublines resistant to Ara-C, guanazole, methyl-glyoxal *bis*(guanylhydrazone), or 4,4-diacetyldiphenylurea *bis*(guanylhydrazone) expressed an increased amount of murine mammary leukemia virus antigen (Strzadala *et al.*, 1981). However, the antigen molecules induced by DTIC have not been identified, although they have been partially characterized. *In vitro* studies showed that the effector cells were T cells and could lyse DTIC-induced variant tumor cells much more efficiently than the parent tumor cells (Testorelli *et al.*, 1978; Fioretti *et al.*, 1978). In addition, DTIC-treated sublines may be less susceptible to killing by natural killer cells (Romani *et al.*, 1983).

The structural requirement of DTIC in inducing the antigenic variants was examined. Four aryltriazene analogues were synthesized and these, as well as DTIC, were compared for *in vivo* induction of antigenic changes of L1210 leukemia cells. The imidazole moiety present in DTIC was not directly responsible for the generation of new antigens, because the four analog triazene derivatives not containing the imidazole ring produced effects on cellular antigenicity similar to those described for DTIC as assayed by transplantability in immunologically competent versus suppressed CD2F$_1$ mice (Fioretti *et al.*, 1981).

DTIC need not be cytotoxic for the tumor cells in order to cause alteration in immunogenicity; a DTIC-resistant subline of L1210 became more immunogenic after DTIC treatment *in vivo* (Fioretti *et al.*, 1981). The appearance of strongly immunogenic variants does not represent the emergence of clones normally repressed except in immunosuppressed (with DTIC) mice because highly immunogenic sublines of L1210 and LSTRA tumors did not emerge in nude mice unless they were treated with DTIC (Campanile *et al.*, 1975). It has been suggested that DTIC treatment of human tumors growing in nude mice could yield useful variants for immunotherapy (Goldin *et al.*, 1980). DTIC has also been found to induce antigenic changes in L1210 *in vitro* (Contessa *et al.*, 1979).

It is not known how much the induction of new antigens on tumor cells by DTIC contributes to the therapeutic effect of DTIC in the tumor-bearing host, but Giampietri *et al.* (1981) concluded that transplantation immunity was so severely depressed in DTIC-treated mice that the increase in tumor antigenicity was probably of no therapeutic value.

3.3. Chemoimmunotherapy

In man, DTIC is not a potent immunosuppressive agent and has been used widely for the treatment of malignant melanoma, a type of cancer that tends to be relatively immunogenic. Several attempts have been made to use a combination of DTIC chemotherapy and some form of immunotherapy, either specific or nonspecific. Currie and McElwain (1975) combined DTIC plus vincristine chemotherapy with a tumor vaccine consisting of irradiated allogeneic melanoma cells and BCG. They observed objective regressions in 17 of 30 patients, but there were no control patients treated with chemotherapy only. However, a vaccine prepared identically but given in combination with DTIC and ICRF 159 did not increase patient survival compared to chemotherapy alone (Newlands *et al.*, 1976). BCG has been reported to improve therapy with DTIC in some studies (Gutterman *et al.*, 1974; Wood *et al.*, 1978) but not in others (Ramseur *et al.*, 1978). The combination of DTIC and *Corynebacterium parvum* has also not proved to be effective (Karakousis *et al.*, 1979).

4. FLUORINATED PYRIMIDINE ANALOGS

The cytotoxic activities of 5FU and 2′-deoxy-5-fluorouridine (FUDR) are caused by the inhibition of thymidylate synthetase, thus inhibiting DNA synthesis by blocking the conversion of deoxyuridine-5′-phosphate (dUMP) to thymidine-5′-phosphate (TMP). 5FU may also act via incorporation of fluorouridine-5′-phosphate into RNA. Two other analogs, N$_1$-(2′-furanidyl)5-fluorauracil (ftorafur) and 5′-deoxy-5-fluorouridine (5DFUR), are inactive until converted to 5FU.

Marked leukopenia after 5FU treatment was evident from its first use as an inhibitor of tumor growth (Curreri *et al.*, 1958). Since that time, a great many reports have documented the immunosuppressive effects of 5FU. A search for analogs that had a better therapeutic index resulted in the development of ftorafur and 5DFUR. Selective rescue of host cells but not tumor cells from 5FU toxicity with allopurinol (Schwartz and Handschumacher, 1979), uridine (Martin *et al.*, 1982), and possibly with interferon or poly I·C (Stolfi *et al.*, 1983) have also been described.

Preferential suppression of antibody responses with conservation of cellular immunity (see the following discussion) has prompted attempts to use 5FU to inhibit the production of blocking or tumor-enhancing activity of serum so that cell-mediated tumor rejection might occur.

4.1. Immunosuppression

An early study utilized two sublines of the Ehrlich ascites tumor, a subline sensitive to 5FU and a subline resistant to 5FU (Lindner *et al.*, 1959). 5FU was administered at 40 mg/kg per day for 6 days beginning 1 day after tumor transplant. Leukopenia developed in tumor-bearing mice following 5FU treatment and was evident by day 1. Untreated tumor-bearing mice developed marked leukocytosis. Cellularity of the bone marrow was greatly reduced in treated mice bearing either the sensitive or resistant tumor. After treatment, bone marrow from mice bearing the 5FU-sensitive subline consisted of 3% immature myeloid cells, 22% immature erythroid cells, 43% mature granulocytes, and 28% lymphocytes, whereas bone marrow from mice bearing the 5FU-resistant subline consisted of 1% immature myeloid cells, 1% immature erythroid cells, 10% mature granulocytes, and 85% lymphocytes. It was not clear whether 5FU differentially affected the bone marrow cells of mice bearing the resistant subline versus the sensitive subline, because the bone marrows from untreated mice bearing the two sublines were also qualitatively different. The data suggest, however, that a drug might be either more or less toxic or suppressive to hosts with different tumors.

Several investigations have determined the effect of 5FU on the response in mice to the T-cell dependent antigen sRBC. In one study, mice injected with sRBC i.v. were treated daily for the next 5 days with 18, 30, or 50 mg/kg of 5FU. Sera were tested for hemagglutination titers on days 7, 14, and 21. All three doses were immunosuppressive (Johnson *et al.*, 1976). Utilizing a plaque-forming cell (PFC) assay, mice treated with 26 mg/kg on days 1–4 after sRBC injection were found to be nonresponsive. Hemolysin titers in the sera of these animals were also severely suppressed. Mice treated with 63 mg/kg on days 1–4 had not recovered hemolysin titers 31 days after injection of sRBC, the last day tested (Ohta *et al.*, 1980). Although the humoral response (PFC) to sRBC was severly depressed by six daily doses of 30 or 60 mg/kg of 5FU, PFC responses to T-cell-independent antigens were not affected (Merluzzi *et al.*, 1982).

Several *in vitro* assays may be used to detect various cellular responses to sRBC in mice. Spleen cells from mice immunized with sRBC were incubated *in vitro* with various drugs before assessment of functional activity. Several antimetabolites, including 5FU, had no effect on complement-dependent cellular cytotoxicity (CDCC), complement-independent cellular cytotoxicity (CICC), antibody-dependent cell-mediated cytotoxicity (ADCC), or phagocytosis of sRBC when spleen cells were treated *in vitro* (Ehrke *et al.*, 1978).

Experiments in mice indicate that 5FU also suppresses cell-mediated responses, including the ability of mice to reject allogeneic tumors (Johnson *et al.*, 1976; Ohta *et al.*, 1980). Lymphoid cells prepared 24 hr after the last injection of 5FU are unable to generate cytotoxic T lymphocytes to allogeneic tumor cells *in vitro* (Merluzzi *et al.*, 1982). However, in some instances 5FU may act in consort with host cells to kill tumor cells. It has been observed that 5FU toxicity for Ehrlich ascites tumors, in the presence of host cells (probably activated macrophages), causes the appearance of diploid tumor cells which are aberrant, dying cells (Connolly *et al.*, 1982). However, 5FU treatment inhibited the inflammatory response and antitumor activity in mice by inhibiting the influx of immature macrophages into the peritoneal cavity (Connolly *et al.*, 1983).

Although 5FU has been found to suppress both humoral and cellular immunity to tumors in man, as determined by leukocyte adherence inhibition (LAI) and serum-mediated blocking of the LAI (Noonan *et al.*, 1977), a recurring observation is that treatment of cancer patients with 5FU preserves or even restores cell-mediated immunity. Development of delayed hypersensitivity to 2,4-dinitrochlorobenzene was depressed in patients treated with 5FU as were primary and secondary antibody responses to *Escherichia coli*, Vi antigen, or tetanus toxoid. In three of six patients, however, 5FU treatment restored DH to PPD, mumps, or trichophyton (Mitchell and DeConti, 1970). Blomgren *et al.* (1965) had reported that both 5FU and FUDR potentiated DH to at least one of the antigens PPD, histoplasmin, trichophyton, or candidin. Another study found that 13 of 17 pancreatic cancer patients remained reactive in LAI assays following administration of 5FU (Dasmahapatra *et al.*, 1982). 5FU did not affect serum Ig levels or titers of blood group antibodies or percent E- and EAC-rosette-forming cells but did cause a decrease in the *in vitro* proliferative response to PHA and PPD; that effect was more pronounced in short-term (less than 6 months) survivors (Nordman *et al.*, 1978). In a study of 19 patients with metastatic carcinoma treated with Adriamycin® followed by 5FU, immunosuppression was also correlated with response of the tumor to chemotherapy (Thatcher *et al.*, 1977). In that study, chemotherapy significantly raised ADCC activity and the percent of E-rosette forming cells in peripheral blood leukocytes (PBLs) from patients whose tumors responded to chemotherapy (i.e., tumor size reduced by 50% or greater) and significantly lowered both natural killer and ADCC activity of PBLs from nonresponders.

The apparent, albeit imperfect, selective abrogation of humoral rather than cellular responses may have its basis in differential enzymatic activities of various lymphocyte populations. A human B-cell leukemic line was found to be more sensitive to 5FU than a T-cell line; the increased sensitivity was caused by increased synthesis of FdUMP via thymidine phosphorylase (Piper and Fox, 1982). B cells were relatively more sensitive to 5FU than T cells (Ohnuma *et al.*, 1978; Ohnuma *et al.*, 1980; Au *et al.*, 1983; Srivastava and Alderfer, 1982) but non-T and non-B cell lines were uniformly insensitive (Ohnuma *et al.*, 1980). Alternatively, the selective immunosuppression need not be caused by differential cytotoxicity of 5FU to effector B or T cells but may be caused by selective elimination of regulatory lymphocytes such as helper cells (Merluzzi *et al.*, 1982).

4.2. Increasing the Therapeutic Index

Attempts to produce pyrimidine analogs with strong antineoplastic activity but with fewer toxic effects have resulted in agents such as ftorafur and 5DFUR. Ftorafur was found to reduce the number of hematopoietic stem cells (spleen colony forming units) in the bone marrow much less than 5FU (Hrsak and Pavicic, 1974). A rebound effect was seen for both agents, but the level above normal was greater for ftorafur than for 5FU. Ftorafur was less toxic to mice than 5FU with several protocols, exhibiting similar myelosuppressive activity at equitoxic doses but suppressing antibody response to sRBC and the rejection of allogeneic tumor cells less than 5FU (Johnson *et al.*, 1976). 5DFUR was much less immunosuppressive than either 5FU or ftorafur in mice to the induction of DH to sRBC, PFC responses to sRBC, development of serum hemolysin titers, and allogeneic tumor rejection (Ohta *et al.*, 1980).

In comparison to 5FU, FUDR, and ftorafur, 5DFUR was found to show equal or better cytostatic activity for Sarcoma S-180, Lewis lung carcinoma, and a squamous cell carcinoma at a lower level of toxicity to the host (Bollag and Hartmann, 1980). Tumor growth was inhibited by 5DFUR with fewer toxic deaths and less depression in white blood cell counts than the other drugs. Bollag and Hartmann suggested that tumors may have higher levels of uridine phosphorylase, the enzyme that converts 5DFUR to 5FU, than do normal cells. Toxicity of 5DFUR *in vitro* to several human tumor cell lines and to human bone marrow was determined and compared to 5FU and FUDR (Armstrong and Cadman, 1983). A therapeutic ratio was defined as the dose of drug that inhibited the ability of bone marrow stem cells to form colonies in soft agar by 25%, divided by the dose of drug that inhibited clonal growth of individual tumor cell lines by 50%. 5DFUR did not preferentially kill human leukemia HL-60 (index of 0.5) but did preferentially kill the two breast cancer lines 47-DN (index 7.5) and MCF-7 (index 6.9), osteosarcoma MG-63 (index 5.9), colon carcinoma HCT (index 1.2), and pancreatic carcinoma (index 1.6). In contrast, neither 5FU or FUDR produced an index greater than 1 to any of these tumor cell lines. A previous study demonstrated that a tumor cell (Ehrlich ascites), but not mouse bone marrow cells, treated with 5DFUR incorporated 5FU into RNA and displayed inhibited thymidylate synthetase activity. No such differential effect was seen if the cells were treated with 5FU or FUDR; 5FU incorporation and thymidylate synthetase inhibition were seen in both tumor and bone marrow cells (Armstrong and Diasio, 1981). Toxicity to bone marrow in the whole animal could nevertheless occur because of conversion of 5DFUR to 5FU by some other tissue. In comparison, ftorafur is apparently not converted to 5FU by either bone marrow or tumor cells but must be converted by other tissue, such as the liver.

An alternative approach to increasing the therapeutic index of 5FU is to selectively rescue host cells. Allopurinol was found to inhibit cytotoxicity of 5FU for some tumor cells (L5178Y, L1210, P388, and Sarcoma 180) but not others (Walker 256 or HeLa cells) *in vitro* (Schwartz and Handschumacher, 1979). The cells rescued by allopurinol probably utilize orotate phosphoribosyltransferase to convert 5FU to 5-fluorouridine 5-phosphate (5FUMP), whereas the cells not rescued by allopurinol most likely convert 5FU to 5FUMP by the sequential action of uridine phosphorylase and uridine kinase. Schwartz and Handschumacher (1979) also stated that allopurinol administration reduced 5FU toxicity *in vivo* in rats and mice. Uridine has also been used to rescue mice treated with high-dose 5FU while preserving antitumor activity (Martin *et al.*, 1982). Interferon or poly I·C also rescues mouse bone marrow cells from 5FU toxicity if given simultaneously (Stolfi *et al.*, 1983), but a differential rescue of bone marrow cells versus tumor cells was not demonstrated.

4.3. Chemoimmunotherapy

Mice cured of a syngeneic plasmacytoma by treatment with 5FU were found to be specifically immune to rechallenge, and anti-θ-sensitive lymphoid cells from cured animals lysed tumor cells *in vitro*. The latter was demonstrable during the therapeutic course as well as after treatment was stopped, but the level was lower, possibly reflecting drug-induced immunosuppression (Teller and Faanes, 1980). Immune activity in treated mice suggests that immunotherapy could enhance the therapeutic effect in combination with 5FU.

In rats bearing a colonic tumor, the response to PHA *in vitro* by PBLs is depressed following surgical removal of the tumor. That depression could be temporarily reversed by treatment with either 4 mg/kg levamisole or 30 mg/kg 5FU. Recovery of lymphocyte transformation activity did not occur if both 5FU and levamisole were given simultaneously. If, however, 5FU was given first, followed a day later by levamisole, recovery was greater and lasted longer (Windle and Bell, 1982).

The effects of BCG on the PFC response to sRBC and on allogeneic skin graft survival in mice treated with a combination of cyclophosphamide, methotrexate, and 5FU (CMF) were found to be very minimal (Sparks *et al.*, 1977). Mice received 20 mg/kg of cyclophosphamide on days 3 and 10 after injection of sRBC i.p. or after skin grafting (BALB/c skin transplanted onto

C57/BL mice), 0.5 mg/kg of methotrexate on days 3–10, and 60 mg/kg of 5FU on days 3, 6, and 10. BCG was given subcutaneously (S.C.) on the day of sRBC injection or skin transplantation and again on days 5 and 10. PFC assays were performed on days, 5, 10, and 14; both CMF and CMF with BCG severely suppressed the primary response at days 5 and 10 with partial recovery evident by day 14. The effects on secondary response to sRBC were determined by giving two injections of sRBC 42 days apart with CMF and BCG treatment started after the second injection. BCG stimulation of PFC formation in the secondary response to sRBC was evident at days 10 and 14 (BCG alone had no effect on the primary response), but both CMF and CMF plus BCG suppressed PFC numbers at days 10 and 14. BCG alone markedly decreased skin graft survival; CMF alone did not affect skin graft survival but did abrogate most of the effect of BCG.

Methanol extraction residue (MER) of BCG was found to restore contact hypersensitivity to 2,4-dinitro-1-fluorobenzene (DNFB) in mice treated with 5FU (Zimbar et al., 1981). In these experiments, MER was given 4 and 3 days prior to sensitization and 5FU (2.5 mg per mouse or about 125 mg/kg) was given 2 days after sensitization. Hypersensitivity on day 5, as assessed by increase in ear thickness, was suppressed by 5FU treatment in mice not pretreated with MER, but MER pretreatment protected the mice from the immunosuppressive affect of 5FU.

Koshimura and Ryoyama (1977) found that OK-432, a streptococcal preparation, but not BCG, enhanced the protection from L1210 provided by 5FU.

Clinical use of 5FU–BCG regimens have been reported with some degree of success claimed. It was found that survival of human colorectal cancer patients after surgery was somewhat improved by 5FU–BCG combined treatment over treatment with BCG only or with no adjuvant therapy (Mavligit et al., 1975). The addition of levamisole and/or BCG to a chemotherapy regimen of 5FU, Adriamycin, and cyclophosphamide significantly increased survival of stage IV breast cancer patients, who responded with an objective remission, but did not alter the overall remission rate compared to chemotherapy alone (Hortobagyi et al., 1978). Patients with resectable gastric cancer treated with 5FU (begun within 4 weeks of surgery: 15 mg/kg on days 1–5, 7, 14, 21, and 28) and BCG (begun at day 7 of the 5FU course and given weekly for 3 months and biweekly thereafter) had a statistically significant prolongation of survival (Popiela et al., 1982).

An important aspect of immunosuppression by 5FU treatment is the depressed response to bacterial challenge. Besides the suppression of antibody response to bacterial antigens described in cancer patients (Mitchell and De Conti, 1970), 5FU also suppressed phagocytic activity of human granulocytes for *Staphytococcus aureus* and *E. coli* (Pruzanski et al., 1983). 5FU-suppressed mice are more susceptible to opportunistic microbial infections (Ishitsuka et al., 1983). Immunotherapy that would restore the patients' resistance to infection might be more important than specific tumor immunotherapy. Ishitsuka et al. (1983) reported that thymosinα_1 treatment of 5FU-suppressed mice protected them from *Candida albicans, Listeria monocytogenes, Pseudomonas aeruginosa,* and *Serratia marcescens.*

5. ANTIFOLATES

Folic acid analogs, of which methotrexate (MTX) is the most widely employed, bind to the enzyme dihydrofolate reductase (DHFR), which converts folic acid to tetrahydrofolate, a coenzyme essential for several enzymes in both purine and pyrimidine metabolic pathways.

The differential toxicity of MTX for different cells can be caused by differences in transport of MTX (Kessel *et al.*, 1968) or the level of DHFR in the cell (Dolnick *et al.*, 1979). In addition, the activities of the enzymes that convert 5-methyltetrahydrofolate and N^5-formyltetrahydrofolate to tetrahydrofolate affect sensitivity of the cell to MTX. Thymidine rescue has been found to increase the therapeutic effectiveness of MTX for tumor cells that rely on *de novo* purine synthesis (Tattersall *et al.*, 1975), and mice bearing tumors that are deficient in the enzyme hypoxanthine-guanine phosphoribosyl transferase (HGPRT$^-$) are rescued from high-dose MTX by a combination of hypoxanthine, thymidine, and allopurinol with a greater antitumor effect than if rescued with citrovorum factor (Abelson and Gorka, 1983).

5.1. Immunosuppression

MTX reduces total cellularity and the number of stem cells in the bone marrow (Vogel, 1961; Pinedo *et al.*, 1976; Pannacciulli *et al.*, 1982) and reduces white blood cell and lymphocyte numbers in the blood (Santos *et al.*, 1964; Hersh *et al.*, 1965). Hersh *et al.* (1965) have shown that 25 mg/m^2 of MTX i.v. every 4th day for 2 weeks was probably as immunosuppressive, based on primary antibody responses to bacterial antigens, as 9–15 mg/m^2 i.v. given on days 1–5 (four of eight patients developing no serum titer versus five of seven developing no titer). Their complete series of 47 patients and six chemotherapy regiments indicated that the degree of immunosuppression induced is antigen dependent. The response to a weak antigen was more easily suppressed than the response to a strong antigen. If the same is true for cell-mediated responses, the conservation of DH to strong antigens, such as PPD or DNFB, probably has little predictive value concerning the simultaneous conservation of cell-mediated immunity (CMI) to weak tumor transplantation antigens.

A series of 20 patients (12 with acute leukemia, 3 with carcinoma, 4 with uveitus, and 1 with hemolytic anemia) were divided into seven treatment groups of 1, 1, 2, 2, 3, 4, and 7 patients and tested for blastogenic response of PBLs to PHA or vaccinia. Because of group sizes, no conclusions regarding any drug, dose, or schedule could be made but, as a group, therapy values were much lower in treated patients than in controls (Hersh and Oppenheim, 1967). Intensive combination therapy (500–1000 mg/m^2 6-MP, plus 7.5–15 mg/m^2 MTX with or without 1000 mg/m^2 prednisolone daily for 5–7 days) produced a rapid appearance (within 3 days) of suppressed immune parameters (leukopenia, blastogenic response), but recovery was equally rapid, occurring in about 3 days after therapy was halted. MTX given intermittently (25 mg/m^2 every 4th day for 40 days) did not cause leukopenia, but inhibited the blastogenic response to the same extent as intensive combination therapy. However, the onset of detectable suppression was delayed from about 3 days to 30 days (Hersh and Oppenheim, 1967).

The antibody response to sRBC is suppressed by MTX treatment in rats (Santos and Owens, 1964) and mice (Uy et al., 1966). Five daily doses of 1 mg/kg MTX severely depresses peak hemagglutinin titers in rats if treatment is begun within 2 days of antigenic challenge. Specificity of the MTX-induced suppression was demonstrated with sRBC and human RBC. MTX treatment begun 2 days after sRBC immunization renders rats unable to respond to sRBC while retaining the ability to respond to human RBC (Santos, 1967). A single 1 mg/kg injection of MTX 2 days after sRBC challenge inhibits PFC (IgM) formation in the mouse (Bareham et al., 1974). MTX inhibited both CDCC and CICC to sRBC in mice given a single dose of 100 mg/kg 2 days after sRBC injection. Complete recovery of activity occurred within 14 days (Medzihradsky et al., 1977). In vitro treatment of spleen cells with MTX inhibited CICC but not CDCC or ADCC (Ehrke et al., 1978).

MTX inhibited the IgG but not the IgM response to Salmonella adelaide in mice at a dose of 2 mg/kg given every 3 days (Blinkoff, 1966). Makulu and Wright (1971) reported that MTX effectively inhibited both the primary and secondary IgG responses to bovine or porcine insulin in guinea pigs but had no effect if given once antibody production had begun. In guinea pigs, 10–15 mg/kg of MTX given i.p. 2 days before, on the same day, 3 days after, and 6 days after immunization with DNFB conjugated with bovine serum albumin (DNFB-BSA) depressed DH and IgM responses slightly but severely depressed IgG$_1$ and IgG$_2$ responses to DNFB-BSA (Harel et al., 1972).

In guinea pigs, MTX selectively blocked the development of a specific population of small lymphocytes present in the draining lymph node once the animal is sensitized to oxazolone (Turk, 1971). Also in the guinea pig, MTX at 5 mg, but not at 1.7 mg, every 48 hr prevented the development of DH to diphtheria toxoid or ovalbumin. Antibody response, as judged by cutaneous anaphylaxis, was also depressed (Friedman et al., 1961). Suppression of DH by MTX is dependent upon the strength of the antigen; a daily dose of 5 mg begun on the day of immunization with BCG and continued until the day of skin testing suppressed the expression of DH but did not block the induction of DH. The guinea pigs became reactive within 7 days after stopping MTX administration (Friedman and Buckler, 1963). It was not clear that antigen was not present after halting MTX treatment, so that induction of DH could have occurred in the 7-day interval before skin testing. MTX, 5 mg/day i.p., could inhibit established DH to PPD. Skin-test-positive strain 2 guinea pigs were treated for 26 days during which time the animals converted from skin test positive to skin test negative. When tested 9 days after MTX treatment was stopped, the guinea pigs were again skin test positive (Friedman, 1964). It was concluded that MTX inhibited the proliferation without producing cytoxic effects on the lymphocytes. However, MTX inhibits DH to BCG in strain 2 guinea pigs much more severely than in Hartley outbred guinea pigs. DH could be totally obliterated by MTX in the former but only partially in the latter (Friedman, 1964; D'Arcy Hart et al., 1968). Such variations in the immunosuppressive potency of MTX might also be expected to occur between patients.

Rejection of an allogeneic tumor may be suppressed by MTX as was demonstrated by the progressive growth of MTX-resistant L1210 variants in allogeneic BALB/c mice treated with 0.75 mg/kg daily for 20 days (Humphreys et al., 1961; Humphreys et al., 1962). Even so, F1 mice compatible with tumor cells at the major histocompatability loci, cured of L1210 by treatment with MTX or halogenated derivatives, were resistant to rechallenge with L1210 cells (Goldin and Humphreys, 1960).

The interaction of host immunity and tumor subpopulations heterogeneous for drug sensitivity in the regulation of tumor growth in drug-treated mice was demonstrated with L1210 and a 3′,5′-dichloromethopterin- (DCM) resistant L1210 variant, M46R (Goldin et al., 1960). Treatment of M46R-bearing mice with DCM had no effect on median survival time. Treatment of L1210-bearing mice with DCM prolonged the median survival from 10 days to 74 days. Treated mice bearing L1210 and M46R were protected from both tumors and survival was equivalent to that of mice bearing L1210 only. One might conclude that the L1210 induced an immune response cross-reactive with M46R that was responsible for host protection, but survival depended upon continued drug administration.

A single LD_{10} dose of MTX was found to be only weakly immunosuppressive to host tumor immunity in a syngeneic mouse lymphoma system (C58 mouse and I_b lymphoma). The secondary antitumor response to a formalin-treated tumor cell vaccine was even more resistant to suppression by MTX, given 24 hr after vaccine, than was the primary response (Martinez et al., 1975).

Generation of cellular cytotoxicity to P815 mastocytoma from allogeneic C57B1/6J mouse spleen cells was inhibited by MTX in vitro. The suppression was dependent on both the dose and timing of the drug. For suppression to occur, 15 nM MTX had to be added within 24 hr of initiating the in vitro sensitizing coculture but 100 nM MTX was effective up to 48 hr later (Bogyo and Mihich, 1980). The same dependence upon drug dose and timing in vivo confounds our analysis of available experimental and clinical data.

5.2. Rescue

Cell killing by antifolates requires their prolonged presence in the cell at high levels; otherwise, the metabolic inhibition is reversible and the cells recover. The differential ability of cells from various tissues to take up and retain antifolates is the basis for the preferential killing of tumor cells over normal tissue cells (Kessel *et al.*, 1968). Thus, in the mouse, L1210 tumor cells are more sensitive to MTX than is intestinal epithelium, which in turn is more sensitive than bone marrow (Sirotnak and Donsbach, 1973; Sirotnak and Moccio, 1980). Other folate analogs have been synthesized in the hope that the differential uptake and retention might be accentuated (Sirotnak *et al.*, 1978). However, a more common course of action has been to preferentially rescue host cells. Citrovorum factor (N^5-formyltetrahydrofolate) (CF) and 5-methyltetrahydrofolate are converted to tetrahydrofolate in the cell; cells with high activity of the enzymes responsible for the conversion to tetrahydrofolate are relatively easy to rescue from MTX (Halpern *et al.*, 1975; Dudman *et al.*, 1982). Indeed, CF rescue after MTX treatment has been used clinically for 25 years (Sullivan *et al.*, 1959; Bertino, 1977).

Bone marrow cells may be rescued from MTX with nucleosides as well. Thymidine was effective in rescuing mice bearing L1210 and treated with MTX without interfering with the antitumor activity (Tattersall *et al.*, 1975; Grindey *et al.*, 1978; Hoglind-Semon and Grindey, 1978).

In these experiments, allopurinol interfered with the increase in survival time of L1210-bearing mice treated with MTX and thymidine. It has been suggested that the preferential rescue by thymidine of normal bone marrow versus L1210 from MTX-induced purine starvation is because of the reliance of the former on purines synthesized by the liver and the latter's reliance on *de novo* purine biosynthesis (Tattersall *et al.*, 1975). Abelson amd Gorka (1983) compared a rescue regimen of hypoxanthine, thymidine, and allopurinol with CF rescue in mice bearing the Dunn osteosarcoma. This tumor is deficient in the enzyme HGPRT, and the injection of MTX, hypoxanthine, thymidine, and allopurinol is an *in situ* simulation of the commonly used selective hypoxanthine–aminopterin–thymidine media, which inhibits $HGPRT^-$ cells but not wild type $HGPRT^+$ cells (Sato *et al.*, 1972). Tumors in mice rescued with hypoxanthine, thymidine, and allopurinol were significantly smaller than tumors in mice rescued with CF. Granulocyte precursor cells were rescued competitively by CF *in vitro*, but rescue by nucleosides was reported to be noncompetive (Pinedo *et al.*, 1976). High-dose MTX (500 mg/kg) severely depressed the cellularity and stem cell content of mouse bone marrow within 2 days and also caused a marked increased in white blood cell and reticulocyte counts in the peripheral blood (Pannancciulli *et al.*, 1982). CF, 14.5 mg/kg given 2 hr after MTX, plus 2.5 mg/kg given 6, 12, 18, and 24 hr after MTX, dramatically rescued bone marrow cells but was much less restorative of the transient suppression of cells in the peripheral blood (Pannaciulli *et al.*, 1982). High-dose MTX with CF rescue has also been found to have little effect on bone marrow and peripheral blood in man (Schreml and Lohrmann, 1979).

CF was able to rescue allogeneic tumor immunity in BALB/c mice treated with MTX (Humphreys *et al.*, 1962) but did not rescue the MTX-induced suppression of DH reactivity in BCG-vaccinated guinea pigs (D'Arcy Hart *et al.*, 1968) nor the MTX-induced suppression of antibody response to a bacterial vaccine in mice (Berenbaum and Brown, 1965). In the latter experiments, rescue with CF redcued mortality and weight loss if given within 8 hr of MTX but did not reverse suppression of the antibody response unless given earlier, 1–2 hr after MTX. Thus, the timing of CF relative to MTX administration, as well as the timing of MTX relative to antigenic insult, are important variables in host suppression. Lysis of sRBC by splenocytes, both with added complement (CDCC) and without added complement (CICC), was reduced by MTX given 2 days after antigen in mice. Maximum suppression was achieved at day 4; recovery began between days 5 and 7 and was complete by day 14. CF could partially rescue CDCC if given simultaneously or up to 5 hr before MTX, but not if given after MTX. CF partially rescued CICC if given 2–5 hours before MTX. Recovery from MTX-induced suppression was greatly enhanced, having returned to normal values by day 7, by CF given as late as 6 hr after MTX. Thus, the primary response to sRBC, as measured by CICC or CDCC, is biphasic, and cells responsible for lysis early in the response (e.g., day 4) can only be spared from MTX by preloading with CF (Medzihardsky *et al.*, 1977). Later information from the same laboratory demonstrated that the optimum timing for CF rescue of CICC (CICC is a T-cell response for EL-4 and P815) and CDCC for tumor cells was tumor dependent. CF reversed CICC inhibition of EL-4 cells (measured at peak activity, which was on day 14) if given 2 hr before, simultaneously, or to a lesser extent, 4 hr after MTX, but not if given 24 hr after MTX (MTX was given 2 days after tumor). Reversal of CICC (at peak activity, day 10) to P815 could be achieved equally well with CF given 2 hr before, 4 hr after, or 24 hr after, but simultaneous administration was less effective (Bogyo *et al.*, 1982). The difference in CF timing required for rescue of these responses may reflect the different kinetics of the immune response to these two tumors; the response to EL-4 peaking at day 14 and the response to P815 peaking at day 10.

Further complications in scheduling decisions arise when combinatiaon chemotherapy is contemplated. If drugs were given 2 days after sRBC injections in mice and the response measured by direct PFC assay, suppression by MTX followed in 1 hr by 5FU was more than additive but 5FU followed by MTX in 1 hr was less than additive (Bareham *et al.*, 1974). Simultaneous administration of MTX and 5FU was additive. Time intervals between MTX and 5FU administration from 30 min to 6 hr were all about equal and caused greater suppression than simultaneous treatment or the use of a 15 min interval. If 5FU was given first, depression of PFC was additive at intervals of 15 min and 6 hr but intermediate intervals (30 min and 1 hr) resulted in less than additive suppression (Bareham *et al.*, 1974). MTX (1 mg/kg on day 2) followed by 5FU (50 mg/kg) in 1 hr did not suppress either allograft rejection (skin grafting) or development of contact hypersensitivity to oxazolone (DiLorenzo *et al.*, 1974).

6. CYTOSINE ARABINOSIDE

Cytosine arabinoside (1-β-D-arabinofuranosyl cytosine) is activated when converted to 1-β-D-arabinofuranosylcytosine 5^1–triphosphate (Ara-CTP) by sequential action of deoxycytidine kinase, deoxycytidylate kinase, and nucleoside diphosphate kinase. Ara-CTP then competitively inhibits DNA polymerase. Deactivation is accomplished in part by cytidine deaminase and deoxycytidylate deaminase. Drug sensitivity of a cell depends upon the activity of the activating and/or degradative pathways within the cell. Sensitivity to Ara-C also depends upon the phase of the cell cycle. Evidence has been presented that Ara-C kills cells in S-phase if the dose given inhibits DNA synthesis for at least 2 hr (Lenaz et al., 1969); otherwise the damage is reversible.

Several reports have described the use of Ara-C to selectively suppress antibody formation without a corresponding suppression of cellular immunity. Since the work of Kaliss (1969), demonstrating the antibody-mediated enhancement of allografts, and the subsequent description of serum "blocking factors" (Hellström et al., 1969), which suppress cellular tumor immunity, it has been feared that immunotherapy might enhance rather than inhibit tumor growth. Mott (1973) hypothesized that "suppression of immune enhancement by chemotherapy may be an important factor in the effective treatment of neoplasia." Several attempts to do just that have utilized Ara-C (Buchman et al., 1979; Griswold et al., 1972; Griswold et al., 1975; Heppner and Calabresi, 1972; Heppner et al., 1974).

Finally, because Ara-C is widely used for the treatment of acute myelogenous leukemia (AML), some consideration will be given to immunosuppression by Ara-C in patients with that disease, in which the immune state may be altered before treatment.

6.1. Immunosuppression

An early report suggested that 400 mg/kg of Ara-C, given in a single dose to mice 1 hr before injection of BGG, enhanced serum antibody titers to BGG determined by 12 days later. The same single dose given 1 day after antigen had no effect on antibody formation, whereas daily injections of 25–50 mg/kg for the 12-day period severely suppressed the primary antibody response to BGG (Buskirk et al., 1965). Rose et al. (1968) gave doses of 2, 20, 40, or 200 mg/kg s.c. at the time of sRBC injections i.p. and daily for 4 days thereafter. Spleen cells were then assayed for PFC, and hemagglutination and hemolysin titers were determined in the sera. Doses of 20 mg/kg and above suppressed PFC numbers, but only 40 mg/kg suppressed antibody titers. Thus, the antibody-forming cells in the treated mice must have produced more antibody per cell. All antibody titers were abolished by 2-mercaptoethanol, indicating that the response was from IgM-producing cells.

A single dose of 2500 mg/kg (estimated to be an LD_{10}) of Ara-C suppressed hemagglutinin titers in mice measured on day 6 of a primary response to sRBC if the drug was given either 48 or 72 hr (but not 24 hr) after antigen. Suppression was transient and serum titers had recovered by day 12 (Harris and Hersh, 1968). If Ara-C was given simultaneously with sRBC, strong suppression of serum titers extended to at least day 75. Spleen PFC were suppressed (4 days after antigen) whether Ara-C was given 24 hr before, simultaneously, or 24, 48, or 72 hr after sRBC. These authors suggested that simultaneously administered Ara-C inhibited differentiation of a monocytic-antigen-processing cell as well as the proliferation of antibody-producing cells (Harris and Hersh, 1968). However, with most protocols, Ara-C seems to be immunosuppressive only while antigen-stimulated lymphocytes are proliferating.

Another contemporary study found that a single dose of Ara-C was maximally suppressive to the humoral response if administered 2 days after sRBC antigen; the same total dose was much more suppressive if split into small doses and given at 3-hr intervals (Gray et al., 1968b). This study used much lower doses of Ara-C than the previous one (60–180 mg/kg rather than 2500 mg/kg) but achieved comparable levels of immunosuppression. Gray et al. (1968b) described the kinetics of the humoral response as determined by both IgG- and IgM-producing PFCs and serum titers of both IgG and IgM. Ara-C diminished and delayed the primary response to sRBC if Ara-C in-jections were not continued past 11 days after sRBC injection. That finding indicates that sufficient antigen to induce a primary response probably per-sisted in the mice for 11 days and that the sRBC/Ara-C treatment did not produce tolerance. Ara-C inhibited both IgM and IgG responses, as measured either by PFC assay or serum titers, after either primary or secondary antigen stimulation. In contrast to the effect on the primary response, however, the secondary response was diminished but not delayed by Ara-C treatment.

The kinetics of the PFC primary response illustrate the importance of the timing of the assay, relative to antigen administration, in assessing the immunosuppressive activity of a drug. When IgM-PFC formation was assayed on day 4 or 5, the immunosuppressive activity was dramatic because the response in untreated mice was at its peak ($>$500 PFC per 10^6 splenocytes) compared to very low numbers of IgM-PFCs in Ara-C-treated mice ($<$10 PFC per 10^6 splenocytes). By day 6, the numbers of IgM-PFCs had fallen to a mean of 72 in the untreated mice and risen to 29 in the treated mice, and by day 7, Ara-C-treated mice had as many IgM-PFC per 10^6 splenocytes as the untreated mice. At that time, a difference in IgG-PFCs was still evident between treated and untreated mice, but that difference was not as dramatic at it was earlier in the response; on day eight, 160 IgG-PFC per 10^6 splenocytes were detected versus 43 for treated, whereas on day 5, there were 256 PFC per 10^6 for untreated versus less than 0.5 per 10^6 for treated mice (Gray et al., 1968b). In these experiments, Ara-C administered prior to sRBC had no effect on the host response regardless of dose or schedule, including 400 mg/kg 1 hr before antigen, a treatment found to enhance serum titers to BGG by Buskirk et al. (1965).

In a companion report, Gray et al. (1968a) found that the graft-versus-host reaction (GVH), as determined by spleen weight in C3HXC57BL F_1 females injected with spleen leukocytes from C57BL male mice, was maximally suppressed if Ara-C was administered 3 days after the donor cells were injected. Again, the same total dose given in smaller, repeated doses was more suppressive than a single bolus. Pretreatment of the donor cells (the effector cells in a GVH) did not suppress the reaction.

In a more recent report, 40 mg/kg of Ara-C, given on days 0–4 to mice, suppressed the humoral response to sRBC and cellular responses to X-irradiated allogeneic L1210 cells. The Ara-C treatment, as measured 7 days after L1210 immunization, decreased cytolytic activity of the splenocytes from 18% to less than 1% in a chromium release assay (CRA) and, when measured 14 days after immunization, decreased killing of tumor cells in a 48-hr clonogenic assay from 70% to 11% (Kan-Mitchell et al., 1980).

In cancer patients, both MTX and Ara-C abolished established DH to candidin, mumps, trichophyton, or PPD but, as administered, Ara-C was much more potent in inhibiting induction of DH to 2,4-dinitrochlorobenzene. In addition, Ara-C completely inhibited the IgG response to bacterial antigens in a primary response but merely delayed the onset of the IgM response (Mitchell et al., 1969).

6.2. Selective Suppression

The primary drug target in cancer chemotherapy is the cancer cell and the occurrence of immunosuppression is an undesireable side effect. However, an argument can be made for the use of chemotherapy to induce selective immunosuppression (Mott, 1973; Heppner et al., 1974). The basis of the argument is that the host response to tumors results in a CMI of tumor cell killing but that the humoral response ultimately inhibits CMI, resulting in what has been termed a "balanced immune response" (Heppner et al., 1974). By selectively inhibiting the humoral (blocking factor) response, the balance might be tipped toward cell-mediated killing and tumor regression. Thus, treatments that preferentially suppress humoral responses might have therapeutic value.

Ara-C suppressed allogeneic skin graft rejections (C57BL graft on C3H host) if 20–40 mg/kg per day were given on days 6–10 after grafting but not if given on days 1–5. Both regimens, however, suppressed antibody-mediated immunity (AMI), as determined by IgG- and IgM-PFC formation against sRBC (Griswold et al., 1972). An Ara-C regimen that selectively inhibited serum-mediated blocking but not cell-mediated cytotoxicity as assessed with the in vitro microcytotoxicity assay inhibited growth of transplanted syngeneic mammary tumors in C3H/HeJ mice (Heppner and Calabresi, 1972). Ara-C was administered daily for the first 5 days following tumor transplantation. The dose was critical. Low doses of 10–20 mg/kg suppressed detectable blocking activity but not CMI and inhibited tumor growth in vivo. The slightly higher doses of 20–40 mg/kg suppressed both CMI and blocking activity and did not inhibit tumor growth in vivo. The dose of 20 mg/kg inhibited CMI as well as AMI but not tumor growth *in vivo* for some transplantable tumors; for other tumors, 20 mg/kg suppressed only AMI, not CMI, and subsequently suppressed tumor growth *in vivo*. Thus, the required dose of Ara-C to cause selective host suppression was tumor specific (Heppner and Calabresi, 1972).

Although many ocogenic viruses, including mouse mammary tumor virus (MMTV) (Blair *et al.*, 1971), cause a general state of immunosuppression, Griswold *et al.* (1975) reported that, compared to virus-free C3H and BALB/c mice, MMTV-infected mice were equally able to respond with a DH reaction to oxazolone. Their lymphocytes also responded more vigorously to PHA stimulation *in vitro*. Treatment of the mice with Ara-C suppressed DH to oxazolone in C3HeB/FeJ (MMTV-free) mice but significantly increased DH to oxazolone in C3H/HeJ (MMTV-infected) mice. A more pronounced enhancement occurred with low-dose Ara-C (10 mg/kg per day) given on days 1–5 after sensitization than with higher doses (20 or 40 mg/kg per day). It was suggested that MMTV induced increased titers of serum blocking activity in untreated mice, thus tipping the balance toward the inhibition of CMI, and that low-dose Ara-C tipped the balance, by inhibiting blocking, back toward the expression of CMI.

The fact that low-dose Ara-C-mediated selective suppression is critically dependent upon the drug dose rather discourages clinical application when tumor kill is sought. However, high-dose Ara-C with 2'-deoxycytidine (CdR) rescue has also been reported to selectively suppress humoral responses in mice (Buchman *et al.*, 1979) and might be more widely useful. In that report, however, the humoral and cellular host responses to the tumor (L1210) were not determined. Toxicity was reduced by CdR without abrogating the antitumor effect in L1210-bearing mice. CdR rescued CMI as determined by prolonged skin allograft survival but did not rescue AMI as determined by a reduced antibody response to sRBC. Buchman *et al.* concluded that "the combined effect of ara-C and CdR ... results in selective destruction of precursor cells with the emphasis on B lymphocytes" (Buchman *et al.*, 1979). Different effector cells in CMI may be selectively rescued from Ara-C-induced immunosuppression by BCG. Ara-C, 20 or 40 mg/kg per day on days 3–7 after immunization of C57BL/6 mice with L1210 cells, suppressed splenocyte CMI in both a 4-hr CRA and a 48-hr microcytotoxicity assay (MCA). BCG rescued CMI as determined by the MCA but not by the CRA (Murahata and Mitchell, 1982). This may reflect the finding that cytotoxicity measured by CRA was T cell mediated while cytotoxicity measured by MCA was B cell mediated for a mouse sarcoma (Leclerc *et al.*, 1973). However, human lymphoid cell lines of B-cell origin are much less sensitive to Ara-C *in vitro* than those of T-cell origin (Ohnuma *et al.*, 1978, 1980). Perhaps the functional subsets of T cells are differentially sensitive to Ara-C, helper cells being killed while killer suppresor cells are spared. Such an event could result in a diminished AMI with an apparent net increase in CMI. Some evidence for this can be found (Athanassiades *et al.*, 1978), but the data are not compelling.

6.3. Drug-Induced Immunosuppression in Acute Myelogenous Leukemia

Ara-C has been found to be the most effective single agent for the treatment of AML but is more often used in combination with an anthracycline, such as daunorubicin or Adriamycin; with 6-TG; or in more complex schedules, which include cyclophosphamide, vincristine, and prednisone.

The synergistic effect of daunorubicin and Ara-C probably results from the Ara-C killing cells in S-phase and blocking other cycling cells at the G_1-S interface; the latter are sensitive to daunorubicin. Thus, Ara-C given before daunorubicin has been found to be the most effective schedule in mice (Edelstein et al., 1974). The killing of L1210 cells was synergistic but the killing of normal bone marrow stem cells was only additive. In AML patients, Ara-C in combination with daunorubicin, or with 6-TG, or with adriamycin, vincristine, and prednisone induced a slight depression in T-cell helper activity initially, which was replaced by a rebound increase in T-cell helper activity. Suppressor activity, by the authors' criteria, was less affected but increased somewhat 2–3 weeks posttherapy (Athanassiades et al., 1978). In a clinical study of 15 patients in remission following treatment with Ara-C, daunorubicin, and 6-TG, mitogen-induced cellular cytotoxicity (MICC) and ADCC were evaluated before and after maintenance therapy courses of Ara-C plus 6-TG or daunomycin (Zighelboim, 1979). AML patients in remission had depressed ADCC and MICC activities, accompanied by a decreased number of Fc-receptor-positive cells in the peripheral blood. This result might have been caused by the initial chemotherapeutic course, because maintenance therapy, including Ara-C as a single agent, caused further reductions in ADCC and MICC, which were maximal after 2–3 weeks and recovered somewhat by the 4th week (Zighelboim, 1979).

A series of 25 patients with AML were treated with several drug regimens. Nineteen patients received a regimen that included Ara-C, 16 of which were treated with cyclophosphamide, vincristine, Ara-C, and prednisone for 5 days after 2 weeks. Immunocompetence before and after treatment was determined by skin testing with a battery of common antigens, in vitro blastogenic responsiveness to PHA and streptolysin 0, and humoral and cellular immune responses to keyhole limpet hemocyanin. Pretreatment immunocompetence correlated with prognosis (86% of competent patients achieved remission but less than half of the immunodeficient patients achieved remission), and immunodeficient patients who converted to a competent state after treatment also achieved remission (Herse et al., 1971).

Although one might expect leukemia patients to have severe generalized immune deficiencies, that is not generally the case. Most patients display DH reactivity to at least some antigens, although it has been observed that patients with acute leukemia (acute lymphocytic leukemia patients as well as AML patients) respond to fewer antigens than normal controls and less often to particular antigens, for example, BCG (Dupuy et al., 1971). In that study, patients were able to produce antibodies in response to a polio vaccine prior to treatment; various therapies suppressed humoral responses.

7. CONCLUSIONS

Despite indisputable evidence that antimetabolite therapy suppresses an array of immunological responses, drug-induced regressions in experimental animals often result in hosts that are immune to rechallenge with tumor cells. DH responses in patients are frequently spared, indeed augmented, by antimetabolite therapy, antigenicity of tumor cells can sometimes be increased by therapy, and the incidence of opportunistic infections does not necessarily increase after therapy.

Metabolite rescue from antimetabolite toxicity has been highly successful in increasing the therapeutic index for many tumors, but success has not necessarily resulted from rescue of the immune system. Rescue often depends upon saving other tissues such as the intestinal epithelium. Antimetabolites have short toxic half-lives and act on proliferating cells. Antigen-stimulated proliferating lymphocytes are sensitive but nondividing stem cells are spared; antimetabolite treatment does not produce tolerance to the stimulating antigen. Thus, application of an antigenic stimulus, or nonspecific stimuli such as BCG, after antimetabolite activity has subsided in the host might be expected to rescue immune function and increase antitumor immunity and/or resistance to infection. Data to support that expectation are disappointing.

The use of antimetabolites to selectively suppress humoral responses so that cellular immunity could more effectively control tumor growth might be possible. However, it is far from clear that "blocking factors" are responsible for tumor growth in any tumor model. The dose of Ara-C required to inhibit tumor growth, apparently by suppressing "blocking factor" production, was dependent upon individual tumors.

Such heterogeneity is typical and is a recurring complication at several levels:

1. Patient population heterogeneity. Antimetabolites are more immunosuppressive for some strains of a species than others. A spectrum of activity should be expected among patients.
2. Heterogeneity of the immune response. The kinetics of the various effector mechanisms in immunity are complex, and studies of immunosuppression induced by antimetabolites stress the importance of (1) the time of drug administration relative to antigenic challenge, (2) the time at which immune function is assessed relative to antigenic challenge, and (3) the time at which immune function is assessed relative to drug administration. The time of effective antigenic challenge in a cancer patients is, of course, unknown.

3. Intertumor heterogeneity. Different types of tumors (e.g., melanoma versus AML) are sensitive to different drugs, and individual tumors of the same type are not uniformly sensitive to the same drug (e.g., Ara-C does not induce remission in all AML patients). Tumors are antigenically heterogeneous, and the degree of antimetabolite-induced suppresion is dependent upon antigenic strength. Tumors may suppress host immunity, some more than others. Thus, the resident host immune cell population upon which antimetabolites act is probably different in every patient.

4. Intratumor heterogeneity. Different subpopulations of an individual tumor are sensitive to different drugs and differ in antigenicity.

These levels of heterogeneity, combined with the "iatrogenic" heterogeneity of doses, schedules, sequences, and various antigens that have been used in the study of antimetabolite-induced immunosuppression make further conclusions unwarranted at this point. The fact remains that, despite their immunosuppressive activities, the use of antimetabolites in various combination chemotherapy regimens is effective in controlling cancers of different types.

ACKNOWLEDGMENTS. The authors wish to thank Ms. Judith McKinley for her skillful and timely typing of this manuscript. The highly critical but helpful suggestions of Dr. Bonnie Miller are greatly appreciated. T. K. was supported in part by a Grant-in-Aid for Cancer Research from the Ministry of Education, Science, and Culture, Japan.

REFERENCES

Abelson, H. T., and Gorka, C., 1983, Absence of hypoxanthine: Guanine phosphoribosyltransferase activity in murine Dunn osteosarcoma, *Cancer Res.* **43**:4098–4101.

Armstrong, R. D., and Cadman, E., 1983, 5′-deoxy-5-fluorouridine selective toxicity for human tumor cells compared to human bone marrow, *Cancer Res.* **43**:2525–2528.

Armstrong, R. D., and Diasio, R. B., 1981, Selective activation of 5′-deoxy-5-fluorouridine by tumor cells as a basis for an improved therapeutic index, *Cancer Res.* **41**:4891–4894.

Athanassiades, P. H., Platts-Mills, T. A. E., Asherson, G. L., and Oliver, R. T. D., 1978, Effect of antileukaemic chemotherapy on helper and suppressor activity of T cells on immunoglobulin production by B cells, *Eur. J. Cancer* **14**:971–976.

Au, R., Rustum, Y. M., Minowada, J., Levenson, C. H., and Srivastava, B. I. S., 1983, Differential selectivity of 5-fluorouracil and its analogs, β-D-4′hydroxy-ftorafur and 5′-deoxy-5-fluorouridine, in cultured human B lymphocytes and mouse L1210 leukemia, *Biochem. Pharmacol.* **32**:541–546.

Ballow, M., and Pantschenko, A. G., 1981, *In vitro* effects of adenosine deaminase inhibitors on lymphocyte mitogen responsiveness in the mouse, *Cellular Immunol.* **64**:29–43.

Bareham, C. R., Griswold, D. E., and Calabresi, P., 1974, Synergism of methotrexate with imuran and with 5-fluorouracil and their effects on hemolysin plaque-forming cell production in the mouse, *Cancer Res.* **34**:571–575.

Barranco, S. C., Ho, D. H. W., Drewinko, B., Romsdahl, M. M., and Humphrey, R. M., 1972, Differential sensitivity of human melanoma cells grown *in vitro* to arabinosylcytocine, *Cancer Res.* **32**:2733–2736.

Barton, R. W., and Goldschneider, I., 1978, 5'-nucleotidase activity in subpopulations of rat lymphocytes, *J. Immunol.* **121:**2329–2334.

Barton, R. W., Martiniuk, F., Hirschhorn, R., and Goldschneider, I., 1979, The distribution of adenosine deaminase among lymphocyte populations in the rat, *J. Immunol.* **122:**216–220.

Berenbaum, M. C., 1969, Dose–response curves for agents that impair cell reproductive integrity: A fundamental difference between dose–response curves of antimetabolites and those for radiation and alkylating agents, *Br. J. Cancer* **23:**426–433.

Berenbaum, M. C., and Brown, I. N., 1965, The effect of delayed administration of folinic acid on immunological inhibition by methotrexate, *Immunology* **8:**251–259.

Berkelhammer, J., Mastrangelo, M. J., and Prehn, R. T., 1977, Effect of treatment with dimentyl triazeno imidazole carboxamide (DTIC, NSC-45388) or 1,3-bis-(2-chloroethyl)-1-nitrosourea (BCNU, NSC-409962) plus vincristine (NSC-67574) on lymphocyte reactivity of melanoma patients, *Cancer Immunol. Immunother.* **2:**119–125.

Bertino, J. R., 1977, "Rescue" techniques in cancer chemotherapy: Use of leucovorin and other rescue agents after methotrexate treatment, *Semin. Oncol.* **4:**203–216.

Blair, P. B., Kripke, M. L., Lappe, M. A., Bonhag, R. S., and Young, L., 1971, Immunologic deficiency associated with mammary tumor virus (MTV) infection in mice: Hemagglutinin response and allograft survival, *J. Immunol.* **106:**364–370.

Blinkoff, R. C., 1966, γ-M and γ-G antibodies in mice: Dissociation of the normal immuno-globulin sequence, *J. Immunol.* **97:**736–746.

Blomgren, S. E., Wolberg, W. H., and Kisken, W. A., 1965, Effect of fluoropyrimidines on delayed cutaneous hypersensitivity, *Cancer Res.* **25:**977–979.

Bogyo, D., and Mihich, E., 1980, Reversal of the *in vitro* methotrexate suppression of cell-mediated immune response by folinic acid and thymidine plus hypoxanthine, *Cancer Res.* **40:**650–654.

Bogyo, D., Ehrke, M. J., and Mihich, E., 1982, Reversal by citrovorum factor of methotrexate-induced suppression of cell-mediated and humoral immune response in mouse model systems, *Biochem. Pharmacol.* **31:**1387–1392.

Bollag, W., and Hartman, H. R., 1980, Tumor inhibitory effects of a new fluorouracil derivative: 5'-deoxy-5-fluorouridine, *Eur. J. Cancer* **16:**427–432.

Bonmassar, E., Bonmassar, A., Vadlamudi, S., and Goldsin A., 1970, Immunological alteration of leukemia cells *in vivo* after treatment with an antitumor drug, *Proc. Natl. Acad. Sci. USA* **66:**1089–1095.

Bonmassar, E., Testorelli, C., Franco, P., Goldin, A., Cudkowicz, G., 1975, Changes of the immunogenic properties of a radiation-induced mouse lymphoma following treatment with antitumor drugs, *Cancer Res.* **35:**1957–1962.

Borel, Y., Fauconnet, M., and Miescher, P. A., 1965, Effect of 6-mercaptopurine (6-MP) on different classes of antibody, *J. Exp. Med.* **122:**263–275.

Bruckner, H. W., Mokyr, M. B., and Mitchell, M. S., 1974, Effect of imidazole-4-carboxamide, 5-(3,3-dimethyl-1-triazeno) on immunity in patients with malignant melanoma, *Cancer Res.* **34:**181–183.

Buchman, V. M., Belyanchikova, N. I., Mkheidze, D. M., Litovchenko, T. A., Lichinitser, M. R., Barkhotkina, M. F., and Svet-Moldavsky, G. J., 1979, 2'-deoxycitidine hydrochloride protection of mice against the lethal toxicity of cytosine arabinoside: Absence of protection of bone marrow lymphocytes, *Cancer Chemother. Pharmacol.* **3:**229–234.

Buskirk, H. H., Crim, J. A., Petering, H. G., Merritt, K., and Johnson, A. G., 1965, Effect of uracil mustard and several antitumor drugs on the primary antibody response in rats and mice, *J. Natl. Cancer Inst.* **34:**747–758.

Campanile, F., Houchens, D. P., Gaston, M., Goldin, A., and Bonmasser, E., 1975, Increased immunogenicity of two lymphoma lines after drug treatment of athymic (nude) mice, *J. Natl. Cancer Inst.* **55:**207–209.

Carson, D. A., Kaye, J., and Wasson, D. B., 1981, The potential importance of soluble deoxynucleotidase activity in mediating deoxyadenosine toxicity in human lymphoblasts, *J. Immunol.* **126:**348–352.

Chanmougan, D., and Schwartz, R. S., 1966, Enhancement of antibody synthesis by 6-mercaptopurine, *J. Exp. Med.* **124**:363–378.

Cohen, A., Lee, J. W. W., Dosch, H. M., and Gelfand, E. W., 1980, The expression of deoxyguanosine toxicity in T lymphocytes at different stages of maturation, *J. Immunol.* **125**:1578–1582.

Connolly, K. M., Armstrong, R. D., Diasio, R. B., and Kaplan, A. M., 1982, Host interactions in the effects of 5-fluorouracil on Ehrlich ascites tumor cells, *Cancer Res.* **42**:4927–4935.

Connolly, K. M., Diasio, R. B., Armstrong, R. D., and Kaplan, A. M., 1983, Decreased immunosuppression associated with antitumor activity of 5-deoxy-5-fluorouridine compared to 5-fluorouracil and 5-fluorouridine, *Cancer Res.* **43**:2529–2535.

Contessa, A. R., Giampietri, A., Bonmassar, A., and Goldin, A., 1979, Increased immunogenicity of L1210 leukemia following short-term exposure to 5(3,3′-dimethyl-1-triazeno)-imidazole-4-carboxamide (DTIC) *in vivo* or *in vitro*, *Cancer Immunol. Immunother.* **7**:71–76.

Curreri, A. R., Ansfield, F. J., McIver, F. A., Waisman, H. A., and Heidelberger, C., 1958, Clinical studies with 5-fluorouracil, *Cancer Res.* **18**:478–484.

Currie, G. A., and McElwain, T. J., 1975, Active immunotherapy as an adjunct to chemotherapy in the treatment of disseminated malignant melanoma: A pilot study, *Br. J. Cancer* **31**:143–156.

D'Arcy Hart, P., Rees, R. J. W., and Niven, J. S. F., 1968, The effect of high dosage of methotrexate associated with folinic acid, on the suppression of tuberculin sensitivity in guinea pigs, *Clin. Exp. Immunol.* **3**:92–98.

Dasmahapatra, K., Goldrosen, M. H., and Douglass, H. O., Jr., 1982, Microplate leukocyte adherence inhibition assay in pancreatic cancer: Effect of chemotherapy on the specific antitumor response, *Cancer Lett.* **16**:307–312.

DeWys, W. D., and Mansky, J. M., 1973, Delayed hematological recovery after cyclophosphamide treatment in the presence of an advanced tumor, *Cancer Res.* **33**:2662–2667.

DiLorenzo, J. A., Griswold, D. E., Bareham, C. R., and Calabresi, P., 1974, Selective alteration on immunocompetence with methotrexate and 5-fluorouracil, *Cancer Res.* **34**:124–128.

Dolnick, B. J., Berenson, R. J., Bertino, J. R., Kaufman, R. J., Nunberg, J. H., and Schimke, R. T., 1979, Correlation of dihydrofolate reductase elevation with gene amplification in a homogeneously staining chromosomal region in L5178Y cells, *J. Cell Biol.* **83**:394–402.

Dosch, H. M., Mansour, A., Cohen, A., Shore, A., and Gelfand, E. W., 1980, Inhibition of suppressor T-cell development following deoxyguanosine administration, *Nature* **285**:494–496.

Drossler, K., Klima, F., and Ambrosius, H., 1983, Kinetics and drug sensitivity of the anti-hapten and anti-carrier IgG1 and IgG2 antibody production in guinea pigs, *Int. Arch. Allergy Appl. Immunol.* **70**:112–117.

Dudman, N. P. B., Slowiaczek, P., and Tattersall, M. H. N., 1982, Methotrexate rescue by 5-methyletrohydrofolate or 5-formyltetrahydrofolate in lymphoblast cell lines, *Cancer Res.* **42**:502–507.

Dupuy, J. M., Kourilsky, F. M., Fradelizzi, D., Feingold, N., Jacquillat, C., Bernard, J., and Dausset, J., 1971, Depression of immunologic reactivity of patients with acute leukemia, *Cancer* **27**:323–331.

Edelstein, M., Vietti, T., and Valeriote, F., 1974, Schedule-dependent synergism for the combination of 1-B-D-arabinofuranosylcytosine and daunorubicin, *Cancer Res.* **34**:293–297.

Ehrke, M. J., Cohen, S. A., and Mihich, E., 1978, Selectivity of inhibition by anticancer agents or mouse spleen immune effector functions involved in responses to sheep erythrocytes, *Cancer Res.* **38**:521–530.

Fioretti, M. C., Romani, L., Taramelli, D., and Goldin, A., 1978, Antigenic properties of lymphoma sublines derived from a drug-treated immunogenic L5178Y leukemia, *Transplantation* **26**:449–451.

Fioretti, M. C., Nardelli, B., Bianchi, R., Nisi, C., and Sava, G., 1981, Antigenic changes of a murine lymphoma by in vivo treatment with triazene derivatives, *Cancer Immunol. Immunother.* **11**:283–286.

Friedman, R. M., 1964, Inhibition of established tuberculin hypersensitivity by methotrexate, *Proc. Soc. Exp. Biol. Med.* **116**:471–475.

Friedman, R. M., and Buckler, C. E., 1963, Methotrexate inhibition of tuberculin hypersensitivity in inbred guinea pigs, *J. Immunol.* **91:**846–850.

Friedman, R. M., Buckler, C. E., and Baron, S., 1961, The effect of amino-methylpteroylglutamic acid on the development of skin hypersensitivity and on antibody formation in guinea pigs, *J. Exp. Med.* **114:**173–183.

Frish, A. W., and Davies, G. H., 1962, Inhibition of hemagglutinin formation by thioguanine : dose–time relationship, *Proc. Soc. Exp. Biol. Med.* **110:**444–447.

Gelfand, E. W., Lee, J. J., and Dosch, H. M., 1979, Selective toxicity of purine deoxynucleosides for human lymphocyte growth and function, *Proc. Natl. Acad. Sci. USA* **76:**1998–2002.

Giampietri, A., Fioretti, M. C., Goldin, A., and Bonmassar, E., 1980, Drug-mediated antigenic changes in murine leukemia cells: Antagonistic effects of quinacrine, an antimutagenic compound, *J. Natl. Cancer Inst.* **64:**297–301.

Giampietri, A., Bonmassar, A., Puccetti, P., Circolo, A., Goldin, A., and Bonmassar, E., 1981, Drug-mediated increase of tumor immunogenicity *in vivo* for a new approach to experimental cancer immunotherapy, *Cancer Res.* **41:**681–687.

Goldin, A., and Humphreys, S. R., 1960, Studies of immunity in mice surviving systemic leukemia L1210, *J. Natl. Cancer Inst.* **24:**283–300.

Goldin, A., Humphreys, S. R., Chapman, G. O., Benditti, J. M., and Chirigos, M. A., 1960, Augmentation of therapeutic efficacy of 3'-5'-dichloroamethopterin against an antifolic-resistant variant of leukemia (L1210-M46R) in mice, *Cancer Res.* **20:**1066–1071.

Goldin, A., Nicolin, A., and Bonmassar, E., 1980, Chemotherapy immunogenicity, *Recent Results Cancer Res.* **75:**185–194.

Gray, G. D., Crim, J. A., and Mickelson, M. M., 1968a, The immunosuppressive activity of ara-cytidine. II. Effects on the graft-versus-host reaction, *Transplantation* **6:**818–825.

Gray, G. D., Mickelson, M. M., and Crim, J. A., 1968b, The immunosuppressive activity of ara-cytidine. I. Effects on antibody-forming cells and humoral antibody, *Transplantation* **6:**805–817.

Grindey, G. B., Hoglind-Semon, J., and Pavelic, Z. P., 1978, Modulation versus rescue of antimetabolite toxicity by salvage metabolites administered by continuous infusion, *Antibiotics Chemother.* **23:**295–304.

Griswold, D. E., Heppner, G. H., and Calabresi, P., 1972, Selective suppression of humoral and cellular immunity with cytozine arabinoside, *Cancer Res.* **32:**298–301.

Grisworld, D. E., Kopp, J. S., Manning, J. S., and Heppner, G. H., 1975, Correction of a murine mammary tumor virus-associated immunological depression by selective immunosuppression with cytosin arabinoside, *Cancer Res.* **35:**2670–2673.

Gusella, J. F., and Housman, D., 1976, Induction of erythroid differentiation *in vitro* by purines and purine analogues, *Cell* **8:**263–269.

Gutterman, J. U., Mavligit, G., Gottlieb, J. A., Burgess, M. A., MacBride, C. M., Einhorn, L., Freireich, E. J., and Hersh, E. M., 1974, Chemoimmunotherapy of disseminated malignant melanoma with dimethyl triazeno imidazole carboxamide and bacillus Calmette-Guerin, *N. Engl. J. Med.* **291:**592–597.

Hakansson, L., and Trope, C., 1974, Cell clones with different sensitivity to cytostatic drugs in methylcholanthrene-induced mouse sarcomas, *Acta Pathol. Microbiol. Scand. (Sect. A)* **82:**41–47.

Halpern, R. M., Halpern, B. C., Clark, B. R., Ashe, H., Hardy, D. N., Jenkinson, P. Y., Chou, S. C., and Smith, R. A., 1975, New approach to antifolate treatment of certain cancers as demonstrated in tissue culture, *Proc. Natl. Acad. Sci. USA* **72:** 4018–4022.

Harel, S., Liacopoulos, P., and Ben-Efraim, S., 1972, Inhibition of immunological components by antigenic competition and other immunodepressing procedures, *Immunology* **22:**515–524.

Harris, J. E., and Hersh, E. M., 1968, The effect of 1-B-D-arabinofuranosylcytosine on the immune response of mice to sheep red blood cells, *Cancer Res.* **28:**2432–2436.

Harrison, S. D., Jr., Giles, H. D., and Denine, E. P., 1980, Antitumor drug toxicity in tumor-free and tumor-bearing mice, *Cancer Chemother. Pharmacol.* **4:**199–204.

Hellström, I., Hellström, K. E., Evans, C. A., Heppner, G. H., Pierce, G. E., and Yang, J. P. S.,

1969, Serum mediated protection of neoplastic cells from inhibition by lymphocytes immune to their tumor specific antigens, *Proc. Natl. Acad. Sci. USA* **62**:362–368.

Heppner, G. H., and Calabresi, P., 1972, Suppression by cytosine arabinoside of serum-blocking factors of cell-mediated immunity to syngeneic transplants of mouse mammary tumors, *J. Natl. Cancer Inst.* **48**:1161–1167.

Heppner, G. H., Griswold, D. E., DiLorenzo, J., Poplin, E. A., and Calabresi, P., 1974, Selective immunosuppression by drugs in balanced immune responses, *Fed. Proc.* **33**:1882–1885.

Heppner, G. H., Dexter, D. L., DeNucci, T., Miller, F. R., and Calabresi, P., 1978, Heterogeneity in drug sensitivity among tumor cell subpopulations of a single mammary tumor, *Cancer Res.* **38**:3758–3763.

Hersh, E. M., and Oppenheim, J. J., 1967, Inhibition of *in vitro* lymphocyte transformation during chemotherapy in man, *Cancer Res.* **27**:98–105.

Hersh, E. M. Carbone, P. P., Wong, V. G., and Freireich, E. J. 1965, Inhibition of the primary immune response in man by anti-metabolites *Cancer Res.* **25**:997–1002.

Hersh, E. M., Whitecar, J. P., Jr., McCredie, K. B., Bodey, G. P., and Freireich, E. J., 1971, Chemotherapy, immunocompetence, immunosuppression, and prognosis in acute leukemia, *N. Engl. J. Med.* **285**:1211–1216.

Hoglind-Semon, J., and Grindey, G. B., 1978, Potentiation of the antitumor activity of methotrexate by concurrent infusion of thymidine, *Cancer Res.* **38**:2905–2911.

Hortobagyi, G. N., Yap, H. Y., Blumenschein, G. R., Gutterman, J. U., Buzdar, A. V., Tashima, C. K., and Hersh, E. M., 1978, Response of disseminated breast cancer to combined modality treatment with chemotherapy and levamisole with or without Bacillus Calmette-Guerin, *Cancer Treat. Rep.* **62**:1685–1692.

Houchens, D. P., Bonmassar, E., Gaston, M. R., Kende, M., Goldin, A., 1976, Drug-mediated immunogenic changes of virus-induced leukemia *in vivo*, *Cancer Res.* **36**:1347–1352.

Hozumi, M., 1983, Fundamentals of chemotherapy of myeloid leukemia by induction of leukemia cell differentiation, *Adv. Cancer Res.* **38**:131–169.

Hrsak, I., and Pavicic, S., 1974, Comparison of the effects of 5-fluorouracil and ftorafur on the haematopoiesis in mice, *Biomedicine* **2**:164–167.

Humphreys, S. R., Chirigos, M. A., Milstead, K. L., Mantel, N., and Goldin, A., 1961, Studies on the suppression of the homograft response with folic acid antagonists, *J. Natl. Cancer Inst.* **27**:259–276.

Humphreys, S. R., Glynn, J. P., Chirigos, M. A., and Goldin, A., 1962, Further studies on the homograft response in BALB/c mice, with L1210 leukemia and a resistant subline, *J. Natl. Cancer Inst.* **28**:1053–1063.

Hunyadi, J., Szegedi, G., Szado, T., Ahmed, A., and Laki, K., 1981, Increased cytotoxic sensitivity of YPC-1 tumor cells from mice treated with nitrosoureas, *Cancer Res.* **41**:1677–1681.

Ishitsuka, H., Umeda, Y., Nakamura, J., and Yagi, Y., 1983, Protective activity of thymosin against opportunistic infections in animal models, *Cancer Immunol. Immunother.* **14**:145–150.

Johnson, R. K., Garibjanian, B. T., Houchens, D. P., Kline, I., Gaston, M. R., Syrkin, A. B., and Goldin, A., 1976, Comparison of 5-fluorouracil and ftorafur. I. Quantitative and qualitative differences in toxicity to mice, *Cancer Treat. Rep.* **60**:1335–1345.

Kaliss, N., 1969, Immunological enhancement, *Int. Rev. Exp. Pathol.* **8**:241–276.

Kan-Mitchell, J., Mitchell, M. S., Lin, T. -S., and Prusoff, W. H., 1980, Comparative analysis of the immunosuppressive properties of two antiviral, iodinated thymidine analogs, 5-iodo-2′-deoxyuridine and 5′-iodo-5′-amino-2′,5′-dideoxyuridine, *Cancer Res.* **40**:3491–3494.

Karakousis, C. P., Didolkar, M. S., Lopez, R., Baffi, R., Moore, R., Holyoke, E. D., 1979, Chemoimmunotherapy (DTIC and *Corynebacterium parvum*) as adjuvant treatment in malignant melanoma, *Cancer Treat. Rep.* **63**:1739–1743.

Kataoka, T., Oh-hashi, F., Sakurai, Y., and Ogihara, K., 1981, Effect of antineoplastic agents on the induction of suppressor macrophages by conconavalin A-bound tumor vaccine, *Cancer Res.* **41**:5151–5157.

Kataoka, T., Akabori, Y., and Sakurai, Y., 1983, 6-mercaptopurine (6-MP)-induced potentiation of active immunotherapy in L1210-bearing mice by eliminating suppressor macrophages, *Proc. Am. Assoc. Cancer Res.* **24**:806.

Kataoka, T., Akabori, Y., and Sakurai, Y., 1984, 6-mercaptopurine-induced potentiation of active immunotherapy in L1210-bearing mice treated with concanavalin A-bound leukemia cell vaccine, *Cancer Res.* **44:**519–524.

Kessel, D., Hall, T. C., and Roberts, D., 1968, Modes of uptake of methotrexate by normal and leukemic human leukocytes in vitro and their relation to drug response, *Cancer Res.* **28:**564–570.

Ketchel, S. J., and Rodriguez, V., 1978, Acute infections in cancer patients, *Semin. Oncol.* **5:**167–179.

Kimball, A. B., Le Page, G. A., Bowman, B., and Herriot, S. J., 1965, Suppression of the homograft response by purinathol nucleosides, *Proc. Soc. Exp. Biol. Med.* **119:**248–252.

Koshimura, S., and Ryoyama, K., 1977, Enhancement of antileukemic effect in the combination of 5-fluorouracil and OK-432, *Cancer Treat. Rep.* **61:**17–27.

Leclerc, J. C., Gomard, E., Plata, F., and Levy, J. P., 1973, Cell-mediated immune reactions against tumors induced by oncornaviruses. II. Nature of the effector cells in tumor-cell cytolysis, *Int. J. Cancer* **11:**426–432.

Lemmel, E., Hurd, E. R., and Ziff, M., 1971, Differential effects of 6-mercaptopurine and cyclophosphamide on autoimmune phenomena in NZB mice, *Clin. Exp. Immunol.* **8:**355–362.

Lenaz, L., Sternberg, S. S., and Philips, F. S., 1969, Cytotoxic effects of 1-B-D-arabinofuranosyl-5-fluorocytosine and of 1-B-D-arabinofuranosylcytosine in proliferating tissues in mice, *Cancer Res.* **29:**1790–1798.

Lindner, A., Santill, D., Hodgett, J., and Nerlinger, C., 1959, Effects of 5-fluorouracil on the hematopoietic system of the mouse, *Cancer Res.* **19:**497–502.

Makulu, D. R., and Wright, P. H., 1971, Effects of methotrexate on insulin antibody production in guinea pigs, *J. Pharmacol. Exp. Ther.* **179:**66–73.

Mantovani, A., Luini, W., Peri, G., Vecchi, A., and Spreafico, F., 1978, Effect of chemotherapeutic agents on natural cell-mediated cytotoxicity in mice, *J. Natl. Cancer Inst.* **61:**1255–1261.

Mantovani, A., Luini, W., Candiani, G. P., and Spreafico, F., 1980, Effect of chemotherapeutic agents on natural and BCG-stimulated macrophage cytotoxicity in mice, *Int. J. Immunopharmacol.* **2:**333–339.

Martin, D. S., Stolfi, R. L., Sawyer, R. C., Spiegelman, S., and Young, C. W., 1982, High-dose 5-fluorouracil with delayed uridine rescue in mice, *Cancer Res.* **42:**3964–3970.

Martinez, D., Lukasewycz, O. A., and Murphy, W. H., 1975, Immune mechanisms in leukemia: Suppression of cellular immunity by drugs and x-irradiation, *J. Immunol.* **115:**724–729.

Massaia, M., Ma, D. D. F., Slywestrowicz, T. A., Tidman, N., Gillprice, G., Janossy, G., and Hoffbrand, A. V. 1982, Enzymes of purine metabolism in human peripheral lymphocyte subpopulations, *Clin. Exp. Immunol.* **50:**148–154.

Mavligit, G. M., Gutterman, J. U., Burgess, M. A., Khankhanian, N., Seibert, G. B., Speer, J. F., Reed, R. C., Jubert, A. V., Martin, R. C., McBride, C. M., Copeland, E. M., Gehan, E. A., and Hersh, E. M., 1975, Adjuvant immunotherapy and chemoimmunotherapy in colorectal cancer of the Dukes' C classification, *Cancer* **36:**2421–2427.

Medzihradsky, J., Ehrke, J., and Mihich, E., 1977, Time limitations in the reversal by citrovorum factor of methotrexate-induced immunosuppression in mice, *Biochem. Pharmacol.* **26:**203–206.

Medzihradsky, J. L., Hollowell, R. P., and Elion, G. B., 1981, Differential inhibition by azathioprine and 6-mercaptopurine of specific suppressor T-cell generation in mice, *J. Immunopharmacol.* **3:**1–16.

Medzihradsky, J. L., Klein, C., and Elion, G. B., 1982, Differential interference by azathioprine and 6-mercaptopurine with antibody-mediated immunoregulation: Synergism of azathioprine and antibody in the control of an immune response, *J. Immunol.* **129:**145–149.

Merluzzi, V. J., Last-Barney, K., Susskind, B. M., and Faanes, R. B., 1982, Recovery of humoral and cellular immunity by soluble mediators after 5-fluorouracil-induced immunosuppression, *Clin. Exp. Immunol.* **50:**318–326.

Mihich, E., 1969a, Combined effects of chemotherapy and immunity against leukemia L1210 in DBA/2 mice, *Cancer Res.* **29:**848–854.

Mihich, E., 1969b, Modification of tumor regression by immunologic means, *Cancer Res.* **29:**2345–2350.

Miller, B. E., Miller, F. R., and Heppner, G. H., 1981, Interactions between tumor subpopulations affecting their sensitivity to the antineoplastic agents cyclophosphamide and methotrexate, *Cancer Res.* **41:**4378–4381.

Miller, B. E., Roi, L. D., Howard, L. M., and Miller, F. R., 1983, Quantitative selectivity of contact-mediated intercellular communication in a metastatic mouse mammary tumor line, *Cancer Res.* **43:**4102–4107.

Mitchell, M. S., and DeConti, R. C., 1970, Immunosuppression by 5-fluorouracil, *Cancer* **26:**884–889.

Mitchell, M. S., Wade, M. E., DeConti, R. C., Bertino, J. R., and Calabresi, P., 1969, Immunosuppressive effects of cytosine arabinoside and methotrexate in man, *Ann. Intern. Med.* **70:**535–547.

Mitchell, M. S., Mejias, E., Daddona, P. E., and Kelley, W., 1978, Purinogenic immunodeficiency diseases: Selective toxicity of deoxyribonucleosides for T cells, *Proc. Natl. Acad. Sci. USA* **75:**5011–5014.

Mitsuoka, A., Baba, M., and Morikawa, S., 1976, Enhancement of delayed hypersensitivity by depletion of suppressor T cells with cyclophosphamide, *Nature* **262:**77–78.

Mott, M. G., 1973, Chemotherapeutic suppression of immune enhancement: A primary determinant of successful cancer therapy, *Lancet* **2:**1092–1094.

Murahata, R. I., and Mitchell, M. S., 1982, Modulation of cell-mediated alloimmunity by BCG. I. Antagonism and potentiation of immunosuppression caused by cytarabine, *J. Natl. Cancer Inst.* **69:**607–612.

Nathan, P., Gonzales, Z. E., Pescovitz, H., Jowles, R. W., and Miller, B. F., 1960, The influence of 6-MP on survival of homologous rabbit kidney transplants, *Fed. Proc.* **19:**216.

Newlands, E. S., Oon, C. J., Roberts, J. T., Elliott, P., Mould, R. F., Topham, C., Madden, F. J. F., Newton, K. A., and Westbury, G., 1976, Clinical trial of combination chemotherapy and specific active immunotherapy in disseminated melanoma, *Br. J. Cancer* **34:**174–179.

Nicolin, A., Vadlamudi, S., and Goldin, A., 1972, Antigenicity of L1210 leukemic sublines induced by drugs, *Cancer Res.* **32:**653–657.

Noonan, F. P., Halliday, W. J., Wall, D. R., and Clunie, G. J. A., 1977. Cell-mediated immunity and serum blocking factors in cancer patients during chemotherapy and immunotherapy, *Cancer Res.* **37:**2473–2480.

Nordman, E., Saarimaa, H., and Toivand, A., 1978, The influence of 5-fluorouracil on cellular and humoral immunity in cancer patients, *Cancer* **41:**64–69.

Ochs, U. H., Chen, S. H., Ochs, H. D., Osborne, W. R. A., and Scott, C. R., 1979, Purine nucleoside phosphorylase deficiency: A molecular model for selective loss of T cell function, *J. Immunol.* **122:**2424–2429.

Ohnuma, T., Arkin, H., Minowada, J., and Holland, J. F., 1978, Differential chemotherapeutic susceptibilty of human T-lymphocytes and B-lymphocytes in culture, *J. Natl. Cancer Inst.* **60:**749–752.

Ohnuma, T., Arkin, H., and Holland, J. F., 1980, Differences in chemotherapeutic susceptibility of human T-, B-, and non-T-/non-B-lymphocytes in culture, *Recent Results Cancer Res.* **75:**61–67.

Ohta, Y., Sueki, K., Kitta, K., Takemoto, K., Ishitsuka, H., and Yagi, Y., 1980, Comparative studies on the immunosuppressive effect among 5′-deoxy-5-fluorouridine, ftorafur, and 5-fluorouracil, *Gann* **71:**190–196.

Orbach-Arbouys, S., and Castes, M., 1979, Augmentation of immune responses after methotrexate administration, *Immunology* **36:**265–269.

Pannacciulli, I., Massa, G., Bogliolo, G., Ghio, R., and Sobrero, A., 1982, Effects of high-dose methotrexate and leucovorin on murine hemopoietic stem cells, *Cancer Res.* **42:**530–534.

Papac, R. J., 1980, Differentiation of human promyelocytic leukemia cells *in vitro* by 6-thioguanine, *Cancer Lett.* **10:**33–38.

Phillips, S. M., and Zweiman, B., 1973, Mechanisms in the suppression of delayed hypersensitivity in the guinea-pig by 6-mercaptopurine, *J. Exp. Med.* **137:**1494–1510.

Phillips, S. M., Catanzaro, P. J., Carpenter, C. B., and Zweiman, B., 1979, Mechanisms in the suppression of delayed hypersensitivity in the guinea pig by 6-mercaptopurine. II. Kinetic and morphologic studies on the monocyte-macrophage component, *Immunopharmacology* **1**:277–299.

Pinedo, H. M., Zaharko, D. S., Bull, J. M., and Chabner, B. A., 1976, The reversal of methotrexate cytotoxicity to mouse bone marrow cells by leucovorin and nucleosides, *Cancer Res.* **36**:4418–4424.

Piper, A. A., and Fox, R. M., 1982, Biochemical basis for the differential sensitivity of human T- and B-lymphocyte lines to 5-fluorouracil, *Cancer Res.* **42**:3753–3760.

Popiela, T., Zembala, M., Oszacki, J., and Jedrychowski, W., 1982, A follow-up study on chemoimmunotherapy (5-fluorouracil and BCG) in advanced gastric cancer, *Cancer Immunol. Immunother.* **13**:182–184.

Prasad, K. N., 1973, Differentiation of neuroblastoma cells induced in culture by 6-thioguanine, *Int. J. Cancer* **12**:631–636.

Pruzanski, W., Saito, S., and DeBoer, G., 1983, Modulatory activity of chemotherapeutic agents on phagocytosis and intracellular bactericidal activity of human polymorphonuclear and mononuclear phagocytes, *Cancer Res.* **43**:1420–1425.

Puccetti, P., Giampietri, A., and Fioretti, M. C., 1978, Long-term depression of two primary immune responses induced by a single dose of 5-(3,3-dimethyl-1-triazeno)-imidazole-4-carboxamide (DTIC), *Experientia* **34**:799–800.

Ramseur, W. L., Richards, F., Muss, H. B., Rhyne, L., Cooper, M. R., White, D. R., Stuart, J. J., and Spurr, C. L., 1978, Chemoimmunotherapy for disseminated malignant malanoma: A prospective randomized study, *Cancer Treat. Rep.* **62**:1085–1087.

Rollinghoff, M., Starzinski-Powitz, A., Pfizenmaier, K., and Wagner, H., 1977, Cyclophosphamide-sensitive T-lymphocytes suppress the *in vivo* generation of antigen-specific cytotoxic T-lymphocytes, *J. Exp. Med.* **145**:455–459.

Romani, L., Migliorati, G., Bonmasser, E., and Fioretti, M. C., 1983, Susceptibility of murine lymphoma cells treated with 5-(3,3-dimethyl-1-triazenyl)-1H-imidazole-4-carboxamide to NK-mediated cytotoxicity *in vitro*, *Int. J. Immunopharmacol.* **5**:299–306.

Rose, N. R., Haber, J. A., and Calabresi, P., 1968, Immunosuppressive effects of selected metabolic inhibitors *in vivo* and *in vitro*, *Proc. Soc. Exp. Biol. Med.* **128**:1121–1128.

Sahiar, K., and Schwartz, R. S., 1964, Inhibition of 19 S antibody synthesis by 7 S antibody, *Science* **145**:395–397.

Santos, G. W., 1967, Immunosuppressive drugs I, *Fed. Proc.* **26**:907–913.

Santos, G. W., and Owens, A. H., 1964, A comparison of selected cytotoxic agents on the primary agglutinin response in rats injected with sheep erythrocytes, *Bull. John Hopkins Hosp.* **116**:384–401.

Santos, G. W., Owens, A. H., Jr., and Sensenbrenner, L. L., 1964, Effects of selected cytotoxic agents on antibody production in man: A preliminary report, *Ann. N.Y. Acad. Sci.* **114**:404–423.

Sato, K., Slesinski, R. S., and Littlefield, J. W., 1972, Chemical mutagenesis at the phosphoribosyltransferase locus in cultured human lymphoblasts, *Proc. Natl. Acad. Sci. USA* **69**:1244–1248.

Schreml, W., and Lohrmann, H. -P., 1979, Effect of high-dose methotrexate with citrovorum factor on human granulopoiesis, *Cancer Res.* **39**:4195–4199.

Schwartz, R. S., and Beldotti, L., 1965, The treatment of chronic murine homologous disease: A comparative study of four immunosuppressive agents, *Transplantation* **3**:79–97.

Schwartz, P. M., and Handschumacher, R. E., 1979, Selective antagonism of 5-fluorouracil cytotoxicity by 4-hydroxypyrazolopyrimidine (Allopurinol) *in vitro*, *Cancer Res.* **39**:3095–3101.

Schwartz, A., Askenase, P. W., and Gershon, R. K., 1978, Regulation of delayed-type hypersensitivity reactions by cyclophosphamide-sensitive T cells, *J. Immunol.* **121**:1573–1577.

Segerling, M., Ohanian, S. H., and Borsos, T., 1975, Enhancing effect by metabolic inhibitors on the killing of tumor cells by antibody and complement, *Cancer Res.* **35**:3195–3203.

Sirotnak, F. M., and Moccio, D. M., 1980, Pharmacokinetic basis for differences in methotrexate sensitivity of normal proliferative tissues in the mouse, *Cancer Res.* **40:**1230–1234.

Sirotnak, F. M., and Donsbach, R. C., 1973, Differential cell permeability and the basis for selective activity of methotrexate during therapy of the L1210 leukemia, *Cancer Res.* **33:**1290–1294.

Sirotank, F. M., DeGraw, J. I., Moccio, D. M., and Dorick, D. M., 1978, Antitumor properties of a new folate analog, 10-deaza-aminopterin, in mice, *Cancer Treat. Rep.* **62:**1047–1052.

Sparks, F. C., Albert, N. E., Andreone, P. A., and Breeding, J. H., 1977, Effect of Bacillus Calmette-Guerin on immunosuppression from cyclophosphamide, methotrexate, and 5-fluorouracil, *Cancer Res.* **37:**2560–2564.

Spiegelberg, H. L., and Miescher, P. A., 1963, The effect of 6-MP and aminopterin on experimental immune thyroiditis in guinea pigs, *J. Exp. Med.* **118:**869–890.

Spreafico, F., 1980, The heterogeneity of the interaction between cancer chemotherapeutic agents and host resistance mechanisms, *Recent Results Cancer Res.* **75:**200–206.

Srivastava, B. I. S., and Alderfer, J. L., 1982, Differential cytotoxicity of some fluorinated derivatives against human leukemic cell lines, *Proc. Am. Assoc. Cancer Res.* **23:**216.

Stolfi, R. L., Martin, D. S., Sawyer, R. C., and Spiegelman, S., 1983, Modulation of 5-fluorouracil-induced toxicity in mice with interferon or with the interferon inducer, polyinosinic-polycytidylic acid, *Cancer Res.* **43:**561–566.

Strzadala, L., Opolski, A., Radzikowski, C., and Mihich, E., 1981, Differential expression of murine leukemia antigen on L1210 parental and drug-resistant sublines, *Cancer Res.* **41:**4934–4937.

Sullivan, R. D., Muler, E., and Sykes, M. P., 1959, Antimetabolite combination chemotherapy: Effects of intraarterial methotrexate–intramuscular citrovorum factor therapy in human cancer. *Cancer* **12:**1248–1262.

Taramelli, D., Romani, L., Bonmasser, A., Goldin, A., and Fioretti, M., 1981, Expression of normal histocompatibility antigens in murine lymphomas treated with 5-(3,3'-dimethyl-1-triazeno)-imidazole-4-carboxamide (DTIC) *in vivo, Eur. J. Cancer* **17:**411–420.

Tarnowski, G. S., Faanes, R. B., Ralph, P., and Williams, N., 1978, Suppression and restoration of cytotoxic T-cell activity during chemotherapy of a mouse T-cell lymphoma and a macrophage tumor, *Cancer Res.* **38:**4540–4545.

Tattersall, M. H. N., Brown, B., Frei, E., III, 1975, The reversal of methotrexate toxicity by thymidine with maintenance of antitumor effects, *Nature* **253:**198–200.

Teller, M. N., and Faanes, R. B., 1980, Association of host immunity with 5-fluorouracil-initiated cure of plasmacytoma LPC-1 in BALB/c mice, *Cancer Res.* **40:**2790–2795.

Testorelli, C., Franco, P., Goldin, A., and Nicolin, A., 1978, *In vitro* lymphocyte stimulation and the generation of cytotoxic lymphocytes with drug-induced antigenic lymphomas, *Cancer Res.* **38:**830–834.

Thatcher, N., Gasiunas, N., Potter, M. R., Crowther, D., and Moore, M., 1977, Effects of intermittent 5-fluorouracil and Adriamycin on various immune parameters on carcinoma patients with reference to the tumour load, *Cancer Immunol. Immunother.* **3:**107–113.

Tsuruo, T., and Fidler, I. J., 1981, Differences in drug sensitivity among tumor cells from parental tumors, selected variants, and spontaneous metastases, *Cancer Res.* **41:**3058–3064.

Turk, J. L., 1971, The effect of immunosuppressive drugs on cellular changes after antigenic stimulation, in: *Immunity, Cancer, and Chemotherapy: Basic Relationships on the Cellular Level* (E. Mihich, ed.), Academic Press, New York, pp. 1–6.

Uy, Q. L., Scrinivasin, T., Santos, G. W., and Owens, A. H., 1966, Effect of selected cytotoxic agents on the primary immune response in mice, *Exp. Hematol.* **10:**4–5.

Van Dijk, H., and Voermans, G. A. G. M., 1978, Cyclophosphamide-like cellular immunostimulation induced by 6-thioguanine, *Immunology* **34:**1077–1081.

Varely, A. M., Lelchuk, R., Hutchings, P., and Cooke, A., 1983, The differential effect of 2-deoxyguanosine on concanavalin A-induced suppressor and cytotoxic activity, *Cellular Immunol.* **81:**99–104.

Vecchi, A., Fioretti, M. C., Mantovani, A., Barzi, A., and Spreafico, F., 1976, The immunodepressive and hematotoxic activity of imidazole-4-carboxamido,5-(3-3-dimethyl-1-triazens) in mice, *Transplantation* **22**:619–624.

Vogel, A. W., 1961, Tumor and marrow damage occurring from methotrexate, monofluoromethotrexate, difluoromethotrexate, and dichloromethotrexate, *Cancer Res.* **21**:743–748.

Windle, R., and Bell, P. R. F., 1982, Lymphoblast transformation following adjuvant treatment of an induced colonic cancer with levamisole and fluorouracil, *Cancer Immunol. Immunother.* **12**:267–271.

Winkelstein, A., 1973, Differentiation effects of immunosuppressants on lymphocyte function, *J. Clin. Invest.* **52**:2293–2299.

Winkelstein, A., Craddock, C. G., and Lawrence, J. S., 1971, Cell replication in the primary hemolysin response: The effect of 6-mercaptopurine, *J. Reticuloendothel. Soc.* **9**:307–322.

Wood, W. C., Cosimi, A. B., and Carey, R. W., and Kaufman, S. D., 1978, Randomized trial of adjuvant therapy for high risk primary malignant melanoma, *Surgery* **83**:677–681.

Wortmann, R. L., Mitchell, B. S., Edwards, N. L., and Fox, I. H., 1979, Biochemical basis for differential deoxyadenosine toxicity to T and B lymphoblasts: Role for 5'-nucleotidase, *Proc. Natl. Acad. Sci. USA* **76**:2434–2437.

Zighelboim, J., 1979, Deficiency of antibody-dependent cellular cytotoxicity and mitogen-induced cellular cytotoxicity effector cell function in patients with acute myelogenous leukemia in remission, *Cancer Res.* **39**:3357–3362.

Zimber, C., Ben-Efraim, S., and Weiss, D. W., 1981, Prevention by the MER tubercle bacillus fraction of immunosuppression induced by cancer chemotherapeutic agents. III. Contact hypersensitivity to dinitrofluorobenzene in mice treated with methotrexate, 5-fluorouracil, or cyclophosphamide, or exposed to dinitrobenzene-sulfonate, *Cancer Immunol. Immunother.* **10**:147–155.

CHAPTER 3

IMMUNOMODULATION BY ANTIBIOTICS

ENRICO MIHICH, M. JANE EHRKE, and
MASAAKI ISHIZUKA

1. INTRODUCTION

The interactions of anticancer drugs with the immune system have often
been considered nonspecific in nature as they appeared to be a consequence
of the antiproliferative action that is at the basis of their antitumor activity
(Mihich, 1979). The majority of anticancer drugs were first shown to have
immunosuppressive potential (Mihich, 1971, 1975; Hersh, 1973, 1974) and
only later it was realized that, under certain conditions, they can also cause
immunoaugmenting effects (Ehrke and Mihich, 1984a,b, 1985; Ehrke *et al.*,
1982). Indeed it is now evident that a number of anticancer agents induce
selective immunomodulating effects as also discussed elsewhere in this volume. A variety of investigations have provided evidence suggesting that
immunomodulation by anticancer drugs depends upon multiple factors, such
as (1) the characteristics of the immunological response; (2) the temporal
relationships between drug action and the regulatory mechanisms of the
immunological response; and (3) the pharmacological characteristics of the
drug. In fact, selectively in immunomodulation by anticancer drugs may
depend both on the multiple biochemical and pharmacological parameters
of drug action that determine their effects in different cell types and on the
intrinsic characteristics of the immunological system, particularly those of
relevant control mechanisms. Increasing knowledge acquired on both of
these sets of factors makes it now possible to obtain basic information on

ENRICO MIHICH and M. JANE EHRKE ● Grace Cancer Drug Center, Roswell Park Memorial
Institute, Buffalo, New York 14263.   MASAAKI ISHIZUKA ● Institute of Microbial Chemistry, Microbial Chemistry Research Foundation, Tokyo 141, Japan.

the selective effects of anticancer drugs on the immune system. Consequently, the rational utilization of these drugs as probes to dissect the mechanism of immunoregulation is becoming feasible, and in fact, desirable. Moreover, it may be possible to increase the therapeutic action of an anticancer drug through the exploitation of its immunomodulating effects; it would seem that remission maintenance may be a phase of treatment that might lend itself optimally to such an approach. Admittedly, to date there is almost a total lack of clinical data relevant to this approach, which is however supported by a large number of observations in animal models.

In this chapter selected examples of immunomodulation provided by certain anticancer antibiotics are discussed. Section 2 is concerned primarily with studies of Adriamycin® that were designed to clarify the multiple interactions of this agent with the various components of host defenses and their regulatory mechanisms. Section 3 is concerned with a review of the effects of several additional antibiotics that also have been studied for their action on immunological responses.

2. IMMUNOMODULATION BY ADRIAMYCIN

The chemistry and antitumor action of Adriamycin (ADM) and its parent anthracycline aminoglycosidic antibiotic, daunorubicin, are well known and have been repeatedly reviewed (Carter, 1980; Young *et al.*, 1981; Muggia *et al.*, 1982; Schwartz, 1983).

2.1. Effects in Tumor Model Systems

A possible involvement of host defense mechanisms in the antitumor effects of ADM was first reported by Schwartz and Grindey (1973). The therapeutic advantage of ADM over daunorubicin against the P288 tumor in the syngeneic DBA/2J mouse was lost if the host had been immunocompromised by sublethal whole body irradiation. Further support of this hypothesis was obtained in studies indicating that ADM had an advantage over daunorubicin in an antigenic but not in an nonantigenic tumor–mouse model system (Giuliani *et al.*, 1974) and in a sham splenectomized but not in a splenectomized host–tumor model system (Schwartz and Kanter, 1975). These results suggested that a relative sparing of host antitumor defenses might contribute to the therapeutic advantage of ADM over daunorubicin.

In a series of experiments utilizing three tumors having different immunogenic characteristics (Mantovani *et al.*, 1979a–c), it was found that the antitumor efficacy of ADM was greater in the model with the greatest potential for host antitumor response. The increased therapeutic effectiveness was lost if the hosts were immunodepressed or adult thymectomized. In further experiments with a L1210Ha leukemia line resistant to 5-(3,3′-dimethyl-1-triazeno)-imidazole-4-carboxamide (DTIC), it was shown that an immunodepressive dose of DTIC significantly reduced the number of cures induced by ADM (Mantovani *et al.*, 1979a). These results, as a whole, suggest that host defenses are instrumental in the antitumor effects of ADM and are consistent with a role of thymus-dependent components in these defenses.

In C57B1/6 mice treated with ADM, followed by subcutaneous (s.c.) inoculation of syngeneic EL4 lymphoma, the spleen cells developed the capability to mount a specific augmented cytolytic activity in response to challenge with the lymphoma in culture in parallel with delayed tumor growth in the host. This cytolytic response did not develop if Thy 1.2^+ cells were removed (Ehrke and Mihich, 1984b). This was the first direct demonstration that ADM-treated mice, in which syngeneic tumor growth was delayed, had increased capacity to develop cytotoxic T-lymphocytes which were specific for the syngeneic tumor.

Cells of the monocyte/macrophage type may also be instrumental in the overall antineoplastic effectiveness of ADM (Mantovani *et al.*, 1979a–c; Riccardi *et al.*, 1979). In fact, the administration of silica or carrageenan markedly reduced the therapeutic effectiveness of ADM in the L1210Ha leukemia and SL2 lymphoma systems but did not modify the action of ADM against the nonimmunogenic L1210Cr leukemia. If 5, 15, or 30 days after drug administration, syngeneic or minor histocompatibility loci incompatible tumors were inoculated 5 to 6 hr after lethal irradiation of the mice, tumor growth inhibitory activity was detected in all groups of ADM-treated mice. Silica and carrageenan were shown to abrogate this antitumor consistent with an involvement of ADM-activated tumoricidal macrophages.

Results obtained using ADM in combination with nonspecific immunostimulants are also consistent with the idea that cells of both the mononuclear phagocytic and thymus-dependent lineages play key roles in the ADM-induced antitumor effects. Thus, the combination of ADM and the macrophage-activating agent, *Corynebacterium parvum*, was better than either alone in increasing the life spans of mice with P388 leukemia or Lewis lung carcinoma but was ineffective in nude mice (Houchens *et al.*, 1976). In the L1210Ha-DBA/2 system, ADM–*C. parvum* was the most active among several combinations tested (Tagliabue *et al.*, 1977). The antitumor activity was shown to be dependent upon dose of ADM and upon the time between ADM and *C. parvum* administration with a 5-day interval resulting in maximum activation. Similar observations were made in the SL-2 lymphoma system (Mantovani *et al.*, 1979b). In studying the kinetics of ADM-induced effects in several host defense systems, a similar dependence between the time of ADM administration, antigen stimulus, and assay was found (Ehrke *et al.*, 1983).

2.2. Modulation of Humoral and Cellular Responses

As summarized in the preceding section, there are strong indications that the antitumor effects of ADM are at least in part a consequence of cooperative therapeutic interactions between the drug and host defenses directed against the tumor. In view of these indications, studies were carried out to evaluate the effects of the antibiotic on humoral and cellular immune responses against xenogeneic and allogeneic antigens to see whether the drugs had only a sparing effect on the defenses of the host, concurrent with its antitumor action, or whether it actually had a modifying effect possibly leading to therapeutically advantageous active immunomodulation.

2.2.1. Effects on Humoral Responses

Daunorubicin and ADM, to a lesser extent, suppressed humoral responses of mice against sheep red blood cells (SRBC) and tumor allografts (Mantovani *et al.*, 1976a,b; Orsini and Mihich, 1975; Vecchi *et al.*, 1976). Under certain conditions, however, augmentation of humoral responses against SRBC and tumor allografts are induced by ADM. In fact, augmented plaque-forming cell (PFC) responses were seen in mice treated with ADM 3 days before sensitization with SRBC (Dimitrov *et al.*, 1978, 1979). Using spleen cells from mice that had been treated with ADM at various times, augmented numbers of direct PFC responses in culture could be seen with cells from day -3 ADM-treated mice, or reduced numbers with cells from day -9- or -1-treated mice, or control levels with cells from day -7- or -5-treated mice (Ehrke *et al.*, 1983). Low concentrations of ADM (1–10 nM) added to primary anti-SRBC/PFC cultures also augmented the number of direct PFC responses (Cohen *et al.*, 1980). In a tumor allograft system, under conditions of near optimal response, ADM given either before (days -3, -1, or 0) or after (days $+1$, $+2$, or $+4$) tumor challenge inhibited the response. In contrast, under conditions of suboptimal response, ADM given 5, 7, or 9 days before tumor challenge augmented the response. These results suggested that ADM can actually cause immunomodulation resulting in opposite effects on the humoral response depending upon conditions.

2.2.2. Effects on Cell-Mediated Cytotoxicity

Higher levels of cell-mediated cytotoxic (CMC) responses were found in the cells of the peritoneal cavity from mice treated with ADM (15 mg/kg) 24 hr prior to tumor allograft than in those from mice treated with daunorubicin; however, a similar difference was not seen with spleen cells (Mantovani *et al.*, 1967a,b). Furthermore, since the level of CMC activity, on a per cell basis in ADM-treated mice was similar to control levels and because of the marked decrease in cellularity induced by ADM, the total lytic units per mouse were lower than in the controls. In contrast to these findings, a drug-induced modulation of the CMC response was seen, however, when a therapeutically effective but lower dose of ADM (5 mg/kg), which did not cause a marked decrease in spleen cellularity, was used (Orsini *et al.*, 1977; Tomazic *et al.*, 1980, 1981; Ehrke *et al.*, 1982, 1983). Under conditions leading to a less than optimal response, ADM given intravenously (i.v.) 5 days before allograft implantation caused augmented levels of cytotoxic T-lymphocyte (CTL) activity to develop in both spleen and peritoneal exudate cell

(PEC) populations. A single injection of ADM on day -13, -11, or -7 also resulted in augmented response, whereas treatment on day -15, -9, -3, or $+2$ did not affect the response and those on day -1 or 0 resulted in decreased responses.

In summary, ADM-induced modulation of both humoral and cellular immune responses was dependent upon: (1) drug dose; (2) antigen dose; (3) time between drug administration, antigen challenge, and evaluation. In general, when conditions resulted in an augmented humoral response, the cellular response was usually not modified, and when the cellular response was augmented, the humoral response was usually inhibited. In almost all systems tested ADM was less suppressive than daunorubicin and immune augmentation by daunorubicin has not been described. Four new ADM analogs were recently studied for their capacity to induce augmentation of the T-cell-mediated cytotoxicity generated in primary mixed lymphocyte tumor cell culture (Mace *et al.*, 1982; Ehrke and Mihich, 1984b). Two of the analogs, 4'-deoxy-ADM and 4'-O-methyl-ADM are active against ADM-resistant colon tumor xenografts in nude mice (Giuliani and Kaplan, 1980). The augmentation of CTL activity induced by the most effective concentration (100 nM) of 4'-epi-ADM was always greater than that induced by ADM. The levels of CTL activity induced by the most effective concentrations of 4'-deoxy-ADM and 4'-O-methyl-ADM were essentially equal to that induced by ADM, whereas 4-demethoxy-ADM had no discernible effect under the conditions tested. The pattern of concentrations most effective for induction of augmented CTL activity was very similar to that reported (Casazza, 1979) for optimum antitumor activity.

2.3. Cellular Basis for the Effects of Adriamycin

In view of the information outlined in Sections 2.1 and 2.2, the effects of ADM on various components of the immune response and related regulatory mechanisms were studied in attempts to identify selective drug actions that would explain the immunomodulation observed. The ADM-induced effects on the T-cell and macrophage systems have been studied in considerable detail, while drug effects on natural killer (NK) activity, antibody-dependent cell-mediated cytotoxicity (ADCC), and soluble mediators have as yet been less completely evaluated.

2.3.1. Effects on T Cells

Augmentation of the generation of CTL induced by ADM occurs under different experimental conditions (Ehrke *et al.*, 1980, 1982; Orsini *et al.*, 1977; Tomazic *et al.*, 1980, 1981). ADM does not seem to affect progenitor cytotoxic T lymphocytes (Ehrke *et al.*, 1984). In fact, (1) when the control CTL response is near optimal, little or no augmentation is seen; (2) spleen cells from control and ADM-treated mice develop comparable CTL in response to heat-treated alloantigen when Interleukin 2 (IL 2) is added; and

(3) the CTL response of nonadherent cells from nontreated and ADM-treated mice is the same upon addition of adherent cells from a single source. Moreover, ADM does not eliminate the cyclophosphamide-sensitive progenitors of culture-induced T suppressor cells (Ehrke *et al.*, 1980; Ryoyama *et al.*, 1981, 1984). In contrast, under specific conditions, ADM seems to reduce the suppression involved in the regulation of humoral responses to SRBC (Cohen *et al.*, 1980; Anaclerio *et al.*, 1980).

In the presence of mature mononuclear phagocytes, the augmented CTL activity is associated with an ADM-induced reduction of Lyt 1^-2^+, adherent T regulatory cells. These cells in the spleen cell population from control mice appear to maintain the developing CTL response at "normal" levels (Ehrke *et al.*, 1984).

2.3.2. Effects on Macrophages

Cells of the monocyte/macrophage type may have a pivotal role in ADM-induced host defense modulations (Mantovani *et al.*, 1976a,b; Mantovani, 1977; Orsini *et al.*, 1977; Tomazic *et al.*, 1980; Ehrke *et al.*, 1982). Mature macrophages are relatively resistant to the cytotoxicity of ADM but more sensitive to daunorubicin (Mantovani, 1982). Similar differences were seen in studies of drug effects, *in vitro*, on macrophage function (Ehrke *et al.*, 1978; Facchinetti *et al.*, 1978; Cohen *et al.*, 1980). After the *in vivo* administration of ADM, monocyte/macrophage-like cells in the spleen were relatively increased as measured by counting phagocytic adherent cells (Mantovani *et al.*, 1976a) or histologically (Orsini *et al.*, 1977). After treatment with ADM under conditions identical to those used for histological evaluation (5 mg/kg, day -5), spleen cells phagocytized SRBC to the same extent as those from nontreated controls on day 0. However, after 5 days in culture, increased phagocytic activity was seen with cells from drug-treated mice (Ehrke *et al.*, 1980; Cohen *et al.*, 1982). This increased activity was derived from a subset of cells likely to be immature cells of the monocyte/macrophage type, which at the initiation of culture was nonphagocytic, insensitive to silica, and nonadherent to plastic but which acquired these characteristics of mature macrophages during culture (Cohen *et al.*, 1982; Ehrke and Mihich, 1985). The phagocytic activity of spleen cells from mice treated with ADM on day -9, -11, or -13 is augmented compared to controls. This time-dependent maturation of the immature macrophage *in vivo* seems similar to that shown to occur during 4 or 5 days of culture; it was also compatible with the time dependence described for the administration of ADM and C. *parvum* to obtain optimal antitumor activity (Mantovani *et al.*, 1979a).

The information obtained in many investigations suggests that macrophages exposed to ADM have augmented tumoricidal activity. It has been proposed that macrophages serve as a drug depot and transfer cytotoxic drug to the tumor target. It was also suggested that ADM activates macrophages to develop direct tumoricidal activity (Stoychkov *et al.*, 1979). Both hypotheses seem to be valid at different times after drug administration. Indeed, within 1–3 days after intraperitoneal (i.p.) administration of the drug, peritoneal macrophages appear to act as drug depots and may be tumoricidal by virture of the transfer of drug to the target cell (Haskill, 1981; Martin *et al.*, 1982). In contrast, 14 days, but not 7 days, after i.v. administration of ADM, alveolar macrophages had tumoricidal activity (Hisano and Fidler, 1982). Moreover, after 15 min exposure to ADM *in vitro*, human cells had augmented monocyte-mediated cytotoxicity only after 3, 4, or 7 days of culture, but not earlier (Kleinerman *et al.*, 1982). Also as recently demonstrated by quantitative spectrofluorometry, while peritoneal cells from mice 1 day after i.p. ADM administration contain concentrations of drug equivalent to that which is toxic for P815 tumor, cells from mice 5 or 7 days after ADM administration do not; these cells, however, have greater cytolytic activity against P815 targets than the former (Salazar and Cohen, 1984).

2.3.3. Effects on Natural Killer Cell Activity

The NK activity of peritoneal cells was augmented after a single i.p. injection of ADM, while that of spleen cells was reduced. This reduction was maximal 3 days after i.p. or i.v. drug treatment and was reversed by removal of cells adherent to plastic (Santoni *et al.*, 1980; Salazar and Cohen, 1984). NK activity of spleen cells from nontreated controls and day −5-ADM-treated mice was not significantly different when assayed on day 0 (Ehrke *et al.*, 1982). After 5 days in culture the cells from ADM-treated mice had reduced NK activity; at this time mature macrophages are increased as are soluble products of macrophage origin. These findings are consistent with the evidence indicating that the activity of NK cells is subject to regulation by macrophages (Cudkowicz and Hochman, 1979) and their soluble factors (Santoni *et al.*, 1980). It is of interest that ADM does not modulate ADCC activity against SRBC, chicken red blood cells, or tumor cells (Ehrke *et al.*, 1978; Cohen *et al.*, 1980; Mantovani, 1982; Mantovani *et al.*, 1976b).

2.3.4. Modification of Soluble Factors

Culture medium (CM) from spleen cells from mice treated with ADM (ADM-CM) 5 days, but not 1 day, before sacrifice has nearly twice the concentration of prostaglandin E_2 (PGE_2) as does CM from nontreated spleen cells (N-CM) (Cohen *et al.*, 1985). While NK activity is sensitive to the addition of indomethacin of PGE_2 to cultures, developing CTL activity is relatively insensitive to PGE_2 changes in this concentration range. An increase in IL-2-like activity also appears to occur with cells from ADM-treated mice. In fact, (1) spleen cells from ADM-treated mice develop CTL in response to heat-treated alloantigen while control spleen cells require an exogenous source of IL 2 to respond (Ehrke *et al.*, 1980, 1982); (2) ADM-CM but not N-CM restores the ability to develop CTL of nontreated spleen cells exposed to either silica treatment or to heat-treated alloantigen (Ehrke *et al.*, 1982); and (3) long-term T-cell cultures can be maintained in ADM-CM but not in

N-CM. The levels of the putative IL 2 inhibitor (Hardt *et al.*, 1981) detectable in the plasma of nontreated and ADM-treated mice were found to be comparable. It is not clear whether the modulation seen in IL 2 production is a primary drug effect or is secondary to ADM-induced modulation of interleukin 1 production by cells of the macrophage lineage; the latter phenomenon occurred with PEC (Cohen *et al.*, 1983). ADM also inhibited the production of migration-inhibitory factor (MIF) by spleen cells (Mantovani, 1982). In conclusion, it would seem that soluble mediators play a major role in the ADM-induced modulation of host defenses.

2.4. Conclusions

It can now be suggested that ADM has unique properties that may be useful when the drug is applied as a probe in basic investigations. For example, following treatment with ADM, one can obtain a spleen cell population enriched for immature cells of the mononuclear phagocyte lineage, and these immature cells provide an enlarged pool of cells for basic investigations of factors affecting macrophage differentiation. Similarly, the ADM sensitivity of the adherent T regulatory cell provides opportunities for the evaluation of this cell and its function. ADM-induced effects on soluble mediators of immune responses provide other opportunities for application of the drug as a probe. In addition, this is an area where there is a further need to establish the relevance of these parameters to the overall antitumor action of the drug.

As outlined above, a multiplicity of functions are affected by ADM, but each appears to be the result of a selective drug–cell interaction. For example, mature macrophages are relatively insensitive to ADM, in contrast to the selective increase in immature mononuclear phagocytes. Similarly, progenitors of and mature cytotoxic T cells as well as progenitors of and mature T suppressor cells are apparently unaffected by ADM, but the drug induces selective elimination of an adherent T regulatory cell. Indeed, the selective interaction of ADM with these two cells subsets, immature mononuclear phagocytes and adherent T regulatory cells, appears to be the site of primary drug immunomodulation.

3. EFFECTS OF ADDITIONAL ANTITUMOR ANTIBIOTICS ON HOST DEFENSES

In addition to ADM a number of antitumor antibiotics have been shown to affect host defenses. In some cases the modifications induced are compatible with the possibility that cooperative interactions between antibiotic and antitumor host defenses are instrumental in determining the therapeutic outcome. The results summarized in this section provide information obtained with a number of antibiotics in studies carried out primarily in Japan.

3.1. Sporamycin

Sporamycin is a polypeptide antibiotic isolated from culture filtrates of *Streptosporangium pseudovulgare* (Komiyama *et al.*, 1977a). This antibiotic is effective against various murine transplantable tumors (Komiyama *et al.*, 1977b). Sporamycin inhibits DNA synthesis and subsequently causes strand scission of cellular DNA (Komiyama and Umezawa, 1978; Okamoto *et al.*, 1979).

Although sporamycin exhibited a strong antitumor effect by daily injections, Komiyama *et al.* (1979) found that a single injection was markedly effective in causing regression of S-180. In fact, when mice bearing S-180 were injected with sporamycin once 3 days after inoculation of the tumor cells, tumor regression was observed within 35 days. Cell-mediated immunity was augmented in mice given sporamycin as indicated by enhancement of MIF activity of spleen cells and delayed-type hypersensitivity to S-180 cells. Augmented cell-mediated antitumor activity of mice treated with sporamycin was also demonstrated by the Winn assay. S-180 tumor cells were mixed with spleen cells derived from sporamycin-treated mice that had been inoculated with S-180 cells, and the mixture was inoculated into normal mice. Tumor growth was markedly inhibited by spleen cells derived from tumor-bearing mice treated with sporamycin as compared to the results obtained with cells from nontreated tumor-bearing controls.

The effect of sporamycin was also studied histopathologically by Kawakubo *et al.* (1980). Degeneration of tumor cells was observed at an early stage after sporamycin treatment, whereas marked infiltration of lymphoid cells in the tissue surrounding the tumor resulted in regression of the tumor at a later stage.

Sporamycin inhibited the growth of syngeneic Meth A fibrosarcoma in Balb/c mice, and cured mice were resistant to reinoculation of the tumor (Umezawa *et al.*, 1981). In this study it was shown that spleen cells from these mice, in a Winn assay, had neutralizing activity against the tumor cells, which was reduced by treatment with anti-Thy 1.2 serum and complement. These results suggested that sporamycin augments antitumor immunity and that this effect involves the activation of T cells.

3.2. Macromomycin and Auromomycin

Macromomycin (Chimura *et al.*, 1968) is a polypeptide antibiotic isolated from culture filtrates of *Streptomyces macromomyceticus*. This antibiotic is effective in inhibiting the growth of various murine tumors (Chimura *et al.*, 1968; Lippman *et al.*, 1975). According to Kunimoto *et al.* (1972), macromomycin binds to the plasma membrane of tumor cells and causes inhibition of DNA synthesis. Lippman *et al.* (1973) suggested that macromomycin was effective in enhancing tumor immunity in mice. A similar effect of macromomycin was also observed in the enhancement of tumor immunity in mice immunized with macromomycin-treated tumor cells (Ishizuka, 1979). Although macromomycin shows favorable activities, it is labile. While searching for more stable and active protein antibiotics, auromomycin was isolated from culture filtrates of the same strain that produced macromomycin (Yamashita *et al.*, 1979). Both antibiotics have a similar molecular weight, isoelectric point, and amino acid composition. Although both exhibit a strong antitumor effect against experimental murine tumors, auromomycin has a stronger antibacterial and antitumor activity, as well as toxicity, than macromomycin. It was reported that the chromophore contained in both antibiotics causes inhibition of DNA synthesis by DNA strand scission (Suzuki *et al.*, 1980). The influence of auromomycin on the transplantability of tumor cells has also been studied (Ishizuka *et al.*, 1980), and the results were described as follows: Murine tumor cells, from the IMC carcinoma which had occurred spontaneously in a CDF_1 mouse and was maintained by serial transplantation into CDF_1 mice weekly, were mixed with different concentrations of auromomycin and then inoculated subcutaneously into mice. Tumor growth was inhibited when more than 0.1 μg/ml of auromomycin was mixed with 5×10^6 tumor cells. Four weeks later, the injected mice were reinoculated with tumor cells, and 30 days thereafter, tumor growth was examined. Mice that had been inoculated with the mixture of 2.5–5 $\times$ 10^6 tumor cells and 0.1 μg of auromomycin were resistant to the reinoculation with 1×10^6 tumor cells. The effect of auromomycin was observed at low concentrations, 0.01–1 μg/ml, whereas mice inoculated with tumor cells treated with concentrations greater than 10 μg/ml could not reject a tumor cell challenge. The resistance was only induced in mice that had been inoculated with the mixture of auromomycin and tumor cells, but not in mice inoculated with tumor cells incubated with and washed free of auromomycin.

It has been observed that macrophages are necessary for induction of resistance. When the mixture was injected into mice treated with silica or trypan blue as inhibitors of macrophage functions, resistance to a rechallenge with tumor cells was not induced. When fractionated lymphoid cell populations from mice that had acquired resistance were examined, the results showed that the T-cell-rich population inhibited tumor growth markedly in the Winn assay.

3.3. Aclacinomycin A

An anthracycline, aclacinomycin, was isolated from culture filtrates of *Streptomyces galilaeus* and its structure determined (Oki *et al.*, 1975). Acalacinomycin has antibacterial activity and antitumor activity against L-1210, P388, and other murine tumors (Hori *et al.*, 1977; Oki *et al.*, 1981). It has less cardiotoxicity than ADM (Oki *et al.*, 1981). This anthracycline antitumor antibiotic is now used for cancer chemotherapy clinically. Employing lymphoblastoma L5178 Y cells and *Escherichia coli*, the mechanism of action was investigated and it was shown that aclacinomycin prevents RNA synthesis through inhibition of RNA polymerase (Yamaki *et al.*, 1978).

The immunomodulating effects of aclacinomycin were studied by Ishizuka *et al.* (1981). The injection of aclacinomycin over a wide dose range (0.05–5 mg/kg) into mice before immunization or at the time of immunization enhanced antibody formation and delayed-type hypersensitivity. Aclacinomycin showed stronger cytotoxicity toward lymphoblasts induced by concanavalin A (ConA), phytohemagglutinin, or lipopolysaccharide than did ADM or mitomycin C (MMC). However, antibody formation in spleen cell cultures was augmented by the addition of aclacinomycin (0.1–10 ng/ml). At the same concentrations as those of aclacinomycin, ADM did not show any stimulatory effect under the conditions tested. The augmentation was observed when the addition was made at the start of the cultures.

The influence of this antibiotic on suppressor cells was examined in mice in which suppressor cells against antibody formation and delayed-type hypersensitivity were induced by injection of high doses of antigen (Lazo *et al.*, 1978). It was reported that the generation of suppressor cells or suppressor activity in mice immunized with high doses of antigen was markedly reduced by aclacinomycin (Ishizuka *et al.*, 1981). Furthermore, aclacinomycin administration to tumor-bearing hosts reduced the ability of cells from these mice to suppress lymphocyte blastogenesis induced by Con A in culture (Ishizuka *et al.*, 1983) (Figure 1). The inhibition of suppressor activity may be one of the possible mechanisms of action with respect to the enhancement of immune responses observed with aclacinomycin. Recent results also indicate that aclacinomycin augments phagocytosis in these cells. Although the mechanism(s) of immunomodulating actions of aclacinomycin in tumor-bearing hosts still remains to be elucidated, the inhibitory effect of the drug on the generation of suppressor functions should prove favorable for cancer therapy.

3.4. Oxanosine

A nucleoside antibiotic, oxanosine, was isolated from culture filtrates of *Streptomyces capreolus* (Shimada *et al.*, 1981). The structure was determined by X-ray crystallographic analysis to be 5-amino-3-β-D-ribofuranosyl-3H-imidazo[4,5-d][1,3]oxazin-7-one (Nakamura *et al.*, 1981) (Figure 2). Oxanosine exhibits weak antibacterial activity and inhibits the growth of tumor cells *in vitro*. Its mode of action was studied by Yagisawa *et al.* (1982). Since its antibacterial activity was antagonized by guanine, guanosine, and guanylic acid, and the inhibitory activity against L-1210 cells was reversed by guanylic acid, oxanosine was considered to be a competitive inhibitor of GMP synthetase.

This nucleoside antibiotic has very low toxicity and 50% of the lethal dose in mice has been estimated to be more than 1 g/kg by the i.v. route. The antitumor activity of oxanosine against murine transplantable tumors such as L-1210, Meth A, and IMC carcinoma has been studied (Nitta, 1983). The i.p. injection of oxanosine at 50–400 mg/kg daily for 10 days from 1 day after the tumor inoculation was effective in prolonging the survival period

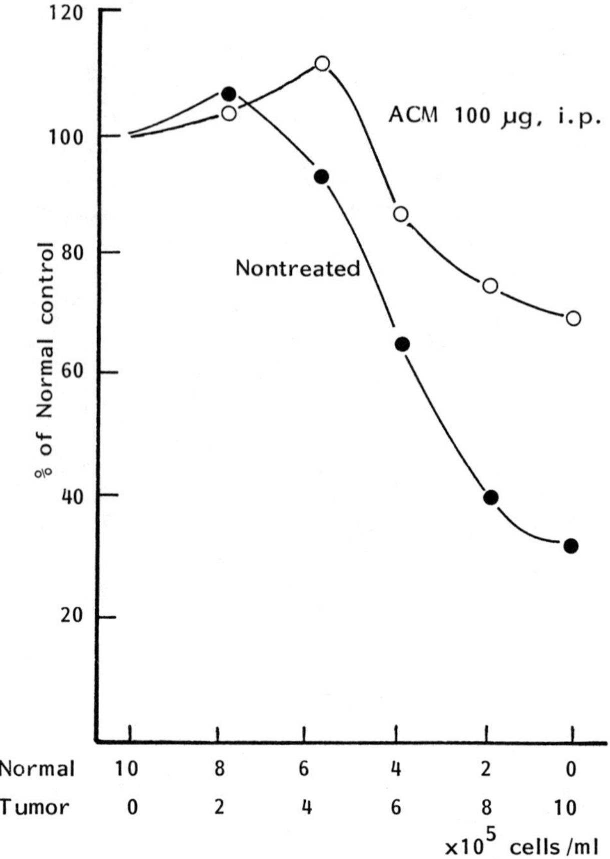

FIGURE 1. Reduction of suppressor activity of spleen cells from tumor-bearing mice treated with aclacinomycin (ACM). CDF$_1$ mice were inoculated with 1×10^6 IMC carcinoma s.c.; 25 days after the tumor inoculation, ACM (100 μg/mouse, i.p.) was injected. Two days thereafter, spleen cells from ACM-treated or nontreated tumor-bearing mice were mixed with spleen cells from normal mice in different ratios as shown in this figure and cultured with Con A (0.5 μg/ml) for 3 days. Result was determined by measuring incorporation of [^{3}H]thymidine into cultured cells.

of mice inoculated with tumor cells. The IC$_{50}$ of oxanosine on cultured L-1210 cells was estimated to be 0.9–1.7 μg/ml.

The influence of oxanosine on immune responses has also been studied by Ishizuka *et al.* (1983), and their results are presented herein in some detail. Oxanosine, even at 200 mg/kg, given at the time of immunization, did not inhibit either antibody formation or delayed-type hypersensitivity to SRBC. At high doses, such as 100–200 mg/kg, the number of IgM-antibody-forming cells was increased significantly. In the case of delayed-type hypersensitivity to SRBC, the response in mice immunized with the optimal dose of antigen (10^5 cells, i.v.) was not affected at doses of less than 100 mg/kg, but in mice immunized with a high dose of antigen (10^8 cells, i.v.),

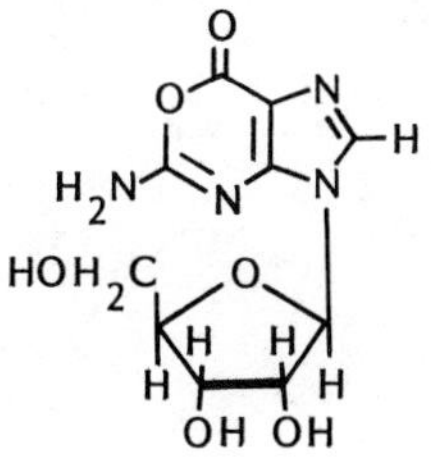

FIGURE 2. Structure of oxanosine.

which has been shown to induce suppression, oxanosine at 25–400 mg/kg augmented the response. Thus, these results suggested that oxanosine may be an inhibitor of suppressor functions. Consequently, the effects of oxanosine on the generation of suppression of delayed-type hypersensitivity was examined. Mice were immunized with a high dose of antigen, and from 2 days from the immunization, oxanosine or another inhibitor such as cyclophosphamide or aclacinomycin was injected daily for 3 days. Five days after immunization, spleen cells were collected as a source of suppressor cells and were transferred to untreated mice. Then the mice were immunized with the optimal dose of antigen, and the response was determined. The results indicated that the daily injection of 50–400 mg/kg inhibited the generation of suppressors of antibody formation and delayed-type hypersensitivity.

The effect of oxanosine on suppressors derived from tumor-bearing mice was also examined. It had been determined in previous experiments that suppressors were induced between 3 and 6 days and from 21 days onward after transplantation of IMC carcinoma. The influence of oxanosine on suppressor functions induced in tumor-bearing mice was examined by giving the agent 2 or 5 days after transplantation of tumor cells; 1 day later (day 3 and day 6, respectively), spleen cells were collected. Populations of spleen cells from tumor-bearing mice were divided into T-cell-rich (nonadherent) and macrophage-rich (adherent) subpopulations. Each cell subpopulation was added to spleen cells from normal mice and the mixture was cultured with Con A; then, the suppressor activity was evaluated in terms of the relative incorporation of [³H]thymidine into the cells. On day 3 suppressor cell activity was observed in both subpopulations from untreated mice although the T-cell-rich population showed stronger activity; oxanosine treatment reduced suppressor activity in both cell populations significantly and the suppressor activity of macrophages was more affected than that of T cells (Table I). Oxanosine treatment on day 5 was more effective in reducing suppressor activity in both cell populations, and the suppressor activity of the macrophage-rich cell population was no longer evident (Table II).

To determine whether the effect of oxanosine is reflected in terms of tumor growth, mice were given oxanosine once 3, 6, or 12 days after implantation of tumor cells. Thirty days after transplantation, tumor growth was assessed by determining tumor weight. The results indicate that injection on day 6 or day 12, but not day 3, resulted in tumor growth inhibition of

TABLE I
Effect of Oxanosine on Suppressors Induced in Tumor-Bearing Mice (Day 3)[a]

	[³H]thymidine incorporation per culture	
Cells with Con A	None	Oxanosine
Normal (N)	38,244	—
Tumor-bearing (TB)	21,387 (44)[b]	22,133 (42)
N + TB	28,883 (24)	29,679 (23)
N + TB non ad.	11,500 (70)	17,526 (54)
N + TB ad.	29,528 (23)	36,076 (6)

[a]CDF$_1$ mice were inoculated with 2 × 10⁶ IMC carcinoma cells. Oxanosine (50 mg/kg) was given 2 days later, 3 days after the tumor inoculation spleen cells were collected. Nylon-wool-column-passed spleen cells were designated as non ad. Plastic adherent cells were designated as ad. Each cell population was mixed with normal spleen cells in ratio of 1 : 1 and cultured with Con A (0.5 μg/ml) for 72 hr.

[b]Numbers in parentheses indicate percent inhibition based on incorporation of N cells with Con A being equal to 100%.

about 40%–60%. The effector cells activated by the injection of oxanosine on day 6 were then examined. Four days after the injection of oxanosine on day 6, spleen cells were collected, and macrophage-depleted and T-cell-depleted cell populations were prepared. Each cell population was mixed with target cells (IMC carcinoma cells, E : T = 100 : 1) and proliferation of tumor cells was determined 16–41 hr after starting the cultures (Figure 3). Comparing each cell population with those from nontreated tumor-bearing mice, cells from the oxanosine-treated mice inhibited tumor cell growth significantly. Among the three cell populations studied, the adherent cell-depleted spleen cells showed the strongest inhibitory effect. T-cell-depleted spleen cells of nontreated mice gave little inhibition, whereas the same cell populations from oxanosine-treated mice still were inhibitory. Therefore, the data suggest that some effectors other than T cells could be activated to become cytotoxic by treatment with oxanosine. The influence of oxanosine

TABLE II
Effect of Oxanosine on Suppressors Induced in Tumor-Bearing Mice (Day 6)[a]

	[³H]thymidine incorporation per culture	
Cells with Con A	None	Oxanosine
Normal (N)	23,836	—
Tumor-bearing (TB)	16,438 (31)[b]	26,284 (0)
N + TB	21,969 (8)	25,622 (0)
N + TB non ad.	15,835 (34)	20,413 (15)
N + TB ad.	26,048 (0)	26,002 (0)

[a]CDF$_1$ mice were inoculated with 2 × 10⁶ IMC carcinoma cells. Oxanosine (50 mg/kg) was given 5 days later, 6 days after the tumor inoculation spleen cells were collected. Nylon-wool-column-passed spleen cells were designated as non ad. Plastic adherent cells were designated as ad. Each cell population was mixed with normal spleen cells in ratio of 1 : 1 and cultured with Con A (0.5 μg/ml) for 72 hr.

[b]Numbers in parentheses indicate percent inhibition based on incorporation of N cells with Con A being equal to 100%.

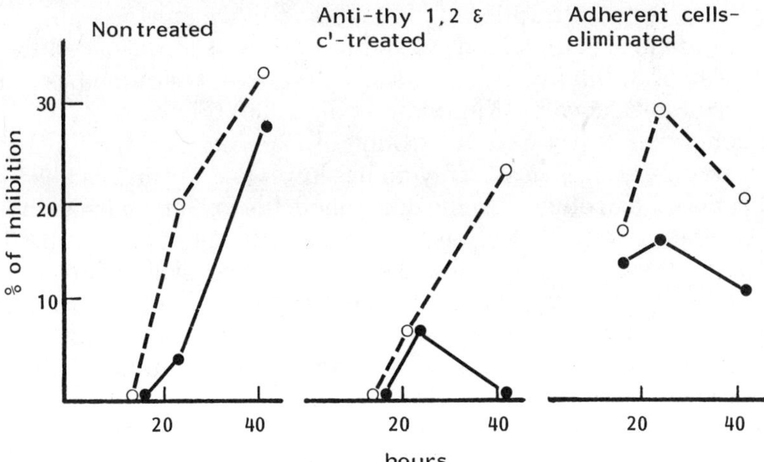

FIGURE 3. Cytotoxicity of spleen cells from IMC-carcinoma-bearing mice given oxanosine against IMC carcinoma cells. (●———●) Nontreated control, (○————○) oxanosine, 50 mg/kg, i.p.

on macrophage functions was also studied. The injection of oxanosine enhanced phagocytosis and PMA-stimulated superoxide anion production by peritoneal macrophages. These results suggest that oxanosine may activate macrophages to become one of the effectors.

In summary, it has been shown that oxanosine acts as an inhibitor of macrophage and/or T-cell suppressors derived from tumor-bearing host; also, it may activate adherent cells to become cytotoxic. The mechanism of action of oxanosine still remains to be elucidated.

3.5. Neothramycin and Mazethramycin

Neothramycin was isolated from culture filtrate of *Streptomyces thioluteus* (Takeuchi *et al.*, 1976). The structure was determined (Figure 4) and shown to be one of the anthramycin group of antibiotics (Miyamaoto *et al.*,

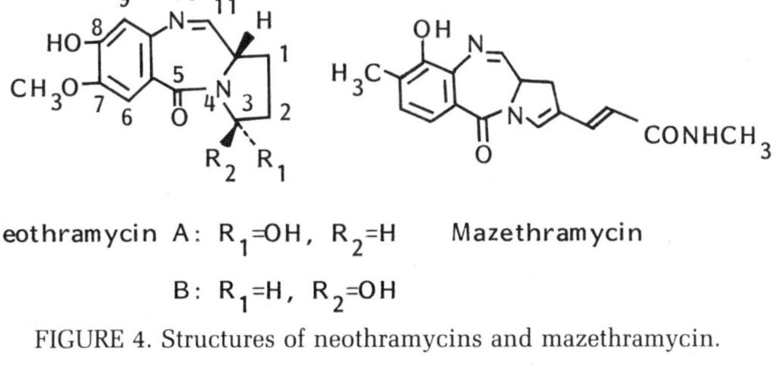

Neothramycin A: R₁=OH, R₂=H   Mazethramycin

B: R₁=H, R₂=OH

FIGURE 4. Structures of neothramycins and mazethramycin.

1977). It is effective in inhibiting L-1210 and other murine transplantable tumors (Hisamatsu *et al.*, 1980). Mazethramycin was also isolated from culture filtrates of *S. thioluteus*, and its structure was determined as a methyl derivative of anthramycin (Kunimoto *et al.*, 1980) (Figure 4).

Among the anthramycin group of antibiotics [the pyrrolo(1,4) benzodiazepine group], neothramycin has lower toxicity and can be injected at higher doses than others. On the other hand, the toxicity of mazethramycin is almost the same as that of anthramycin. Although these antibiotics are effective in inhibiting lymphoid leukemias, they do not show myelotoxicity in mice (Hisamatsu *et al.*, 1980). The mechanism of action of neothramycin in inhibiting tumor growth has been shown to involve its covalent binding to guanine residue of DNA, thus causing inhibition of cellular DNA synthesis (Maruyama *et al.*, 1981).

The influence of neothramycin and mazethramycin on immune responses has been studied, and it was found that these antibiotics did not suppress the immune responses, but augmented them (Ishizuka *et al.*, 1983). When mice were injected with neothramycin or mazethramycin at the time of immunization, IgM antibody formation and delayed-type hypersensitivity to SRBC were enhanced over a wide dose range. In testing the effect of mazethramycin on antibody formation by spleen cell cultures, the addition of 0.01–1 ng/ml of this antibiotic to cultures was found to increase the number of antibody-forming cells.

The effect of these antibiotics on macrophage functions has also been studied. Phagocytosis by peritoneal macrophages was stimulated following the injection of neothramycin and mazethramycin. These results were compatible with the possibility that these antibiotics may activate macrophages to become cytotoxic. Therefore, the effect of neothramycin and mazethramycin on phorbol myristate acetate (PMA)-induced superoxide anion production by macrophages (an indicator of activated macrophages) was examined. It was found that the PMA-stimulated superoxide anion production by macrophages from mice that had received these antibiotics was about three times greater than that resulting from PMA stimulation alone. The effect of mazethramycin is shown in Figure 5.

Mice were given neothramycin or mazethramycin, and 1–5 days later, they were inoculated with L-1210, S-180, or IMC carcinoma. Their survival time was then determined. In this test system, the injection of these antibiotics before implantation of tumor cells prolonged the survival time of the mice markedly, whereas the effect was reduced in mice treated with silica or trypan blue. Thus, these findings further suggest that these antibiotics may activate cell- or macrophage-mediated cytotoxicity. After treatment of mice with the drugs, the cytotoxicity of peritoneal macrophages or of spleen cells was tested. It was observed that peritoneal macrophages were cytotoxic, but not whole spleen cells. These results indicate that the intraperitoneal injection of neothramycin or mazethramycin activates macrophages to become cytotoxic. Thus the immunoenhancing effect of these antibiotics on

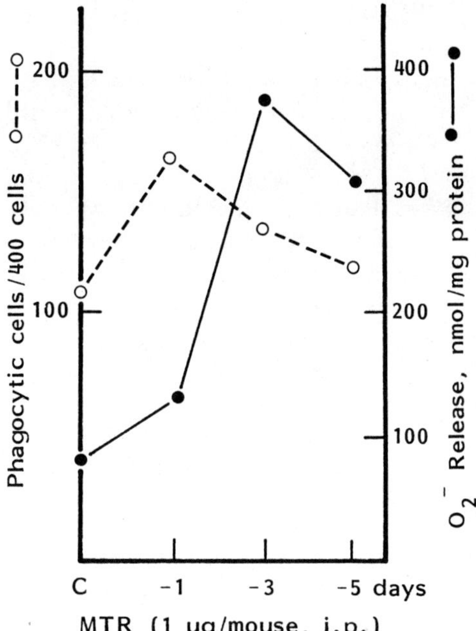

FIGURE 5. Effect of mazethramycin (MTR) on phagocytosis of yeasts and O_2^- release by macrophages.

antibody formation and delayed-type hypersensitivity may be caused by macrophage-mediated effects.

3.6. Mitomycin C

The antitumor activities of MMC in experimental tumor systems and in humans are well known. This antibiotic has acquired considerable interest in clinical practice especially when used in combination with other agents.

There are a few reported studies that indicate the probable immuno-modulating potential of MMC. The agent was shown to augment resistance to subsequent challenge with live tumor when administered in conjunction with a Con-A-bound L-1210 vaccine; 50% were long-term survivors (LTS) in a group given 1.23 mg/kg of MMC plus vaccine versus 3% LTS in a group given vaccine alone (Kataoka *et al.*, 1978, 1980). The augmentation was specific for L-1210 leukemia and was found to be dependent on the timing of antibiotic and vaccine administration with a clear indication that the effect was not directly related to a drug-induced inhibition of tumor growth. It was shown that the suppressor functions of peritoneal cells induced by the vaccine were inhibited by the antibiotic in a polyclonal *in vitro* spleen cell blastogenesis assay. The administration of MMC (1 mg/kg) or a protein-bound polysaccharide preparation, PS-K (500 or 1000 mg/kg), 1 or 5 days, respectively, after P388 transplantation resulted in little effect on the tumor growth;

however, when the treatments were combined, significant numbers of LTS resulted. Similar effects were not seen with cyclophosphamide, 5-fluorouracil, or 6-mercaptopurine in combination with PS-K (Oh-Hashi *et al.*, 1978). Peritoneal exudate cells from rats that had received MMC (200 μg/200 g rat) 1 or 4 days earlier were found to have tumoricidal activity *in vitro* (Ogura *et al.*, 1980). Human peripheral blood lymphocytes, from normal healthy donors, that were treated with MMC (100 μg/ml per 10^7 cells) for 30 min at 37°C and then incubated for 18 hr were found to have reduced spontaneous and interferon-boosted NK activity; however, following only a 1-hr incubation, both activities were augmented above those of nontreated control cells (Ortaldo *et al.*, 1980). Finally, several reports suggest that "nonspecifically" induced T suppressor cells are MMC sensitive (Nadler and Hodes, 1977; Lomnitzer and Rabson, 1982) while antigen-induced T suppressor cells are MMC insensitive (Nadler and Hodes, 1977; Argyris, 1979). All of these findings are consistent with the possibility that MMC, under defined conditions, may selectively modulate host defense mechanisms.

4. CONCLUDING REMARKS

As discussed in this chapter a number of anticancer antibiotics are capable of modifying host defense mechanisms in a way that may be therapeutically advantageous. In some cases the modification seems to be exerted at the level of the mechanisms of control of the immune system; this would suggest that such agents actually have immunomodulating capabilities. Indeed with the rapid increase of knowledge about the network of circuits involved in immune responses, acquisition of basic information about selective drug effects on immune systems has become possible. The potential of these agents as exquisitely selective probes in basic investigations of immunoregulation is being realized. It is also possible to propose the potential of increasing the therapeutic efficacy of a drug with protocols designed to optimize the drug's immunomodulating characteristics without unduly compromising its direct antitumor toxicity. At this time there are almost no clinical observations relevant to this approach. However, as indicated by the examples obtained in the studies of antibiotics discussed herein, it is evident that in animal model systems immunomodulation by anticancer agents may in fact be instrumental in determining cooperative interactions with drug-induced antineoplastic action toward achieving therapeutic results. Clarification of the potential of this approach in humans seems to be worthy of intensive clinical investigation.

REFERENCES

Anaclerio, A., Conti, G., Goggi, G., Honorati, M. C., Ruggeri, A., Moras, M. L., and Spreafico, F., 1980, Effect of cytotoxic agents on suppressor cells in mice, *Eur. J. Cancer* **16**:53–58.
Argyris, B. F., 1979, Suppressor activity in the spleen of tumor-bearing mice, in: *Mitomycin C:*

Current Status and New Developments, (S. K. Carter, S. T. Cooke, and N. A. Alder, eds.), Academic Press, New York, pp. 61–67.

Carter, S. K., 1980, The clinical evaluation of analogs. III. Anthracyclines, *Cancer Chemother. Pharmacol.* **4:**5–10.

Casazza, A. M., 1979, Experimental evaluation of anthracycline analogs, *Cancer Treat. Rep.* **63:**835–844.

Chimura, H., Ishizuka, M., Hamada, M., Hori, S., Kimura, K., Iwanaga, J., Takeuchi, T., and Umezawa, H., 1968, A new antibiotic, macromomycin, exhibiting antitumor and antimicrobial activity, *J. Antibiotics* **21:**44–49.

Cohen, S. A., Ehrke M. J., and Mihich, E., 1980, Selective imbalances of cellular immune responses by Adriamycin, in: *Advances in Enzyme Regulation* (G. Weber ed.), Pergamon Press, New York, pp. 335–346.

Cohen, S. A., Ehrke, M. J., Ryoyama, K., and Mihich, E., 1982, Augmentation of the phagocytic activity of murine spleen cell populations induced by Adriamycin, *Immunopharmacology* **5:**75–83.

Cohen, S. A., Salazar, D., and Wicher, J., 1983, Adriamycin-induced activation of NK activity may initially involve LAF production, *Cancer Immunol. Immunother.* **15:**188–193.

Cohen, S. A., Salazar, D., Wicher, J., and Ehrke, M. J., 1985, Adriamycin-induced effects on cultured murine splenic natural killer-like activity, *Cancer Res.* (submitted).

Cudkowicz, G., and Hochman, P. S., 1979, Do natural killer cells engage in regulated reaction against self to ensure homeostasis? *Immunol. Rev.* **44:**13–41.

Dimitrov, N. V., Denny, T. N., and LaVigne, R., 1978, Immune responses during administration of Adriamycin and *Corynebacterium parvum*, *Clin. Immunol. Immunopathol.* **9:**177–183.

Dimitrov, N. V., Denny, T. N., Weisman, M. F., and Cameron, D. G., 1979, Effect of Adriamycin and *Corynebacterium parvum* in tumor-bearing mice: Modulation of response to sheep red blood cells, *J. Natl. Cancer Inst.* **63:**423–426.

Ehrke, M. J., and Mihich, E., 1984a, Immunological effects of anticancer drugs, in: *Clinical Chemotherapy*, Volume 3 (H. P. Kuemmerle, K. Karrer, G. Mathe, and P. Periti, eds.), Georg Thieme Verlag, Stuttgart, pp. 475–499.

Ehrke, M. J., and Mihich, E., 1984b, Adriamycin and other anthracyclines, in: *Clinics in Immunology and Allergy*, Volume 4, No. 2 (J. Fahey and M. Mitchell, eds.), W. B. Saunders, London, pp. 259–277.

Ehrke, M. J., and Mihich, E., 1985, Immunoregulation by cancer chemotherapeutic agents, in: *The Reticuloendothelial System: A Comprehensive Treatise*, Volume 8: *Pharmacology* (J. W. Hadden and A. Szentivanyi, eds.), Plenum Press, New York, pp. 309–347.

Ehrke, M. J., Cohen, S. A., and Mihich, E., 1978, Selectivity of inhibition by anticancer agents of mouse spleen immune effector functions involved in responses to sheep erythrocytes, *Cancer Res.* **38:**521–530.

Ehrke, M. J., Ryoyama, K., Tomazic, V., Cohen, S. A., and Mihich, E., 1980, Selective imbalances of cellular immune responses by Adriamycin, in: *Recent Results in Cancer Research*, Volume 75 (G. Mathe and F. M. Muggia, eds.), Springer-Verlag, Berlin, pp. 195–199.

Ehrke, M. J., Cohen, S. A., and Mihich, E., 1982, Selective effects of Adriamycin on murine host defense systems, in: *Immunological Reviews*, Volume 65 (G. Moller, ed.), Munksgaard, Copenhagen, pp. 55–78.

Ehrke, M. J., Tomazic, V., Ryoyama, K., Cohen, S. A., and Mihich, E.; 1983, Adriamycin-induced immunomodulation: Dependence upon time of administration, *Int. J. Immunopharmacol.* **5:**43–48.

Ehrke, M. J., Ryoyama, K., and Cohen, S. A., 1984, Cellular basis for Adriamycin-induced augmentation of cell-mediated cytotoxicity in culture, *Cancer Res.* **44:**2497–2504.

Facchinetti, T., Raz, A., and Goldman, R., 1978, A differential interaction of daunomycin, Adriamycin and N-trifluoroacetyl Adriamycin 14-valerate with mouse peritoneal macrophages, *Cancer Res.* **38:**3944–3949.

Giuliani, F. C., and Kaplan, N. O., 1980, New doxorubicin analogs active against doxorubicin-resistant colon tumor xenografts in nude mouse, *Cancer Res.* **40:**4682–4687.

Giuliani, F., Casazza, A. M., and DiMarco, A., 1974, Virologic and immunologic properties and response to Daunomycin and Adriamycin of a non-regressing mouse tumor derived from MSV-induced sarcoma, *Biomedicine* **21**:435–439.

Hardt, C., Rollinghoff, M., Pfizenmaier, K., Mosmann, H., and Wagner, H., 1981, Lyt-23$^+$ cyclophosphamide-sensitive T cells regulate the activity of an Interleukin 2 inhibitor *in vivo*, *J. Exp. Med.* **154**:262–274.

Haskill, J. S., 1981, Adriamycin-activated macrophages as tumor growth inhibitors, *Cancer Res.* **41**:3852–3856.

Hersh, E. M., 1973, Modification of host defense mechanism, in: *Cancer Medicine* (J. F. Holland and E. Frei, III, eds.), Lea and Febiger, Philadelphia, pp. 681–699.

Hersh, E. M., 1974, Immunosuppressive agents, in: *Antineoplastic and Immuno-suppressive Agents I* (A. C. Sartorelli and D. G. Johns, eds.), Springer-Verlag, New York, pp. 577–617.

Hisamatsu, T., Uchida, S., Takeuchi, T., Ishizuka, M., and Umezawa, H., 1980, Antitumor effect of a new antibiotic, neothramycin, *Gann* **71**:308–312.

Hisano, G., and Fidler, I. J., 1982, Systemic activation of macrophages by liposome-entrapped muramyl tripeptide in mice pretreated with the chemotherapeutic agent Adriamycin, *Cancer Immunol. Immunother.* **14**:61–66.

Hori, S., Shirai, M., Harano, S., Oki, T., Inui, T., Tsukagoshi, S., Ishizuka, M., Takeuchi, T., and Umezawa, H., 1977, Antitumor activity of new anthracycline antibiotics, aclacinomycin-A and its analogs, and their toxicity, *Gann* **68**:685–690.

Houchens, D. P., Johnson, R. K., Ovejera, A., Gaston, M. R., and Goldin, A., 1976, Effects of *Corynebacterium parvum* alone and in combination with Adriamycin in experimental tumor systems, *Cancer Treat. Rep.* **60**:823–828.

Ishizuka, M., 1979, Influence of inhibitors against enzymes located on the cell surface on immune responses and its antitumor effect, *Jpn. J. Cancer Chemother.* **5**(Suppl. 1):165–174.

Ishizuka, M., Fukasawa, S., Masuda, T., Sato, J., Kanbayashi, N., Takeuchi, T., and Umezawa, H., 1980, Antitumor effect of bactobolin and its influence on mouse immune system and hematopoietic cells, *J. Antibiotics* **33**:1054–1062.

Ishizuka, M., Takeuchi, T., Masuda, T., Fukasawa, S., and Umezawa, H., 1981, Enhancement of immune responses and possible inhibition of suppressor cells by aclacinomycin A, *J. Antibiotics* **34**:331–340.

Ishizuka, M., Takeuchi, T., and Umezawa, H., 1983, Immunomodulating effects of the antitumor antibiotics, aclacinomycin, oxanosine, neothramycin, and mazethramycin, *Sapporo Cancer Sem. Abstr.* **3**:9.

Kataoka, T., Kobayashi, H., and Sakurai, Y., 1978, Potentiation of concanavalin A-bound L1210 vaccine *in vivo* by chemotherapeutic agents, *Cancer Res.* **38**:1202–1207.

Kataoka, T., Ogihara, K., and Sakurai, Y., 1980, Immunoprophylactic and immunotherapeutic response by concanavalin A-bound tumor vaccine enhanced by chemotherapeutic agents eliminating possible suppressors, *Cancer Res.* **40**:3839–3845.

Kawakubo, Y., Komiyama, K., Umezawa, I., and Nishiyama, Y., 1980, Histopathological studies on antitumor effect of sporamycin, *Cancer Chemother. Pharmacol.* **5**:113–118.

Kleinerman, E. S., Zwelling, L. A., Schwartz, R., and Muchmore, A. V., 1982, Effect of L-phenylalanine mustard, Adriamycin, actinomycin D, and 4′-(9-acridinylamino) methanesulfon-m-anisidide on naturally occurring human spontaneous monocyte-mediated cytotoxicity, *Cancer Res.* **42**:1692–1695.

Komiyama, K., and Umezawa, I., 1978, Tissue pharmacokinetics and inhibition of synthesis in mice treated with sporamycin, *J. Antibiotics* **31**:473–476.

Komiyama, K., Sugimoto, K., Takeshima, H., and Umezaswa, I., 1977a, A new antitumor antibiotic, sporamycin, *J. Antibiotics* **30**:202–208.

Komiyama, K., Takeshima, H., and Umezawa, I., 1977b, Antitumor activity of a new antibiotic, sporamycin, *Gann* **68**:213–219.

Komiyama, K., Umezawa, I., Akiyama, T., and Hata, T., 1979, Immunological studies on sporamycin-treated animals, *J. Antibiotics* **32**:1201–1206.

Kunimoto, T., Hori, M., and Umezawa, H., 1972, Macromomycin: An inhibitor of the membrane function of tumor cells, *Cancer Res.* **32**:1251–1256.

Kunimoto, S., Masuda, T., Kanbayashi, N., Hamada, M., Naganawa, H., Miyamoto, M., Takeuchi,

T., and Umezawa, H., 1980, Mazethramycin, a new member of anthramycin group antibiotics, *J. Antibiotics* **33**:665–667.

Lazo, P. S., Tsolas, O., Sun, S. C., Pontremoli, S., and Horecker, B. L., 1978, Modification of fructose bisphosphatase by a proteolytic enzyme from rat liver lysosomes, *Arch. Biochem. Biophys.* **188**:308–314.

Lippman, M. M., and Abbott, B. J., 1973, Modification of transplantability and tumor growth following treatment of L1210 leukemia and Ta3Ha cells with macromomycin (NSC-170105), *Cancer Chemother. Rep.* **37**:501–503.

Lippman, M. M., Laster, W. R., Abbott, B. J., Benditti, J., and Baratta, M., 1975, Antitumor activity of macromomycin B (NSC-170105) against murine leukemias, melanoma, and lung carcinoma, *Cancer Res.* **35**:939–945.

Lomnitzer, R., and Rabson, A. R., 1982, Induction of suppressor cells after activation of human peripheral blood mononuclear cells with sodium periodate, *Immunology* **45**:7–11.

Mace, K., Schlaefli, E., Ehrke, M. J., and Mihich, E., 1982, Effects of Adriamycin analogs on the development of a cell mediated cytotoxicity response generated *in vitro*: Comparison with Adriamycin, *Proc. Am. Assoc. Cancer Res.* **23**:253.

Mantovani, A., 1977, *In vitro* and *in vivo* cytotoxicity of Adriamycin and daunomycin for murine macrophages, *Cancer Res.* **37**:815–820.

Mantovani, A., 1982, The interaction of cancer chemotherapy agents with mononuclear phagtocytes, in: *Advances in Pharmacology and Chemotherapy* (S. Garattini, A. Goldin, and F. Hawking, eds.), Volume 19, Academic Press, New York, pp. 35–66.

Mantovani, A., Tagliabue, A., Vecchi, A., and Spreafico, F., 1976a, Effects of Adriamycin and daunomycin on spleen cell populations in normal and tumor allografted mice, *Eur. J. Cancer* **12**:381–387.

Mantovani, A., Vecchi, A., Tagliabue, A., and Spreafico, F., 1976b, The effects of Adriamycin and daunomycin on antitumoral immune effector mechanisms in an allogeneic system, *Eur. J. Cancer* **12**:371–379.

Mantovani, A., Candiani, P., Luini, W., Salmona, M., Spreafico, F., and Garattini, S., 1979a, Effects of chemotherapeutic agents on host defense mechanisms: Its possible relevance for the antitumoral activity of these drugs, in: *Current Trends in Tumor Immunology* (S. Ferrone, S. Gorini, R. B. Herberman, R. A. Reisfeld, eds.), Garland Press, New York, pp. 139–154.

Mantovani, A., Polentarutti, N., Luini, W., Peri, G., and Spreafico, F., 1979b, Role of host defense mechanisms in the antitumor activity of Adriamycin and daunomycin in mice, *J. Natl. Cancer Inst.* **63**:61–66.

Mantovani, A., Vecchi, A., Tagliabue, A., and Spreafico, F., 1979c, The effect of chemotherapeutic agents on host defense mechanisms: Its relevance for chemoimmunotherapy combinations, in: *Tumor-Associated Antigens and Their Specific Immune Responses* (F. Spreafico and R. Arnon, eds.), Academic Press, New York, pp. 271–286.

Martin, F., Caignard, A., Olsson, O., Jeannin, J. F., and Leclerc, A., 1982, Tumoricidal effect of macrophages exposed to Adriamycin *in vivo* or *in vitro*, *Cancer Res* **42**:3851–3857.

Maruyama, I. N., Tanaka, N., Kondo, S., and Umezawa, H., 1981, Fluorospectrometric studies on neothramycin and its relation with DNA, *J. Antibiotics* **34**:427–435.

Mihich, E., 1971, Preclinical evaluation of the interrelationships between cancer chemotherapy and immunity, in: *Prediction of Response in Cancer Chemotherapy and Immunity* (T. C. Hall, ed.), NCI Monograph 34, U.S. Government Printing Office, Washington, pp. 90–102.

Mihich, E., 1975, Immunosuppression in cancer therapeutics, *Transplantation Proc.* **7**:275–278.

Mihich, E., 1979, Drug selectivity in the suppression of the immune response, in: *Drugs and Immune Responsiveness* (J. L. Turk and D. Parker, eds.), Macmillan Press, London, pp. 25–39.

Miyamaoto, M., Kondo, S., Naganawa, H., Maeda, K., Ohno, M., and Umezawa, H., 1977, Structure and synthesis of neothramycin, *J. Antibiotics* **30**:340–343.

Muggia, F. M., Young, C. W., and Carter, S. K., 1982, *Anthracycline Antibiotics in Cancer Therapy*, Martinus Nijhoff, The Hague.

Nadler, L. M., and Hodes, R. J., 1977, Regulatory mechanisms in cell-mediated immune responses. II. Comparison of culture-induced and alloantigen-induced suppressor cells in MLR and CML, *J. Immunol.* **118:**1886–1895.

Nakamura, H., Yagisawa, N., Shimada, N., Takita, T., Umezawa, H., and Iitaka, Y., 1981, The X-ray structure determination of oxanosine, *J. Antibiotics* **34:**1219–1221.

Nitta, K., 1983, A new approach to cancer immunochemotherapy, *Jpn. J. Cancer Chemother.* **10:**1117–1128.

Ogura, T., Shindo, H., Namba, M., and Yamamura, Y., 1980, Tumoricidal activity of peritoneal exudate cells from rats treated with Mitomycin C, *Gann* **71:**920–921.

Oh-Hashi, F., Kataoka, T., and Tsukagoshi, S., 1978, Effect of combined use of anticancer drugs with a polysaccharide preparation, Krestin, on mouse leukemia P388, *Gann* **69:**255–257.

Okamoto, M., Komiyama, K., Takeshima, H., Yamamoto, H., and Umezawa, I., 1979, The mode of action of a new antitumor antibiotic, sporamycin, *J. Antibiotics* **32:**386–391.

Oki, T., Matsuzawa, Y., Yoshimoto, A., Numata, K., Kitamura, I., Hori, S., Takamatsu, A., Umezawa, H., Ishizuka, M., Naganawa, H., Suda, H., Hamada, M., and Takeuchi, T., 1975, New antitumor antibiotics, aclacinomycins A and B, *J. Antibiotics* **28:**830–834.

Oki, T., Takeuchi, T., Oka, S., and Umezawa, H., 1981, New anthracycline antibiotic aclacinomycin A: Experimental studies and correlations with clinical trials, *Recent Results Cancer Res.* **76:**21–39.

Orsini, F., and Mihich, E., 1975, Immunosuppression by Adriamycin (AM) and daunorubicin (DM), *Proc. Am. Assoc. Cancer Res.* **16:**130.

Orsini, F., Pavelic, Z., and Mihich, E., 1977, Increased primary cell-mediated immunity in culture subsequent to Adriamycin or daunorubicin treatment of spleen donor mice, *Cancer Res.* **37:**1719–1726.

Ortaldo, J. R., Phillips, W., Wasserman, K., and Herberman, R. B., 1980, Effects of metabolic inhibitors on spontaneous and interferon-boosted human natural killer cell activity, *J. Immunol.* **125:**1839–1844.

Riccardi, C., Puccetti, P., Santoni, A., Herberman, R. B., and Bonmassar, E., 1979, Adriamycin-induced antitumor response in lethally irradiated mice, *Immunopharmacology* **1:**211–220.

Ryoyama, K., Ehrke, M. J., and Mihich, E., 1981, Cell–cell interaction in the generation of "nonspecific" suppressor cells in culture and its modification by anti-cancer drugs, in: *Proceedings of the EORTC Symposium on Immunopharmacologic Effects of Radiotherapy,* (J. Dubois, B. Serrou, and C. Rosenfeld, eds.), Raven Press, New York, pp. 23–27.

Ryoyama, K., Ehrke , M. J., and Mihich, E., 1984, Induction of suppressor T cells in culture. II. Modification by Adriamycin, *Int. J. Immunopharmacol.* **6**(5):521–527.

Salazar, D., and Cohen, S. A., 1984, Multiple tumoricidal effector mechanisms induced by Adriamycin, *Cancer Res.* **44:**2561–2566.

Santoni, A., Riccardi, C., Sorci, V. and Herberman, R., 1980, Effects of Adriamycin on the activity of mouse natural killer cells, *J. Immunol.* **124:**2329–2335.

Schwartz, H. S., 1983, Mechanisms of selective cytotoxicity of Adriamycin, daunorubicin, and related anthracyclines, in: *Molecular Aspects of Anticancer Drug Action: Topics in Molecular and Structural Biology,* Volume 3 (S. Neidle and M. J. Waring, eds.), Macmillan, New York.

Schwartz, H. S., and Grindey, G. B., 1973, Adriamycin and daunorubicin: A comparison of antitumor activities and tissue uptake in mice following immunosuppression, *Cancer Res.* **33:**1837–1844.

Schwartz, H., and Kanter, P., 1975, Cell interactions: Determinants of selective toxicity of Adriamycin and daunorubicin, *Cancer Chemother. Rep.* **6:**107–114.

Shimada, N., Yagisawa, N., Naganawa, H., Takita, T., Hamada, M., Takeuchi, T., and Umezawa, H., 1981, Oxanosine: A novel nucleoside from actinomycetes, *J. Antibiotics* **34:**1216–1218.

Stoychkov, J. N., Schultz, R. M., Chirigos, M. A., Pavlidis, N. A., and Goldin, A., 1979, Effects of Adriamycin and cyclophosphamide treatment on induction of macrophage cytotoxic function in mice, *Cancer Res.* **39:**3014–3017.

Suzuki, H., Miura, K., Kumada, Y., Takeuchi, T., and Tanaka, N., 1980, Biological activities of non-protein chromophores of antitumor protein antibiotics: Auromomycin and neocarzinostatin, *Biochem. Biophys. Res. Commun.* **94:**255–261.

Tagliabue, A., Polentarutti, N., Vecchi, A., Mantovani, A., and Spreafico, F., 1977, Combination chemo-immunotherapy with Adriamycin in experimental tumor systems, *Eur. J. Cancer* **13:**657.

Takeuchi, T., Miyamaoto, M., Ishizuka, M., Naganawa, H., Kondo, S., Hamada M., and Umezawa, H., 1976, Neothramycins A and B: New antitumor antibiotics, *J. Antibiotics* **29:**93–96.

Tomazic, V., Ehrke, M. J., and Mihich, E., 1980, Modulation of the cytotoxic response against allogeneic tumor cells in culture by Adriamycin, *Cancer Res.* **40:**2748–2755.

Tomazic, V., Ehrke, M. J., and Mihich, E., 1981, Augmentation of the development of immune responses of mice against allogeneic tumor cells after Adriamycin treatment, *Cancer Res.* **41:**3370–3376.

Umezawa, I., Komiyama, K., Kawakubo, Y., Koyanagi, N., Arai, H., and Nishiyama, Y., 1981, Immunological studies on the antitumor effect of sporamycin, *Gann* **72:**598–603.

Vecchi, A., Mantovani, A., Tagliabue, A., and Spreafico, F., 1976, A characterization of immunosuppressive activity of Adriamycin and daunomycin on humoral antibody production and tumor allograft rejection, *Cancer Res.* **36:**1222–1227.

Yagisawa, N., Shimada, N., Takita, T., Ishizuka, M., Takeuchi, T., and Umezawa, H., 1982, Mode of action of oxanosine: A novel nucleoside antibiotic, *J. Antibiotics* **35:**755–759.

Yamaki, H., Suzuki, H., Nishimura, T., and Tanaka, N., 1978, Mechanism of action of aclacinomycin A. I. The effect on macromolecular syntheses, *J. Antibiotics* **31:**1149–1154.

Yamashita, T., Naoi, N., Hidaka, T., Watanabe, K., Kumada, Y., Takeuchi, T., and Umezawa, H., 1979, Studies on auromomycin, *J. Antibiotics* **32:**330–339.

Young, R. C., Ozols, R. F., and Myers, C. E., 1981, The anthracycline antineoplastic drugs, *N. Engl. J. Med.* **305:**139–153.

CHAPTER 4

EFFECTS OF ALKYLATING AGENTS ON IMMUNOREGULATORY MECHANISMS

HOWARD OZER

1. INTRODUCTION

The bifunctional alkylating agents include a broad range of clinically useful and experimental inhibitors of nucleic acid synthesis, among which are the nitrogen mustard melphalan, the nitrogen mustard derivative chlorambucil, as well as cyclophosphamide and its numerous derivatives, thiotepa, and busulfan. As cytotoxic agents for rapidly proliferating cells, these compounds play an important clinical role in the therapy of certain leukemias and lymphomas, of multiple myeloma, and of a variety of solid tumors as well. Unfortunately, from the standpoint of their therapeutic efficacy, their cytotoxic effects extend to rapidly dividing normal cells as well, particularly those of the hematopoietic system, including erythroid stem cells, megakaryocytes, and immunocompetent lymphoblast precursors of both the T- and B-cell series. In the clinic, these cytotoxic effects on hematopoietic cells are viewed as noxious side effects, causing dose-limiting granulocytopenia, anemia, and thrombocytopenia and leading to systemic infections as well as localized candidiasis and herpes zoster as a result of their interference with normal B- and T-cell maturation and function.

The predominant effects of the bifunctional alkylating agents on nucleic acid synthesis led initially to their classification as immunosuppressants of antibody formation, and attempts were made in the early literature to subcategorize these compounds as either class 1, class 2, or class 3 agents depending on whether their predominant immunosuppressive effects were

HOWARD OZER • Tumor Immunology Laboratory, Department of Medical Oncology, Roswell Park Memorial Institute, Buffalo, New York 14263.

noted when the drugs were given prior to antigen administration, after antigen administration, or both. Nitrogen mustard was demonstrated by Spurr (1947) to completely inhibit the antibody response in the rabbit to typhoid vaccine when given as a single injection immediately prior to vaccination. Green (1958) further characterized this effect by demonstrating that depression of immunoglobulin production was most effective when four daily injections of nitrogen mustard were given simultaneously with, 2 days before, or 4 days prior to immunization. If nitrogen mustard treatment was initiated 2 days after antigen injection, an extension in the peak antibody titer from 5 to 21 days was demonstrated. In contrast, Berenbaum (1962, 1967) found that a single injection of nitrogen mustard suppressed murine antibody titers to typhoid–paratyphoid A and B vaccines most effectively only when given 2 days after antigen administration and not before.

Although considerably less toxic than nitrogen mustard, cyclophosphamide was shown to inhibit antibody production in a similar fashion. Stender (1961) observed suppression of antibody production against *Brucella militensis* in rats receiving a single injection of cyclophosphamide between 24 hr before and 4 days after immunization. Dietrich and Dukor (1968) reported that the murine hemagglutinin response to sheep erythrocytes was inhibited by cyclophosphamide injections at 1 and 2 days after antigen administration, and Kawaguchi (1970) demonstrated that a single injection of cyclophosphamide 2 to 4 days after immunization eliminated the response to bovine gamma globulin. Santos (1967) described the selective suppression of IgG antibody synthesis in rats immunized with sheep erythrocytes. In these experiments, a cyclophosphamide course of five daily injections was utilized, and the suppression was only observed when the course was initiated 2 days after antigen administration.

The suppressive effects of cyclophosphamide on antibody formation were first utilized to alter immunoregulation of the murine response to sheep erythrocytes in the experiments of Aisenberg (1967), Aisenberg and Davis (1968), and Dietrich and Dukor (1968) in which tolerance to subsequent antigenic challenge could be induced by a single injection of cyclophosphamide simultaneously with or 2 days after the initial immunization. Tolerance was best elicited in these experiments with the use of high antigenic doses and antigens that were only weakly immunogenic. Since each of these factors are characteristic of directly induced B-cell tolerance, however, they did not necessarily imply an effect of alkylating agents on T–B cell immunoregulatory interactions.

Direct histological evidence of the inhibitory effects of the alkylators nitrogen mustard and cyclophosphamide on B-cell differentiation and proliferation was first provided by van den Broek (1971) using a rabbit model. The two agents were found to have qualitatively similar effects on nonantigenically stimulated B-derived lymphoid areas causing interphase death of marginal zone cells within germinal centers and of follicular small lymphocytes. It was concluded that the immunological effects of these substances, when given prior to antigenic challenge, were dependent upon the degree of direct histological damage to the nonthymus-derived, follicular lymphocytes and marginal zone cells. No direct destruction of mature plasma cells was noted, suggesting that the agents provoked suppression of antibody synthesis by blocking differentiation of B cells and plasmablasts toward mature plasma cells.

van den Broek (1971) also examined the effects of both nitrogen mustard and cyclophosphamide on a cell-mediated response, skin allograft rejection in rabbits. Following single doses that abrogated antibody synthesis (nitrogen mustard, 2 mg/kg; cyclophosphamide, 100–200 mg/kg), he observed no effects on allograft survival when the drugs were administered either 24 hr prior to, simultaneously with, or 4–7 days after grafting. Similar negative results in allograft rejection were reported by McQuarrie et al. (1960), who found no prolongation of skin graft survival in either rats or rabbits following doses of nitrogen mustard by a variety of schedules, which were sufficient to cause prolonged leukopenia. In contrast, a prolongation of skin allograft survival times from 11 days in controls to 25 days was observed by Jones et al. (1963) in rabbits receiving daily injections of cyclophosphamide, 25 mg/kg. Gordon et al. (1970) also reported suppression of cell-mediated immune responses in a different experimental system in which a xenogeneic graft-versus-host reaction in rats was reduced by pretreatment with cyclophosphamide.

These early experimental data thus unequivocally demonstrated a profound inhibitory effect of bifunctional alkylators on antibody synthesis to specific antigens when the drugs were administered before, simultaneously, or immediately following immunization. The data of van den Broek (1971) suggested that these observations were the result of direct cytotoxic effects on the antibody-producing cell population rather than from any indirect effect on immunoregulation. Further, only inhibitory suppressive effects were described and the effects of these agents on cell-mediated immunity were either considered to be minor or nonexistent. The results that demonstrated the unique immunoenhancing properties of cyclophosphamide and other alkylators were yet to be described. However it was these latter data that were to set the stage for the use of cyclophosphamide as an immunological probe specific for regulatory cell function in the immune system.

2. THE EFFECTS OF ALKYLATING AGENTS ON B-CELL SUPPRESSION AND AUGMENTATION OF DELAYED HYPERSENSITIVITY

These early studies with cyclophosphamide had thus established that it was a potent immunosuppressive agent in experimental animals (Maguire et al., 1961; Jones et al., 1963) and humans (Santos et al., 1964). However, during studies of the effect of cyclophosphamide on allergic contact dermititis in guinea pigs, Maguire and Ettore (1967a,b) came upon the surprising finding that when given at an appropriate time cyclophosphamide augmented the development of allergic contact dermatitis rather than suppressed it. In the early 1970s, Turk and Poulter (1972) confirmed that cyclophosphamide, which by then had become the model alkylating agent for *in vivo* studies, had a selective effect in depleting the B-lymphocyte-dependent areas of lymphoid tissues of mice and guinea pigs when given in a single dose of 300 mg/kg. In further murine experiments, Poulter and Turk (1972) showed that cyclophosphamide had a preferential effect in causing a relative increase in the proportion of T lymphocytes in these tissues. The functional implications of these observations were followed up in a study (Turk *et al.*, 1972) in which it was found that pretreatment of guinea pigs with cyclophosphamide given in a single dose of 300 mg/kg 3 days before sensitization with 2,4-dinitrofluorobenzene (DNFB) increased the intensity of contact reactions in animals tested 7 days later. This was associated with a decreased production of humoral antibody to dinitrophenylated protein and the preferential depletion of B lymphocytes from the spleen and lymph nodes similar to that previously observed. As a result of these findings and experiments involving partial reconstitution of function by splenic tissue from normal sensitized donors, it was suggested that in contact sensitivity in the normal animal T-lymphocyte function was modulated by B-lymphocyte function. Depletion of B lymphocytes by cyclophosphamide was therefore thought to have the effect of producing an appearance of increased T-cell activity. However, in these experiments it was found that there was no increase in tuberculin reactivity in animals treated similarly with cyclophosphamide. This was interpreted as indicating that B-cell modulation of T-cell function was not a typical feature of delayed hypersensitivity, in contrast to the generally accepted tenets of the time.

In a subsequent study, Turk and Parker (1973) demonstrated that melphalan also produced an augmentation of delayed hypersensitivity to certain antigens but failed to result in a similar depletion of B-derived lymphoid tissue to that observed with cyclophosphamide. Two other alkylating agents, chlorambucil and busulfan, as well as methotrexate and procarbazine were also examined. They were not found, however, to enhance contact sensitivity significantly when used in the same way as cyclophosphamide. As with cyclophosphamide, the other drugs effective in enhancing contact sensitivity did so without any evidence of increased proliferation of lymphocytes in the draining lymph nodes during the early phase of sensitization. Despite the lack of histological evidence of B-cell depletion with melphalan, Turk and Parker (1973) postulated that the apparent increase in T-cell activity in these cell-mediated reactions was similar to that observed with cyclophosphamide, and was a result of the *functional* suppression of B-cell activity by this agent.

Katz *et al.* (1974) extended this hypothesis with the suggestion that B cells were acting as suppressor cells in the regulation of contact sensitivity. Lagrange *et al.* (1974b) subsequently suggested that the regulatory influence of B cells on T-cell function might be mediated directly by antibody. In their study, cyclophosphamide-treated mice developed high levels of delayed type hypersensitivity to sheep red blood cells with doses of sheep red blood cells that resulted in tolerance of T-cell activity in mice not treated with the alkylating agent. They suggested that cyclophosphamide thus enhanced delayed-type hypersensitivity in direct proportion to its release of T-cell mediated responses from the feedback inhibition accompanied by antibody formation. They also emphasized the point that cyclophosphamide had already been suggested to exert differential suppressive effects on T-cell function as well as on B cells (Santos and Owens, 1965). They demonstrated that timing of the dose of administered cyclophosphamide critically affected the immunosuppression of delayed-type hypersensitivity in their murine system. A single dose of cyclophosphamide that augmented the level of delayed-type hypersensitivity when given as much as 10 days prior to immunization caused a profound, if transient, depression of T-cell activity when given 2 days following immunization. Still later in the immune response, when delayed-type hypersensitivity was already established, cyclophosphamide had little apparent effect on T-cell activity apart from its negative influence on monocyte precursor differentiation.

They suggested that these differential effects of timing of the cyclophosphamide injection on T-cell immunity were the result of both the mechanism of action of cyclophosphamide and of the physiological state of participating lymphocyte populations before and after becoming engaged by an antigenic stimulus. The proliferative response of the popliteal lymph node cells was delayed for 48 hr in mice immunized and treated simultaneously with cyclophosphamide. This indicated an upper limit of 2 days on the duration of the cytostatic action of cyclophosphamide in the mouse. Yet animals treated 4, 6 or even 8 days before immunization developed abnormally high levels of delayed-type hypersensitivity by day 4. This indicated a long-lasting regulatory influence of cyclophosphamide on the cells responsible for the inhibition of T-cell-mediated responses. Moreover, the drug-affected cells were clearly distinct from those that mediated delayed-type hypersensitivity in being continuously susceptible to a drug that was known to be active only at certain stages of the mitotic cycle (DeWys and Kight, 1969) and were therefore clearly derived from rapidly replicating precursors.

Although an origin in rapidly replicating precursors provided an explanation as to why bone-marrow-derived B cells and germinal center cells should be so vulnerable to the toxic action of cyclophosphamide (Howard and Shand, 1979), and why the T-cell-potentiating effect of the drug should be accompanied by a delay in the appearance of antibody-forming cells in regional lymph nodes and of hemagglutinins in the serum, Lagrange et al. (1974b) also emphasized the point that cyclophosphamide exerts a more depressive effect on antibody production if given after antigenic stimulation (Santos, 1967). They attributed this inhibition to a direct interference of cyclophosphamide with T-cell-mediated helper activity. This implied either that helper cells and the mediators of delayed-type hypersensitivity belonged to the same cell population or that regulatory helper activity was necessary for both antibody production and delayed cellular immunity, with both responses being inhibited by the suppressive effects of cyclophosphamide given 1–3 days after antigen on this positive regulatory cell population. Although resting or differentiated T cells were apparently unaffected by cyclophosphamide, those mediating delayed-type hypersensitivity were clearly affected at the time point of antigen induction, thus suggesting that dividing precursors of the effector populations were the sensitive target of these agents.

The extreme susceptibility of dividing cells to the toxicity of cyclophosphamide in this study was demonstrated by the abrupt cessation of thymidine incorporation by responding regional nodes when cyclophosphamide was given 2 days following immunization. As a result, antibody-forming cells failed to appear in the regional node, antibody could not be detected in serum, and delayed responses were absent on day 4 when they should have been reaching a peak. This latter effect was mainly caused by destruction of specific effector cells, as illustrated by adoptive transfer experiments. T-cell-mediated immunity did, however, recover from the severe depression caused by cyclophosphamide: cells began proliferating and ultimately resulted in a high level of delayed hypersensitivity by day 8. The observation of greatest importance that Lagrange *et al.* (1974b) made was that animals administered cyclophosphamide at or within 48 hr of immunization demonstrated significant *enhancement* in the ultimate level of delayed-type hypersensitivity. They suggested that this enhancement resulted from the drug's effect on the normal "feedback inhibition" of delayed-type hypersensitivity effectors, although they also ascribed this "feedback inhibition" to the drug's effects in suppressing antibody formation and thereby allowing the release of T-cell immunoregulatory control. Of particular interest, however, was their demonstration that, when cyclophosphamide and a subcutaneous injection of antigen were given synchronously, maximum augmentation of delayed-type hypersensitivity occurred in the absence of any suppression of antibody formation. They interpreted these data to indicate that, although not suppressed, antibody formation was prevented, providing more time for proliferation of T cells expressing specific cellular immunity. These data, although misinterpreted in light of the current data presented in the following text; thus provided the fundamental observations regarding the ability of cyclophosphamide, when specifically timed and in selective doses, to both augment and suppress immune responses. Coupled with the then emerging evidence of the critical regulatory role of suppressor T lymphocytes in immune responses, these data provided the foundation for the demonstration that the immunoenhancing activity of cyclophosphamide is the result of T-suppressor-cell blockade.

3. THE EFFECTS OF CYCLOPHOSPHAMIDE ON SUPPRESSOR T LYMPHOCYTES

At this point, several investigators had been able to demonstrate that immunization of mice with low doses of sheep red blood cells, which were known to be suboptimal for antibody responses, led to sensitization for delayed foot pad reactions within 4 days (Kettman, 1972; Lagrange *et al.*, 1974a; Mackaness *et al.*, 1974). These delayed-type hypersensitivity reactions cannot be elicited in mice that have been immunized with larger doses of sheep red blood cells that are more optimal for antibody responses (Mackaness *et al.*, 1974). Previous investigators had suggested that B-cell responses to high-dose immunization caused suppression of T-cell-mediated delayed foot pad reactions (Mackaness *et al.*, 1974). In support of this notion was the observation that animals pretreated with B-cell-depleting doses of cyclophosphamide (2–300 mg/kg) had markedly suppressed antibody responses and augmented delayed reactions (Turk *et al.*, 1972; Turk and Parker, 1973; LaGrange *et al.*, 1974b). Using larger than optimal doses of sheep red blood cells as antigen, Askenase *et al.* (1975) demonstrated that a very low dose of cyclophosphamide (20 mg/kg) could augment the delayed reactions elicited by injection in the foot pads of mice immunized with greater than optimal doses of antigen. These small doses of cyclophosphamide had no detectable suppressive effect on the production of hemagglutinating antibodies at the time of testing for delayed hypersensitivity. They thus suggested that, if cyclophosphamide augmented delayed-type hypersensitivity responses by removing a suppressor influence, this effect was not solely the result of depression of antibody responses. Whereas other workers had shown that higher doses of cyclophosphamide could both potentiate delayed reactions and concomitantly depress antibody responses, Askenase *et al.* (1975) first suggested that the association of these two effects of cyclophosphamide were not causally related. In fact, in several instances they found that delayed foot pad reactions and antibody responses were both augmented by cyclophosphamide pretreatment. In addition, mice immunized with suboptimal doses of sheep red blood cells produced no detectable antibodies at 4 days yet did have delayed responses that were augmented by cyclophosphamide. They speculated that this low zone suppression of delayed-type hypersensitivity, which was uncovered by cyclophosphamide pretreatment, was similar to low zone tolerance for antibody production. Mice immunized with high doses of sheep red blood cells, when pretreated with 200 mg/kg of cyclophosphamide, similar to antigen modification, displayed complete antibody tolerance (the mice made no antibody at day 10 after priming on day 0 and challenge on day 4) although good delayed responses could be elicited.

These data meshed well with the emerging evidence that regulatory T cells could have both augmentative and suppressive effects on other T-cell responses as well as on antibody formation. Askenase *et al.* (1975) pointed out that those doses of antigen that are optimal for antibody production by B cells might induce regulatory T cells to produce one type of immunity and concomitantly suppress another. Those doses of antigen that are optimal for antibody production by B cells could also induce regulatory T cells to suppress delayed hypersensitivity responses independently of the ensuing antibody response. Thus, the previously described reciprocal relationship between antibody formation and delayed hypersensitivity was shown to be regulated by T cells directly, without indirect participation of feedback signals from target cells (i.e., antibody). Although earlier reports had indicated that cyclophosphamide selectively depleted nonthymus-dependent areas of lymphoid tissues, depressed antibody responses, and was not toxic for T cells, more contemporary information had indicated that subpopulations of T cells were indeed rapidly dividing (Moorehead and Claman, 1974) and thus were probably sensitive to cyclophosphamide (Polak and Turk, 1974).

Although these data therefore demonstrated that low-dose cyclophosphamide pretreatment failed to produce reductions in hemagglutinating antibody titers, they did not exclude the possibility that subpopulations of B cells producing antibodies of specialized classes or other B-cell products could have been affected by cyclophosphamide. Although small quantities or local production of certain B-cell products were still in the running as candidates for the target of low-dose cyclophosphamide treatment, gross changes in the delayed hypersensitivity response were clearly produced by low-dose cyclophosphamide pretreatment without the production of concomitant gross alterations in the antibody response.

If these findings were correct, it was apparent that previous investigations showing that cyclophosphamide pretreatment enhanced contact sensitivity inadvertently used supraoptimal doses of antigen. Sy *et al.* (1977) subsequently performed experiments in which they sought to confirm Askenase's findings that cyclophosphamide enhancement of sensitization requires supraoptimal doses of antigen and whether the suppression produced by supraoptimal doses of antigen was mediated by suppressor T cells sensitive to low doses of cyclophosphamide. Because cyclophosphamide had already been shown to inhibit suppressor T cells (Polak and Turk, 1974; Mitsuoka *et al.*, 1976), they utilized this agent in examining contact sensitization to dinitrofluorobenzene in BALB/c mice. Cyclophosphamide given at 200 mg/kg was found to have no effect on the development of specific delayed responses to immunizing doses when injected before optimal sensitization, indicating that the mice had precursors of specifically immunocompetent cells that were resistant to cyclophosphamide and that cyclophosphamide-sensitive suppressor cells were not actively inhibiting responses to optimal antigen doses. By contrast, the depression of sensitization in supraoptimally immunized (antigen-overloaded) mice and the reversal of this depression by prior injection of cyclophosphamide indicated that the cellular immune response involves a balance between the competing activities of two populations of cells. Sy *et al.* (1977) went on to suggest that the precursors of the specifically sensitized effectors were cyclophosphamide resistant, whereas the suppressor population generated by antigen overload has precursors that are cyclophosphamide sensitive. Alternative data from other sources regarding the physiology of suppressor cell precursors had already suggested that they were short lived, rapidly dividing cells (Taylor and Basten, 1976; Pierce and Kapp, 1976). The data provided by Sy *et al.* (1977) demonstrated that suppressor cells were capable of rapid regeneration and that mice treated with cyclophosphamide could again demonstate normal suppressor function when sensitized with supraoptimal doses of antigen 7–14 days after drug treatment.

These conflicting data regarding the effects of cyclophosphamide on T-cell-mediated responses and dependency on both the timing of drug dosage and the dose of antigen utilized were subsequently resolved by Schwartz *et al.* (1978). It was clear from previous work that pretreatment of animals with high doses of cyclophosphamide (300 mg/kg) or other alkylators could depress positive components of T-cell-mediated responses, including helper function (Addison 1973; Anderson *et al.*, 1974; Willers and Sluis, 1975), delayed-type hypersensitivity in certain systems (Jokipii and Jokipii, 1973; Turk *et al.*, 1972; Kerckhaert *et al.*, 1974a,b), and *in vitro* DNA synthetic responses (Milton *et al.*, 1976). This left open the possibility that the augmenting effects of low doses of cyclophosphamide were the result of its "specifically" depleting a suppressor population without affecting helper or amplifier cells. Even at low doses (50 mg/kg), however, cyclophosphamide had also been shown to kill a normal T-cell subpopulation in lymph nodes and spleen, and render the remaining T cells less capable of inducing graft-versus-host responses (Schwartz *et al.*, 1976). Schwartz *et al.* (1978) resolved these apparently opposing effects by demonstrating that the effect of cyclophosphamide pretreatment on delayed hypersensitivity depends primarily on the level of immune response induced in control mice, rather than on the type of antigen or the cyclophosphamide dose employed. Thus delayed responses both to sheep erythrocytes and to major histocompatibility antigens could be inhibited and low-level responses enhanced by cyclophosphamide pretreatment.

At least certain participating cell subsets, including delayed hypersensitivity inducer T cells (Huber *et al.*, 1976; Vadas *et al.*, 1976) and effector cells such as macrophages (Lubaroff and Waksman, 1968), that comprise the major cellular components of the effector arm of delayed responses were relatively resistant to cyclophosphamide. Thus the primary targets of cyclophosphamide pretreatment appeared to be the regulatory cell components, both suppressor and amplifier, whose interactions led to the observed net immune response to a given antigen. The concept that both positive and negative regulatory cell functions could be affected by cyclophosphamide paved the way for understanding the influence of alkylating agents on the immune system and also provided a tool for further dissection of cellular immunological function.

The effects of cyclophosphamide on T lymphocytes regulating delayed responses were subsequently extended in studies that demonstrated the drug's effects on cellular regulatory components of the humoral immune response. Ramshaw *et al.* (1976) had previously established that T cells from mice with humoral immunity against horse red blood cells could specifically suppress the induction of delayed-type hypersensitivity to this antigen. In these experiments, high levels of delayed-type hypersensitivity were induced by treating mice with cyclophosphamide 24 hr after immunization with a large dose of horse red blood cells. In subsequent experiments (Ramshaw *et al.*, 1977), they examined the concomitant ablation of the antibody response to horse red blood cells in this experimental situation. Four lines of evidence indicated that this unresponsive state was maintained by active T-cell suppression. First, the cellular basis of the unresponsive state was demonstrated in adoptive transfer experiments to reside in the T-cell rather than the B-cell population. Second, when normal spleens were transferred into the unresponsive animals, they were unable to break the unresponsive state. Third, the induction of unresponsiveness was antagonized by anti-T-cell serum. Finally, T cells from unresponsive mice specifically suppressed the anti-horse-red-blood-cell antibody response of normal spleen cells when these were recombined and injected into irradiated recipients.

The experiments demonstrating that T cells rather than B cells from unresponsive mice are incompetent in mounting a humoral response confirmed that cyclophosphamide-induced antibody unresponsiveness is mediated by specific regulatory T cells and is accompanied by high levels of delayed hypersensitivity when animals are sensitized in the presence of excess antigen. These two sets of observations suggested that the inverse relationship between humoral and cell-mediated immunity was mediated by different types of suppressor T cells, which differed in their inductive requirements (antigen timing and dose) and in their sensitivity to cyclophosphamide.

Further evidence that cyclophosphamide-induced unresponsiveness could be the result of an active suppressor-T-cell function was provided in a murine tumor allograft model by Bonavida (1977). Mice sensitized against a tumor allograft and given cyclophosphamide (120 mg/kg) 6 days later failed to generate a cytotoxic immune response to the allograft. Spleen cells derived from these mice suppressed the generation of a cytotoxic T-cell response by normal spleen cells in mixed leukocyte cultures. The cyclophosphamide-resistant suppressor cells were not, however, antigen specific since suppression was obtained with stimulating agents of murine H-2 halotypes different from those used for priming. The suppressor cells were further found to be radioresistant, mitomycin C resistant and were inactivated with specific anti-T-cell serum, confirming their T-cell derivation.

These data provided two possible explanations of the mechanisms of cyclophosphamide-induced immunosuppression. The first possibility was that the drug was directly cytotoxic for immunocompetent lymphocytes, particularly those that have undergone antigenic differentiation and division. Bonavida's data (1977) also bolstered the theory of inhibition by active suppression, however, without ruling out direct cytoxicity. The suppressor cells in their model required both antigenic sensitization and cyclophosphamide treatment to develop since mice treated with cyclophosphamide alone or antigen alone did not suppress. Although antigen was needed for activation of suppressor cells, the suppressor cells were not specific to the sensitizing antigens. Once generated, the suppressor cells did not require proliferation to exert their suppressive effect as demonstrated by resistance both to irradiation and to the DNA inhibitor mitomycin C.

These data also emphasized that sensitivity and resistance of suppressor cells to cyclophosphamide were critically dependent on the time of cyclophosphamide administration relative to the antigenic stimulation. As described previously, suppressor function was primarily sensitive when the drug was administered either prior to or immediately following antigenic stimulation. Bonavida (1977) demonstrated that cyclophosphamide administration 6 days after antigenic stimulation results in the appearance of cyclophosphamide-resistant suppressor cells. It could thus be inferred from these data that nonantigen-stimulated suppressor cells were cyclophosphamide sensitive, whereas antigen-activated suppressor cells were cyclophosphamide resistant. Clearly the effects of alkylating agents on immunoregulation were multifaceted and could be manipulated in a highly selective manner.

The finding that these drugs directly interfered with the normal homeostatic regulatory mechanisms by their inhibition of suppressor cell function (Askenase *et al.*, 1975) was extended by Rollinghoff *et al.* (1977), who observed induction of cytotoxic lymphocytes in mice to hapten-conjugated syngeneic cells after treatment with cyclophosphamide. This suggested that another potential effect of alkylating agents on normal immunoregulatory mechanisms might be to release control of autoreactive cytotoxic T cells. L'Age-Stehr and Diamantstein (1978) confirmed this hypothesis in mice injected with a single dose of cyclophosphamide at 125 mg/kg. At various time intervals, isolated splenic T cells were injected subcutaneously into the foot pads of syngeneic recipients, and the resulting local graft-versus-host reaction was determined in the draining lymph nodes. Autoreactive cells could be detected in the spleens of donors with a peak 6 days after cyclophosphamide treatment. Spleen cells treated with anti-T-cell serum and complement failed to induce a graft-versus-host reaction, indicating a T-cell derivation of the autoreactive cells. As in local graft-versus-host reactions induced by allogeneic cells, the autoreactive graft-versus-host reaction induced by cyclophosphamide was dependent upon cells of host origin. This was shown by the failure of irradiated spleen cells of cyclophosphamide-treated recipients to give a reaction when injected with autoreactive cells 1 day after either treatment. T cells derived from donors 8–9 days after cyclophosphamide treatment did not elicit a graft-versus-host reaction. Moreover, these cells, mixed with autoreactive cells, abolished the graft-versus-host reaction, but if the donors were intravenously injected 20 hr after cyclophosphamide with 5×10^7 syngeneic thymocytes, autoreactive cells were not detectable. Splenic T cells of these animals collected 5 days after thymocyte injection suppressed the activity of autoreactive cells, indicating cyclophosphamide sensitivity of suppressor cell precursors.

4. DEMONSTRATION OF IMMUNOREGULATORY EFFECTS *IN VITRO* BY ACTIVATION OF CYCLOPHOSPHAMIDE WITH LIVER MICROSOMES AND BY ACTIVE METABOLITES

The immunoregulatory effects of cyclophosphamide had, until this time, been demonstrable only *in vivo* because the drug itself was an inactive precursor that required activation by liver microsomes. A sequence of enzymatic and/or spontaneous changes leads to the formation of several intermediary and terminal metabolites, some of which have been identified as cytotoxic in experimental tumor systems (Connors *et al.*, 1974; Takamizawa *et al.*, 1975). This activation sequence can be reproduced *in vitro* using isolated rat liver microsomes and cofactors (Brock and Hohorst, 1963; Connors *et al.*, 1970). Spleen cells treated *in vitro* with microsomally activated cyclophosphamide were examined for their immune responsiveness following transfer to lethally irradiated syngeneic recipients, for their ability to regenerate surface immunoglobulin receptors and to generate graft-versus-host reactivity by Shand (1978). The pretreatment of spleen cells with activated cyclophosphamide at a concentration of 30–50 μg/ml abolished the ability of spleen cells both to respond to sheep red blood cells 1 day after transfer and to regenerate surface immunoglobulin receptors. These effects could not be ascribed to cytotoxicity by this concentration of activated cyclophosphamide because (1) the transfer of congenic CBA (Iglb) pretreated spleen cells into irradiated CBA (Igla) recipients resulted in the appearance of donor-derived immunoglobulin in the serum of recipient mice 14 days after transfer, and (2) no difference in residual cell viability was detectable between activated cyclophosphamide-treated and control spleen cells even following 24 hr of culture.

Induction kinetics in the *in vitro* system revealed that (1) a minimum exposure time was required between activated cyclophosphamide and spleen cells, and (2) suppression was not evident when pretreatments were performed for 1 hr at 0°C. These results implicate a metabolic event involving the transport of metabolites from the extracellular fluid to the nucleus. Immunocompetence began to recover in transferred drug-treated spleen cells after 7 days, suggesting that B cells or their precursors (and presumably the immediate precursors of helper T cells) were not irreversibly inhibited. Although this recovery is rather longer than the 3–4 days seen after cyclophosphamide is administered *in vivo* (Bach, 1975, 1976), it is not known to what extent cell recruitment might play a role in the latter situation.

Shand and Howard (1978, 1979) subsequently compared a number of cyclophosphamide metabolites and other alkylating agents for their ability to induce *in vitro* and *in vivo* immunosuppression and to inhibit B-cell receptor regeneration. They found that, following the injection of cyclophosphamide *in vivo* at 150 mg/kg but not the other alkylators melphalan or chlorambucil, splenic B cells were for several days unable to regenerate their surface immunoglobulin receptors subsequent to capping with antiimmunoglobulin serum and culture *in vitro*. Similarly, *in vitro* induction of immunosuppression and inhibition of B-cell receptor regeneration were inhibited primarily by the most active alkylating metabolites of cyclophosphamide [4-hydroperoxycyclophosphamide (4-HC) and phosphoramide mustard] but also by the potent alkylator melphalan, which was inactive *in vivo* (Shand and Howard, 1978, 1979). Although these inhibitory activities on immunoregulation were found to be restricted to those molecules with demonstrable alkylating activity, they are nonetheless entirely reversible and not dependent on events leading to cytotoxic cell death, consistent with the previous *in vivo* evidence that inhibition of suppressor function or augmentation of nonspecific suppression by cyclophosphamide were reversible effects.

5. THE EFFECTS OF CYCLOPHOSPHAMIDE ON THE IMMUNOREGULATION OF ANTITUMOR RESPONSES

A variety of investigators using *in vivo* and *in vitro* systems had thus provided evidence demonstrating a differential effect of cyclophosphamide on T-cell functions. On the one hand, cyclophosphamide-sensitive suppressor T cells had been described both in cell-mediated and humoral immune responses (Askenase *et al.*, 1975; Debre *et al.*, 1976; Rollinghoff *et al.*, 1977). Other T-cell functions, like cytotoxic T-cell responses against allogeneic cells as well as delayed-type hypersensitivity reactions, were found to be relatively resistant to cyclophosphamide (Ferguson and Simmons,1978; L'Age-Stehr and Diamantstein, 1978; Gill and Liew, 1978). Cytotoxic T cells are generated in response to allogeneic cells but may also result from exposure to major-histocompatibility-complex- (MHC) identical cells expressing either viral antigens, chemically added haptens, or minor histocompatibility antigens (Doherty *et al.*, 1976; Shearer *et al.*, 1976; Bevan, 1975). Efficient lysis is obtained only when the cytotoxic T cells and targets are syngeneic at the MHC. This kind of MHC-restricted cytotoxicity may play an important role especially in the control of tumor development and viral diseases. Hurme (1979) compared the cyclophosphamide sensitivity of allogeneic cytotoxic T responses and two types of murine-major-histocompatibility-restricted cytotoxic T-cell responses: the *in vitro* primary response to trinitrophenyl TNP coupled syngeneic cells and the *in vitro* cytotoxic response of female cells to male spleen cells (H-Y antigen), in which *in vivo* priming is required. Allogeneic cytotoxic T-cell function was found to be relatively resistant, whereas MHC-restricted cytotoxicity was readily depressed with a low dose of cyclophosphamide, suggesting a further dichotomy of cyclophosphamide sensitivity between precursors of cytotoxic cells responding to MHC-compatible and -incompatible antigens.

The sensitivity of suppressor function regulating MHC-restricted cytotoxicity or cytotoxicity for virally induced tumors has similarly been found highly sensitive to low doses of cyclophosphamide. Glaser (1979) found that when the drug was administered to mice prior to immunization with syngeneic SV40-transformed cells the specific cytotoxic immune response elicited was stronger and lasted longer when compared to the response generated in noncyclophosphamide-treated mice. The augmentation effect of the drug was dependent on the cyclophosphamide concentration being optimal at 100 mg/kg and on the time of drug administration in relation to antigen being optimal at 2 days before antigen immunization. Transfer of T cells from normal syngeneic mice to drug-treated animals abolished the cyclophosphamide-induced augmentation of the immune response. These results implied that cyclophosphamide-sensitive T cells suppressed the in vivo generation of specific effector T cells against SV40-induced tumor-associated antigens.

This situation was analogous to that previously described by Fujimoto et al. (1976a,b) and Greene et al. (1979), in which mice bearing nonviral tumors that were known to be antigenic could not reject them because of the presence of specific suppressor T cells. When these cells were adoptively transferred to immune animals bearing the same tumor, rejection of the tumor was also prevented. Yu et al. (1980) examined a model in which mice bearing large methylcholanthrene-induced fibrosarcomas lost the ability to respond in vitro to mitogen stimulation and to specifically neutralize autologous tumor cells in vivo. This depressed immune capability was caused by active suppression, since spleen cells from advanced tumor-bearing mice could supress the mitogen response to normal spleen cells and could inhibit tumor rejection when adoptively transferred to mice previously immunized against the tumor. Treatment with cyclophosphamide (100 mg/kg) was found to affect the immune capability of the host, in addition to having a direct effect on the tumor. When cyclophosphamide was administered 1 day after tumor inoculation, the treated animals developed the ability to neutralize tumor at the same time as untreated controls but retained this capability as the tumors became advanced. Treatment with a single dose of cyclophosphamide as late as 11 or 20 days after tumor inoculation maintained or restored the tumor-neutralizing capacity of spleen cells. Cyclophosphamide thus appears to alter the antitumor response of the host by inhibiting both cytotoxic and suppressor cells, but the cytotoxic cells recover rapidly, whereas the suppressor cells do not.

Ideally, one would like to separate the direct cytotoxic effects of cyclophosphamide on tumor growth from any indirect effect mediated by changes in the immune response. The studies described by Yu et al. (1980) provided initial evidence that the therapeutic effects were at least partially caused by alteration of the immune response. Tumor-bearing mice developed neutralizing spleen cells by 9 days but then lost their neutralizing capacity after 22 days. Similar mice treated with cyclophosphamide 1 day after tumor inoculation also developed tumor-neutralizing spleen cells, but these animals retained their neutralizing capacity until they died of their tumors after 4–5 weeks. Although tumors appeared more slowly in mice treated with cyclophosphamide, comparison of treated and untreated animals with tumors of the same size suggested that the effect of the drug on the immune response was probably direct and not caused by differences in duration of tumor burden or in size of tumors.

Other investigators also provided early evidence that supported the hypothesis that part of the effect of cyclophosphamide on tumors was mediated indirectly by altering the immune response. Cyclophosphamide has been found to have much less effect on tumor growth if the immune capability of the host is depressed (Lubet and Carlson, 1978; Mathe *et al.*, 1977). In addition, in other immune tumor systems, cyclophosphamide has been postulated to eliminate tumor-induced suppressor cells (Glaser, 1979; Greene, *et al.*, 1979; Hellström and Hellström, 1978). Benacerraf (1978) reported that two distinct populations of suppressor cells could be identified in immunoregulation of tumor rejection, one of which was functionally characterized as initiating suppressor cell differentiation and the other as an effector suppressor cell. He found that only initiating suppressor cells, but not effector suppressor cells, were sensitive to cyclophosphamide and that therefore optimal efficacy was obtained only if the drug were administered prior to immunization.

Greenberg *et al.* (1981), utilizing an adoptive transfer assay, demonstrated that cyclophosphamide could improve tumor immunity in combination with specifically immune cells. Mice bearing disseminated Friend-virus-induced leukemia could be successfully treated by a combination of cyclophosphamide (180 mg/kg) and adoptive transfer of syngeneic immune lymphocytes. Therapeutic efficacy in this model was largely dependent on the presence of phenotypically helper T cells, whereas cells cytotoxic to the leukemia *in vitro* were derived from the cytotoxic/suppressor subset. In these models, the cyclophosphamide has a direct tumoricidal effect (Greenberg *et al.*, 1981), as well as potentially facilitating effects on host tumor immunity, and therapy with immune cells without cyclophosphamide has no apparent *in vivo* antitumor effect (Fefer *et al.*, 1976).

Utilizing another adoptive transfer model, however, Boyer *et al.* (1982) have been able to demonstrate an independent beneficial effect of cyclophosphamide on tumor immunity in the absence of direct cytotoxic effects. Peritoneal exudate T lymphocytes from rats immune to the 13762A rat mammary tumor conferred specific tumor rejection immunity on normal naive recipients. The efficiency of systemic adoptive transfer of tumor rejection immunity with immune peritoneal exudate T cells was improved by cyclophosphamide pretreatment of recipients prior to tumor cell inoculation. Optimal potentiation was obtained with a dose of cyclophosphamide as low as 50–100 mg/kg given the day prior to transfer of immune T cells. Cyclophosphamide pretreatment of recipients was effective 1–3 days prior to transfer. The cyclophosphamide-potentiating effect was lost with longer intervals between cyclophosphamide administration and transfer indicating recipient recovery. Cyclophosphamide pretreatment enabled recipients to reject greater numbers (100 times) of tumor cells and inhibited tumor challenge established before systemic adoptive transfer. The drug-induced potentiation of systemic transfer of tumor immunity was reversed by intravenously administered normal spleen cells. These observations are consistent with the conclusion that a cyclophosphamide-sensitive suppressor cell is capable of restricting the expression of adoptive immunity. Cyclophosphamide-induced inhibition of these suppressor cells allows increased efficacy of cytotoxic effector T lymphocytes in this system.

Cyclophosphamide in very low doses that are not sufficiently cytotoxic to kill all tumor cells directly have also been shown to cure animals by eliminating suppressor T cells (Hancock and Kilburn, 1982; Larson and Sparck, 1983; Livingston *et al.*, 1983). As might be expected, the timing of drug administration following tumor inoculation was found to be critical for successful therapy of MOPC-315-tumor-bearing mice (Hengst *et al.*, 1980). Following inoculation with 3.5×10^8 viable tumor cells, a single intraperitoneal injection of cyclophosphamide at 15 mg/kg cured most mice when administered at 1–2 weeks but only a few mice when given at day 4. The time interval between tumor inoculation and cyclophosphamide administration rather than the tumor size was critical for successful therapy since mice bearing nonpalpable tumors 12–13 days postinoculation with 10^5 viable tumor cells were cured by cyclophosphamide therapy. Furthermore, cyclophosphamide therapy of mice bearing large tumors was not curative for mice that had been treated previously when their tumors were nonpalpable. A curative injection of cyclophosphamide into mice bearing large tumors results in an augmented ability of their spleen cells to mount a cytotoxic antitumor response upon *in vitro* immunization with mitomycin-C-treated stimulator tumor cells. Since depletion of glass-adherent cells from tumor-bearer spleens prior to *in vitro* immunization was shown to result in greater augmentation of antitumor cytotoxicity than that obtained by depletion of tumor cells, these data suggested that in addition to the drug's tumoricidal activity, it also eliminated other suppressor elements in the spleen. Mice cured of tumors following cyclophosphamide therapy exhibited a high degree of antitumor immunity as induced *in vivo* by their ability to reject a large tumor challenge and *in vitro* by the ability of their spleen cells to mount a secondary antitumor response upon *in vitro* stimulation.

In a subsequent report, Hengst *et al.* (1981) bolstered the evidence that the curative effect of low-dose cyclophosphamide was not solely caused by tumoricidal activity of the drug, because 3 or 4 days after therapy, when the cyclophosphamide had been cleared from the circulation, viable proliferating tumor cells were present in the subcutaneous tumor site. That the curative effect of 15 mg/kg of cyclophosphamide for mice bearing large tumors required the presence of T-cell-dependent antitumor immunity was indicated by the fact that tumor regression was abrogated by treatment of the tumor bearers with antithymocyte serum. Mokyr and Dray (1983) and Mokyr *et al.* (1982) compared high (200 mg/kg) with low-dose (15 mg/kg) cyclophosphamide in treating MOPC-315 and demonstrated that tumor eradication with low doses required the combination of the toxic effects of the drug and of T-cell dependent antitumor immunity. Tumor eradication by the high dose of drug does not require the participation of antitumor immunity but depends primarily on the tumoricidal activity of the drug. Spleen cells from tumor-bearing mice treated with low-dose cyclophosphamide exhibit an augmented antitumor immune potential, whereas spleen cells from tumor-bearing mice treated with the high dose of cyclophosphamide exhibit suppressed antitumor immunity. More importantly, tumor-bearing mice treated with the low dose of drug are able to reject a challenge with 300 times the minimal lethal tumor dose given 1, 6, or 31 days after cyclophosphamide therapy, whereas mice treated with the high dose of drug are unable to reject such a challenge given within the same time intervals after cyclophosphamide therapy. Moreover, when mice bearing a large tumor are treated with a high dose of cyclophosphamide and subsequently challenged again with tumor cells to establish a day-4 nonpalpable tumor, this tumor was less responsive to cure by combined chemoimmunotherapy than were day-4 tumors in normal mice. Thus, although the higher doses of cyclophosphamide can cure most mice bearing a large MOPC-315 tumor, they not only do not result in antitumor immunity, but actually reduce the effectiveness of chemoimmunotherapy for a second tumor challenge. In contrast, mice cured with the low dose of cyclophosphamide exhibit long-lasting potent antitumor immunity.

6. THE EFFECTS OF CYCLOPHOSPHAMIDE ON T-LYMPHOCYTE SUBSET FUNCTION

As early as 1978, Benacerraf (1978) had proposed that the differential effects of cyclophosphamide dosage and timing, whether in relation to antigenic or tumor challenge, could be explained by postulating two different populations of suppressor T cells, an *initiating suppressor cell* and an *effector suppressor cell*. Only the initiating suppressor cell was cyclophosphamide sensitive, explaining the fact that augmented immunity was obtained only when the drug was administered before or in the immediate postimmunization period. Subsequent reports by other investigators described similar or related observations, which ultimately confirmed the speculation that the suppressor precursors were the sensitive population, although such a conclusion was not immediately apparent from the published data.

The sensitivity of suppressor precursors, which are responsible for establishing allograft unresponsiveness to cyclophosphamide, was described by Wood and Monaco (1979) utilizing three models of specific unresponsiveness to skin allografts in adult mice immunosuppressed with antilymphocyte serum. In the first model, mice were thymectomized, treated with antilymphocyte serum, and injected with 300×10^6 hybrid lymphoid cells. These mice accepted donor skin grafts permanently and became lymphoid cell chimeras. In the second model, nonthymectomized, antilymphocyte-serum-treated mice were injected with 25×10^6 nonhybrid, homozygous allogeneic bone marrow cells. Although survival of skin allografts was prolonged in this model, it was not permanent and the recipients were not chimeras. In the third model, recipients were thymectomized before treatment with antilymphocyte serum and injection of 25×10^6 allogeneic cells. A majority of these mice maintained donor skin grafts for over 100 days and 40% survived permanently, although they were not chimeras. The effect of cyclophosphamide on induction of unresponsiveness was studied in these models. Cyclophosphamide was given before lymphoid transfer and skin graft survival was compared in drug-treated versus untreated mice. Cyclophosphamide reduced the enhancing effect of lymphoid cells only in non-thymectomized, antilymphocyte-serum-treated mice. In contrast, cyclophosphamide had no effect on the induction of unresponsiveness in either thymectomized model. These results suggested that thymocyte-derived precursors of suppressor effector cells were required for the induction and/or maintenance of unresponsiveness to skin allografts and could be blocked from differentiation by cyclophosphamide.

Other contemporary studies also suggested that suppressor precursors were sensitive to cyclophosphamide. Rollinghoff et al. (1977) showed that the in vivo generation of cytotoxic activity to TNP-conjugated syngeneic lymphocytes in mice is normally suppressed by some mechanism that is sensitive to cyclophosphamide. Treatment of mice with cyclophosphamide before immunization augments the cytotoxic effect and the effect of cyclophosphamide can be abolished by the transfer of normal syngeneic T cells. Mitsuoka et al. (1976) found that there was a marked enhancement of the delayed hypersensitivity response to human serum albumin in mice given cyclophosphamide 1 day before sensitization. This enhancing effect could be eliminated by the transfer of syngeneic thymus cells, but not spleen cells, suggesting that cyclophosphamide blocked suppressor precursors from maturing into antigen-specific effectors. Ferguson and Simmons (1978) suggested that two subpopulations of T cells, cytotoxic and suppressor cells, have different sensitivities to cyclophosphamide. In their experiments, normal spleen cells cultured for 5 days produced a population of cells that suppressed cell-mediated cytotoxicity. They showed that if the spleen cell donors are treated with cyclophosphamide 24 hr before their spleens are removed and used for culture, the cells generated in culture cannot suppress cell-mediated cytotoxicity. However, these cells are still capable of developing into cytotoxic cells.

Similar data have been obtained in other experimental autoimmune systems. Lando et al. (1979) have described a model in which protection against experimental allergic encephalomyelitis was induced in susceptible mice by supraoptimal immunization with either spinal cord homogenate or myelin basic protein. Unresponsiveness was found to be mediated by splenic suppressor T cells (following induction) and could be adoptively transferred to normal syngeneic recipients. Low-dose cyclophosphamide (20 mg/kg) administered 2 days before the encephalitogenic challenge abrogated the unresponsiveness to experimental allergic encephalomyelitis and reverted the protected mice sensitive to disease induction. Low-dose cyclophosphamide was also active on adoptively transferred unresponsiveness; thus donors that had been treated with cyclophosphamide were unable to further transfer unresponsiveness. The site of action of cyclophosphamide in this system was suppressor-T-cell function identified by the use of anti-T-cell sera. Cyclophosphamide was optimally effective when injected 2 days before disease induction, i.e., 11 days after the prevention injection that induces the suppressor cells. This appears to argue against a block of early suppressor precursors, although it is entirely possible that the suppressor population in this system undergoes continual renewal caused by the continued stimulus of the antigen in incomplete Freund's adjuvant. The fact that cyclophosphamide was not effective in abrogating unresponsiveness when administered 5 days after disease induction further suggests that suppressor cells are active only at the induction phase of sensitization.

Mitsuoka *et al.* (1979) compared effector and suppressor cell functional sensitivity to cyclophosphamide in a delayed hypersensitivity response in young and aged mice. Delayed hypersensitivity to methylated human serum albumin could be enhanced with cyclophosphamide in young mice but not in aged animals. The enhancement resulted from the elimination of suppressor cells, although delayed hypersensitivity effectors were partially sensitive as well, albeit only transiently. They suggested that the suppressor T function that was cyclophosphamide sensitive represented a central regulatory, antigen-nonspecific cell population, whereas mature T effector cells were much less sensitive.

Similar conclusions have been reached in comparing cyclophosphamide with other alkylating agents. Paul *et al.* (1982) compared several alkylating agents in blocking adoptive T-suppressor-cell function following supraoptimal immunization of mice with sheep red blood cells. None of the alkylating agents injected 2 days prior to supraoptimal immunization prevented the induction of suppressor cell effectors capable of exerting suppression in the secondary host. When injected 2 days following supraoptimal immunization, both cyclophosphamide and carmustine (BCNU) caused a dramatic reduction in the capability of donor splenocytes to induce suppression in the secondary host. Cyclophosphamide and BCNU, but not lomustine, semustine, or melphalan, when injected 5 days after supraoptimal immunization, severely curtailed the expression of suppressor activity when spleen cells were transferred on day 14. T suppressor precursor cells were more sensitive to cyclophosphamide than to BCNU. As suppressor cells differentiated and matured after supraoptimal immunization, their sensitivity to cyclophosphamide gradually diminished. These results thus indicate that equally potent alkylating agents can have diverse effects on the induction and expression of suppressor function and their specific action may depend on the time of administration in relation to antigenic challenge.

Although both administration of cyclophosphamide with antigen and adoptive transfer experiments had therefore strongly suggested that the immunoaugmenting effects of the drug on humoral and cellular immunity were a result of its effects on suppressor precursors, more direct proof was lacking because cyclophosphamide was inactive *in vitro*. Although Shand and Howard (1979) and Shand (1978) had shown that microsomally activated cyclophosphamide and certain derivatives were immunosuppressive *in vitro*, no equivalent *in vitro* model of suppressor cell blockade had been described. Diamantstein *et al.* (1979) first described such a model utilizing the *in vitro* active 4-HC and the mitogenic response of murine spleen cells to dextran sulfate. As measured in a [^{3}H]thymidine uptake assay, spleen cells of mice injected 7 days previously with a 125 mg/kg single dose of cyclophosphamide gave an enhanced response to dextran sulfate, a diminished response to lipopolysaccharide (LPS), and a normal response to concanavalin A (Con A). Addition of syngeneic thymocytes to spleen cells inhibited the enhanced response of the cells to dextran sulfate and slightly enhanced their response to LPS. Pretreatment of thymocytes by 4-HC *in vitro* abrogated the effect of thymocytes on the dextran sulfate response but not on the LPS response. Pretreatment of spleen cells by small doses of 4-HC (0.1–1.0 μg/ml) *in vitro* enhanced the capacity of the cells to respond to dextran sulfate but either did not affect or even diminished their capacity to respond to LPS. The enhancement of the dextran sulfate response by 4-HC treatment could not be detected using spleen cells depleted of T cells or lacking functioning T cells. 4-HC concentrations greater than 3 μg/ml diminished or abolished the capacity of the spleen cells to respond to LPS as well as their capacity to respond to dextran sulfate.

These results showed (1) that in contrast to the LPS-reactive B-lymphocyte subset, the proliferative capacity of dextran-sulfate-reactive cells is negatively controlled by a cyclophosphamide and 4-HC-sensitive T-cell subset and (2) that these T suppressor cells are more sensitive to cyclophosphamide and 4-HC than B lymphocytes or T cells performing other immunological functions.

Kaufmann *et al.* (1980) subsequently extended their system to determine the relative susceptibilities of functional murine T-cell subsets involved in a delayed-type hypersensitivity response to sheep red blood cells *in vitro*. They demonstrated that T suppressor precursors were more sensitive to 4-HC than were antigen-activated T suppressors of delayed hypersensitivity obtained 4 days after sensitization. On the other hand, antigen-activated T suppressors proved to be more sensitive to 4-HC than were effectors of delayed hypersensitivity. Using microsomally activated cyclophosphamide, Shand and Liew (1980) confirmed that effectors of delayed hypersensitivity are more resistant to cyclophosphamide than are suppressor T cells. Differential sensitivity of T subsets in delayed-type hypersensitivity in comparison to humoral immune responses has also been postulated. Diminished humoral responses caused by specific suppressors in mice injected with a high dose of antigen have been demonstrated in adoptive transfer experiments (Whisler and Stobo, 1978). In contrast to induced unresponsiveness in delayed hypersensitivity that can be broken by cyclophosphamide when given after antigen, however, the same cyclophosphamide application regimen induces permanent tolerance at the humoral level, presumably caused and maintained by antigen-specific suppressor cells (Ramshaw *et al.*, 1977). Thus, based on these *in vivo* data, it has been postulated (Whisler and Stobo, 1978) that T suppressors of humoral and delayed responses differ in their sensitivity to cyclophosphamide. Diamantstein *et al.* (1981) confirmed this hypothesis *in vitro* with the demonstration that T suppressors of humoral responses were more resistant *in vitro* to 4-HC than were T suppressors of delayed responses.

This observation led Diamantstein *et al.* (1981) to propose the following schema of cyclophosphamide's immunoregulatory interactions: Injection of a high dose of heterologous erythrocytes, besides B-cell proliferation and differentiation, will induce responses from both helper and suppressor T regulatory populations controlling humoral and cellular responses. The outcome of the measurable response depends on interactions of these cells within regulatory circuits (Cantor and Gershon, 1979). Cyclophosphamide injected after a high dose of antigen preferentially abolishes the activity of B cells, T suppressors of delayed responses, and T helpers for humoral responses. Choosing a dose that eliminates these cell functions without affecting T suppressors of humoral responses or delayed hypersensitivity effectors will break delayed-type unresponsiveness and render the animals tolerant at the humoral level and thus lead to the observed inverse relationship between humoral and cellular immunity. Because little is yet known about whether any correlation exists between phenotypically defined murine subsets (e.g., Ly, Qa, IJ) and their susceptibility to cyclophosphamide, Diamantstein *et al.* (1981) went on to propose that the T-cell subset of a given regulatory circuit with the highest sensitivity to cyclophosphamide determines whether help or suppression prevails in the final outcome.

Our own data have partially confirmed these postulates in the murine response to alloantigens using an *in vitro* cell-mediated cytotoxicity assay and 4-HC (Cowens *et al.*, 1984). Treatment of spleen cells with 4-HC inhibited the development of suppressor function in culture but did not prevent the development of cytotoxicity to alloantigens. The effects of 4-HC pretreatment at a concentration of 15 μM were found to be specific for Thy-1.2$^+$ suppressor cells and inhibited suppressor function in a dose-dependent fashion (50% effective dose = 7.86 $\pm$ 0.28 μM). The 4-HC-sensitive suppressor precursor population is most likely Lyt 1$^+$2$^+$, whereas differentiated suppressor cells are of the Lyt 1$^-$2$^+$ phenotype.

In the T-cell regulation of B-cell function, regulator cells are easily distinguished from effector cells because they bear different surface determinants. In the T-cell regulation of T effector function, however, the characterization of the cells involved is not complete. Cantor and Boyse (1975) and Jadinski *et al.* (1976) have suggested that the Lyt 2$^+$3$^+$ subset contains both the precursors and the differentiated effector cells for suppression (Con-A-induced) and cytotoxicity in the T-cell-mediated response to alloantigens. Hathcock and Hodes (1982) have recently reported that, when T suppressors are developed by short-term culture, the Lyt 1$^+$2$^-$ subset contains the precursors and differentiated cells for suppression, whereas the precursors of the T cytotoxic cells in the cytotoxic T-lymphocyte response to alloantigen are in the Lyt 1^+2^+ subset. The experiments with anti-Lyt antibody (Cowens et al., 1984) show that development of mature T suppressor function is dependent upon cells expressing Lyt 1- and Lyt 2-defined antigens before differentiation. This may indicate that the suppressor precursor is Lyt 1^+2^+ or, alternatively, that an Lyt 1^+2^- inducer cell (which may be 4-HC sensitive) is required for the maturation of Lyt 2^+ suppressor effector cells. In addition, the ability of 4-HC-pretreated 4-day-cultured cells to develop a cell-mediated cytotoxic response was dependent upon T cells sensitive to anti-Lyt 1 and anti-Lyt 2 antibodies. The selectivity of 4-HC that has been demonstrated in our study allows T lymphocytes to be fractionated into 4-HC-sensitive (T suppressor precursors) and -resistant (T cytotoxic precursors) subsets without the use of Lyt antibody. Because the preponderance of evidence is that the precursors of T suppressors and T cytotoxic cells are different cells, 4-HC may be useful in isolating them for further study of their properties.

7. THE EFFECTS OF CYCLOPHOSPHAMIDE AND *IN-VITRO*-ACTIVE COMPOUNDS ON HUMAN IMMUNOREGULATORY FUNCTION

Despite the repeated demonstration of the enhancement of both cellular and humoral immunity in a variety of animal systems, the only clearly defined effect of cyclophosphamide on lymphocyte function in man prior to 1980 was the description of its potent immunosuppressive activity, primarily on B-cell function (Santos et al., 1964). Stevenson and Fauci (1980) employed high doses of standard formulation cyclophosphamide *in vitro* (some variable *in vitro* activity of the drug is present in standard formulations) to examine the effects on mitogen-induced anti-sheep-red-blood-cell immunoglobulin secretion in a plaque assay. It was found that the plaque-forming B cells in this system were sensitive to cyclophosphamide over a wide concentration range, including concentrations that have a minimal effect on overall cell viability (Cupps et al., 1982). Kinetic experiments revealed that cyclophosphamide exerted its inhibitory effect on the plaque response only if added very early in culture. Thus, it appeared that *in vitro* cyclophosphamide may exert its inhibitory influence on an early phase of polyclonal B-cell activation. When T-cell-enriched populations were incubated overnight with high concentrations of cyclophosphamide and then added back in coculture to fresh autologous B cells, significant enhancement of plaque responses was observed, suggesting a selective inhibition or elimination of a regulatory suppressor cell population found in lymphocyte preparations. Helper T cells are relatively resistant to the inhibitory actions of cyclophosphamide. Thus, human B cells appear to be most sensitive to cyclophosphamide, followed in sensitivity by the suppressor cell population in the T-cell fraction, with relative resistance of the helper T cells.

These preliminary *in vitro* results and the availability of a well-characterized *in-vitro*-active cyclophosphamide compound led us to examine in detail the effects of 4-HC on defined human immunoregulatory lymphocyte subsets. We examined the *in vitro* sensitivity of functional human T-cell subsets to 4-HC in a polyclonal B-cell differentiation assay and in the generation of mitogen-induced suppressor cells for effector B-cell function. Con-A-induced T suppression of B-cell differentiation is completely abrogated by a 1 hr pretreatment of T cells at very low concentrations of between 10^{-2} and 20 μM, whereas inducer T-cell function is sensitive only to concentrations $\geq$ 40 μM. The effects of 4-HC on suppressor T cells appear to occur at concentrations that do not result in DNA cross-linking or decreased blastogenesis. Con-A-induced T suppressors are generated from within the OKT4$^+$, OKT8$^-$ subset and are sensitive to low-dose 4-HC only before activation, whereas differentiated suppressor cells are resistant to concentrations in excess of 80 nmol/ml. Low-dose 4-HC pretreatment of the B-cell population results in abrogation of immunoglobulin secretion when treated B cells are cocultured with unfractionated T cells, however, this effect is completely reversible if pretreated B cells are cocultured with T cells devoid of suppressor activity. These results demonstrate that human presuppressor cells for B effector function differentiate in response to Con A from the OKT4$^+$, OKT8$^-$ subset and are exquisitely sensitive to low concentrations of 4-HC, whereas mature suppressor and inducer functions are resistant to all but very high concentrations *in vitro*. The differential sensitivity of functional T- and B-cell subsets to 4-HC *in vitro* can thus be a very useful probe in dissecting immunoregulatory interactions in both mouse and man.

We next examined the effects of 4-HC on regulatory T–T interactions in mixed lymphocyte culture (MLC) responses and for allospecific cytotoxic T lymphocyte (CTL) responses (Smith *et al.*, 1985). Induction of cytotoxic lymphocytes and MLC proliferation were both sensitive to $\geq$40 μM 4-HC, whereas CTL effectors were resistant to $\geq$80 μM. CTL were restricted to the OKT4$^-$,8$^+$ subset and the cells showing sensitivity to $\geq$40 μM 4-HC were apparently OKT4$^+$,8$^-$ and possibly OKT4$^-$,8$^+$ helper inducer T cells. Secondary MLC and CTL responses displayed a similar 4-HC concentration dependent inhibition that was only detected at suboptimal responder-to-stimulator ratios. This suggests the mechanisms of CTL activation in primary and secondary MLC responses are similar.

Pretreatment of T cells with $\leq$20 μM 4-HC for 1 hr prior to Con A activation abrogated suppression of both MLC and CTL. In contrast, treatment with 80 μM 4-HC following Con A induction was without effect on differentiated T suppressor activity. Studies utilizing monoclonal antibody/complement depletion demonstrated that the suppressor precursor and differentiated suppressors for T effector function were restricted to the OKT4$^+$,8$^-$ subset. These results support the hypothesis that regulatory T-cell (inducer and suppressor) function is more sensitive to the inhibitory effects of 4-HC than cytotoxic precursor/effector function (Varkila and Hurme, 1983). Con-A-inducible suppressor cell precursors therefore have the greatest sensitivity to 4-HC ($\leq$20 μM) followed by inducers of primary and secondary CTL (40–60 μM). Differentiated primary and secondary CTL and suppressor effectors were resistant to the inhibitory effects of up to 100 μM 4-HC.

Relatively limited data are available on the *in vivo* effects of cyclophosphamide (or other alkylating agents, for that matter) on the regulatory function of human lymphocyte subsets. Berd *et al.* (1982) examined the induction of delayed-type hypersensitivity and andtibody to keyhole limpet hemocyanin (KLH), and delayed-type hypersensitivity to 1-chloro-2,4-dinitrobenzene (DNCB) in 22 patients receiving cyclophosphamide for metastatic cancer, 12 with melanoma and 10 with colorectal carcinoma. Sixteen days before cyclophosphamide, half the patients received KLH and half received DNCB; 3 days after cyclophosphamide, they received KLH and DNCB, whichever they had not received initially. Blood was drawn for antibody titer and/or skin testing was performed 14 days after administration of antigen. For each antigen, the responses of precyclophosphamide patients were compared with those of postcyclophosphamide patients.

They found that pretreatment of patients with cyclophosphamide significantly augmented the development of delayed-type hypersensitivity to KLH. The delayed-type hypersensitivity reactions of patients given KLH 3 days after cyclophosphamide were significantly greater than those of patients given KLH without cyclophosphamide (medians: KLH alone = 0, KLH after cyclophosphamide = 18 mm; p = 0.025). With cyclophosphamide pretreatment, 11 of 11 patients developed a delayed-type hypersensitivity response of greater than 5 mm, compared with 4 of 11 without cyclophosphamide (p = 0.002). No patient developed delayed-type hypersensitivity to DNCB when it was given without cyclophosphamide, whereas 3 of 11 developed delayed-type hypersensitivity when DNCB was given 3 days after cyclophosphamide (p = 0.82). Cyclophosphamide pretreatment neither augmented nor suppressed the antibody response to KLH. The proportion of patients with antibody 14 days after antigen was 2 of 11 without cyclophosphamide and 4 of 11 with cyclophosphamide pretreatment (p = 0.24).

In a related follow-up study, Berd *et al.* (1984) administered cyclophosphamide (1000 mg/m^2) to 19 patients with advanced, metastatic cancer and monitored the compositional and functional changes in their peripheral blood mononuclear cells. Within 2 days of administration of cyclophosphamide, the lymphocyte count fell significantly (mean decrease = 26.0%) and remained significantly depressed through day 14 with recovery beginning by day 21. T and B lymphocytes were depleted to about the same degree at each time point. Moreover, there was no selective depletion of the Leu 2$^+$ (suppressor cytotoxic) or Leu 3$^+$ (helper inducer) subsets of T lymphocytes. Proliferative responses to mitogens (phytohemagglutinin, Con A, pokeweed mitogen) and to allogeneic cells fell significantly within 1 day of administration of cyclophosphamide and continued to be diminished on day 2. However, these responses recovered to pretreatment levels by day 3 and, in some cases, exceeded pretreatment levels on day 7. Concanavalin-A-inducible suppressor activity was also diminished on day 1 (mean decrease,

23.4%) and day 2 (mean decrease, 39.2%). However, in contrast to the proliferative responses, suppressor activity continued to be significantly impaired on day 3 (mean decrease, 31.6%) and only partially recovered by day 7 (mean decrease, 22.1%). Both Con-A-inducible suppression and proliferative responses declined again on days 14 and 21. Thus, between 3 and 7 days after administration of cyclophosphamide, there appeared to be impairment of nonspecific T-cell-mediated suppressor activity of peripheral blood lymphocytes that was not merely a reflection of impaired lymphocyte function in general. This could account for the augmented delayed-type hypersensitivity responses of cyclophosphamide-treated patients.

Similar results have been described by Bast *et al.* (1983) in experiments characterizing the cell surface phenotype of peripheral mononuclear cells after intravenous injection of cyclophosphamide and prednisolone. Low doses of cyclophosphamide (100–600 mg/m^2) temporarily decreased levels of circulating B lymphocytes. Slightly higher doses of cyclophosphamide (200–600 mg/m^2) produced transient depression of T8-, M1-, and Ia-positive cells. After doses of 200–400 mg cyclophosphamide/m^2, T4-positive cells were spared, resulting in a transient elevation of the T4/T8 ratio. With higher doses of cyclophosphamide (greater than or equal to 600 mg/m^2), all T cells were affected and the T4/T8 ratio declined to pretreatment levels. By contrast, intravenous injection of prednisolone at 40 mg/m^2 reduced the T4/T8 ratio. Levels of both T4 and T8 cells declined, but T4 cells were affected more markedly than T8 cells.

Finally, the original suggestion by our group that low-dose cyclophosphamide would selectively block presuppressor T activity for both cellular and humoral immune function (Ozer *et al.*, 1981) has been confirmed *in vivo* by D. Berd, H. C. Maguire, and M. J. Mastrangelo (unpublished data). In a very recent study, 18 patients with advanced metastatic cancer were alternately assigned to one of two groups. Sixteen days before cyclophosphamide, one group received KLH and the other group received DNCB. Cyclophosphamide (300 mg/m^2) was given as an intravenous bolus on day 0. Three days after cyclophosphamide, the patients received KLH or DNCB, whichever they had not received initially. Blood was drawn for antibody titer and skin-testing was performed 14 days after administration of KLH or DNCB. In addition, skin tests to microbial recall antigens were made 2 days before and 17 days after cyclophosphamide.

Pretreatment with low-dose cyclophosphamide resulted in significant augmentation of delayed-type hypersensitivity to KLH; thus, the median delayed-type hypersensitivity responses were: KLH alone = 10 mm; KLH after cyclophosphamide = 27 mm; p < 0.01. Cyclophosphamide pretreatment also resulted in augmentation of the antibody response to KLH. The median total antibody titers (log$_2$ of reciprocal of dilution) were as follows: KLH alone = <1; KLH after cyclophosphamide = 3; p < 0.01. All nine cyclophosphamide-pretreated subjects, but only 4 of 9 controls developed measurable anti-KLH antibody titers. Cyclophosphamide pretreatment neither augmented nor suppressed the 48-hr challenge reaction to DNCB. Moreover, cyclophosphamide had no effect on delayed-type hypersensitivity responses to the recall antigens, dermatophytin, *Candida*, and mumps.

8. CONCLUDING REMARKS: IMPLICATIONS IN HUMAN IMMUNOREGULATION

Cyclophosphamide is a broad spectrum antitumor agent that was the product of a search to improve the selectivity of alkylating agents. The common side effects of cyclophosphamide (nausea, vomiting, alopecia, and hemorrhagic cystitis) are mild compared to the profound myelosuppression of nitrogen mustard, the first alkylating agent to undergo clinical trial.

The mechanisms by which cyclophosphamide and 4-HC exert their immunoregulatory effects vary with relative time of antigen administration and drug concentration. Previous studies have shown that cross-linking of DNA is not apparent until exposure equals or exceeds 20 μM (M. Colvin, unpublished data). Experiments reported by our group (Ozer *et al.*, 1982) have ascertained that *in vitro* there is no impairment of [³H]thymidine incorporation in response to mitogens with concentrations less than 10 μM. These studies also show impairment of suppressor cell development by 25% at concentrations as low as 1 μM suggesting that a mechanism other than DNA cross-linking is responsible for the immunomodulation of 4-HC. On a molecular level, the activity of activated cyclophosphamide or 4-HC need not be directed against nucleic acids alone. The alkylation of nucleophilic proteins and peroxidation of lipids secondary to glutathione depletion are also possible mechanisms of drug action.

L'Age-Stehr and Diamantstein (1978) proposed that cyclophosphamide treatment induced the appearance of new antigenic sites that resulted in the induction of autoreactive cytolytic cells. These authors postulated that the neoantigen was the product of a reactivated virus or an antigen found on a more primitive precursor cell. While there was no direct evidence presented to support their claim, the theory of cell surface modification by 4-HC is worthy of consideration. The actual mechanism of cyclophosphamide modification of the cell membrane may be debated, but if the HLA-D/DR gene products were to be modified by 4-HC, then the suppressive activity of these cells would be compromised. This would result from their inability to interact specifically with their target cell.

Experiments in which 4-HC was added at the initiation of culture show, not surprisingly, that the drug, at appropriate concentrations, inhibits the incorporation of [³H]thymidine by responding lymphocytes as well as the induction of cytotoxic effector cells (Ozer *et al.*, 1982; Smith *et al.*, 1982). There is remarkable agreement between the dose–response curves of the mixed lymphocyte response (MLR) and the cell-mediated lympholysis (CML) assay with the 50% effective dose of both responses being approximately 5 μM. In the murine system, different cell subpopulations are involved in the proliferative and the cytotoxic responses. Ly 1^{+},2,3^{-} helper/inducer cells have been shown to respond with proliferation to alloantigen while the Ly $1^-,2,3^+$ serves as precursor to the cytotoxic cell. In the murine model, the helper cell plays a role in both the MLR and the CML. The Ly 1 subpopulation proliferates as well as helps the Ly 2,3 cell by the elaboration of interleukin 2. Inhibition of this single cellular subpopulation could explain the close correlation between the MLR and CML dose–response curves.

Investigators studying the cellular interactions of the immune response have, for the past 5 years, utilized monoclonal antibody and radiation sensitivity to dissect the various components. A model for the regulation of the human cellular response to allogeneic cells has been constructed based on available data (Figure 1).

Ozer *et al.* (1982) reported that T helper cells in pokeweed mitogen- (PWM) induced immunoglobulin production were only sensitive to 4-HC concentrations exceeding 40 μM. Thomas *et al.* (1980) reported that OKT4$^+$ helper activity for PWM-driven immunoglobulin production was sensitive to irradiation with 1250 R. The radiosensitivity of OKT4$^+$ help for the induction of cytotoxic effectors was not studied specifically. Merluzzi and co-workers (1980) reported that murine cytotoxic lymphocytes could be generated from cyclophosphamide-treated mice if Ly 1$^+$ cells are added to the MLC. This indicates that the T helper cell is the more sensitive cell. Studies in both human and murine systems have found that the regulatory cells (suppressor and inducer/helper) are generally more sensitive to cyclophosphamide, 4-HC, or irradiation than effector cells. This general rule is further supported by our own data (Ozer *et al.*, 1981; Cowens *et al.*, 1984; Smith *et al.*, 1982).

The most sensitive of the lymphocyte functions examined during the

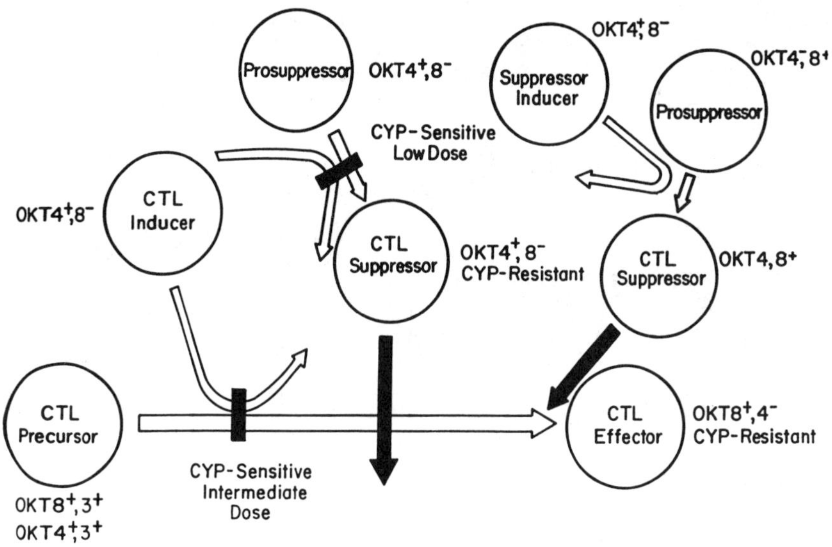

FIGURE 1. Hypothetical regulation of cytotoxic function.

course of our own studies with 4-HC was the incubation of Con A suppressor cells (Ozer *et al.*, 1982; Smith *et al.*, 1982). This is in agreement with the findings of Diamantstein *et al.* (1981). We reported that treatment of suppressor cell precursors or suppressor inducer cells with 10 μM 4-HC prior to Con A activation abrogated the development of suppression of PWM-driven IgG and IgM production. Diamantstein *et al.* (1979) reported that pretreatment of murine T lymphocytes with 4-HC inhibited the development of suppressor cells with the ability to depress splenic B-cell responses to dextran sulfate. In a subsequent publication Kaufmann *et al.* (1980) reported that presuppressor T cells participating in murine delayed responses were also sensitive to very low concentrations of 4-HC. In experiments reported by our laboratory (Ozer *et al.*, 1982; Smith *et al.*, 1982), 25% inhibition of suppressor cell activity was seen at a concentration of 1 μM of 4-HC; a concentration with no effect on the induction of cytotoxic lymphocytes. Inhibition of suppressor cell development was maximal at concentrations of $\geq$20 μM. Unfortunately, the functional subpopulation of cells sensitive to these very low concentrations is unknown, but a hypothetical schema of humoral immunoregulation is presented in Figure 2.

Evidence reported to date indicates that cooperation between two subpopulations of T lymphocytes is necessary for the development of human suppressor cells (Whydehaag *et al.*, 1979; Broder *et al.*, 1981). Morimoto and co-workers (1982) recently reported that OKT4[+] suppressor inducer cells are required to activate the OKT8[+] presuppressor cell to become suppressive to the primary antibody response. The OKT4[+] suppressor inducer cell was

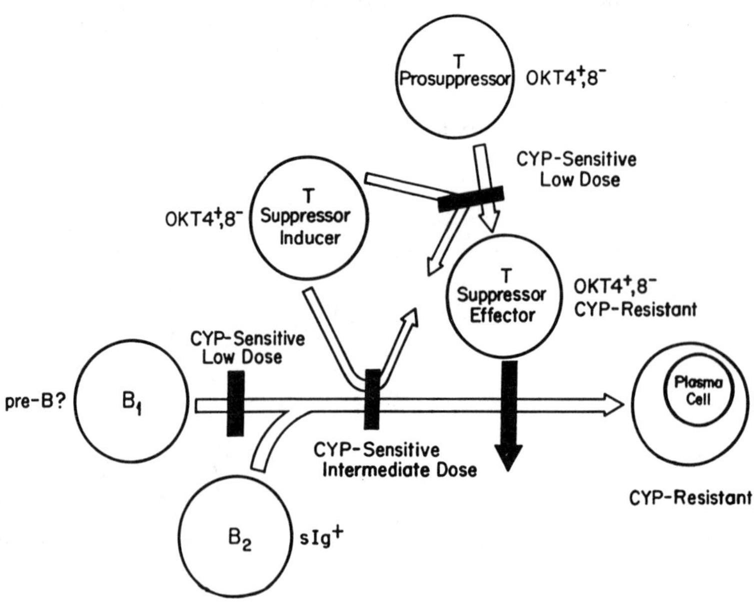

FIGURE 2. Hypothetical regulation of mitogen-induced B-cell differentiation.

also shown to bear Ia antigen (Yachie *et al.*, 1982). This OKT4$^+$ inducer activity was sensitive to X irradiation at a dose of 1500 R. This was an extension of earlier work of this group where they reported the OKT8$^+$ subpopulation to be suppressive when the separation of cells took place following the induction of the suppressor cells (Reinherz *et al.*, 1980).

Results reported from our laboratory and elsewhere (Ozer *et al.*, 1982; Thomas *et al.*, 1980) have described inducible suppressor cell precursors in the OKT4$^+$,8$^-$ subset. This is a controversial point as, prior to 1981, all reports indicated that suppressor cells bore the OKT8 marker. Many of these early studies utilized fluorescence sorting methodology to separate the various subpopulations and the separation occurred following the induction of the cell. Ozer *et al.* (1981) reported that OKT4 monoclonal antibody plus complement produced a cell population that was >95% OKT3$^+$, >90% OKT8$^+$, and <4% OKT4$^+$ by FACS II analysis. The profile of the OKT8 monoclonal antibody plus complement treatment was >90% OKT3, >90% OKT4, and <4% OKT8$^+$. The three publications reporting suppressor cell precursors in the OKT4$^+$ population utilized complement-mediated lysis to prepare lymphocyte subpopulation. The finding of an OKT4$^+$ suppressor is not a contradiction of the earlier reports but rather the description of a new subpopulation, the suppressor precursor. More recent investigations using the method of complement lysis have confirmed the presence of an OKT8$^+$ suppressor cell (Morimoto *et al.*, 1980).

Thomas *et al.* (1981) reported that OKT4$^+$ precursors to suppressor cells were radiosensitive and bore an antigen, OKT17, which was shared with a radioresistant helper of B-cell differentiation. If the radioresistant OKT4$^+$,17$^+$ helper also serves as the suppressor inducer cell, then indeed the presuppressor cell will be the actual radiosensitive and 4-HC-sensitive component of inducible suppression. As of yet the precise target of 4-HC is uncertain, so in the models presented in Figures 1 and 2, the site of 4-HC activity is a process rather than a particular cell.

As mentioned earlier, the inhibition of suppressor cell development at concentrations lower than 20 μM cannot be explained by inhibition of proliferation by DNA cross-linking. One hypothesis is that cell surface markers necessary for cooperation between the suppressor cell and its target are modified by the drug (Shand, 1978). Engleman and McDevitt (1978) described a patient with a functional suppressor cell leukemia whose lymphocytes would only suppress lymphocytes isolated from donors matched at the HLA-D locus. 4-HC may modify these specificities, so while the suppressor cell is generated, it cannot function. This hypothesis is contradicted by two pieces of our own data (Smith *et al.*, 1985). First, 4-HC treatment with concentrations as high as 100 μM was unable to modify antigenicity as detected by sensitized lymphocytes. Secondly, and more convincing, in our experiments we have found no inhibition of suppressor cell activity when preformed Con-A-activated cells were treated with 4-HC. Presumably, these cells already bear the Class II gene products necessary for interaction with their target cell. This would argue against 4-HC-induced impairment of suppressor–target interaction. This does not rule out drug-induced modification of the interaction between the suppressor inducer and the presuppressor, should it be required in this system.

The ability of cyclophosphamide to modify suppressor development is not solely the product of the antiproliferative effect of the drug. A number of agents, including Adriamycin®, vincristine, vinblastine, cytosine arabinoside, and 5-fluorouracil have all been shown to have no effect on the induction of the Con A suppressor cell. Thus, cyclophosphamide and its derivatives are unique among this group of agents for their ability to inhibit the induction of suppressor cells. Studies reported here further underscore the novelty of cyclophosphamide and certain other alkylating agents. The interest in cyclophosphamide as an immunomodulating agent dates back to 1967 when Maguire and Ettore (1967a,b) reported enhancement of DNCB contact sensitivity with cyclophosphamide pretreatment. As the cellular basis of enhancement has become known, interest has shifted from simple explanation of a biological curiosity to the use of cyclophosphamide and 4-HC as biological probes. As more is learned about this highly selective and powerful alkylating agent's effects on immunoregulation, cyclophosphamide's potential application in modifying specific immunological abnormalities may move it from its current role as a cytoreductive drug to that of a specific biological response modifier.

REFERENCES

Addison, I. E., 1973, Immunosuppression with busulphan: The effect on spleen, marrow, and thymus cells of mice, *Eur. J. Immunol.* **3**:419–424.

Aisenberg, A. C., 1967, Studies on cyclophosphamide-induced tolerance to sheep erythrocytes, *J. Exp. Med.* **125**:833–845.

Aisenberg, A. C., and Davis, C., 1968, The thymus and recovery from cyclophosphamide-induced tolerance to sheep erythrocytes, *J. Exp. Med.* **128**:35–46.

Anderson, H. R., Dresser, D. W., and Wortis, H. H., 1974, The relationship between the immunoglobulin class of B-cell precursors and the degree of synergism obtained from the presence of T cells, *Clin. Exp. Immunol.* **16**:393–400.

Askenase, P. W., Hayden, B. J., and Gershon, R. K., 1975, Augmentation of delayed-type hypersensitivity by doses of cyclophosphamide which do not affect antibody responses, *J. Exp. Med.* **141**(3):697–702.

Bach, J. F., 1975, The mode of action of immunosuppressive agents, in: *Frontiers of Biology*, Volume 41, North-Holland, Amsterdam, New York.

Bach, J. F., 1976, The pharmacological and immunological basis for the use of immunosuppressive drugs, *Drugs* **11**(1):1–13.

Bast, R. C., Jr., Reinherz, E. L., Maver, C., Lavin, P., and Schlossman, S. F., 1983, Contrasting effects of cyclophosphamide and prednisolone on the phenotype of human peripheral blood leukocytes, *Clin. Immunol. Immunopathol.* **28**(1):101–114.

Benacerraf, B., 1978, Suppressor T-cells and suppressor factor, *Hosp. Pract.* **13**:65–75.

Berd, D., Mastrangelo, M. J., Engstrom, P. F., Paul, A., and Maguire, H., 1982, Augmentation of the human immune response by cyclophosphamide, *Cancer Res.* **42**:4862–4866.

Berd, D., Maguire, H. C., and Mastrangelo, M. J., 1984, Impairment of concanavalin A-inducible suppressor activity following administration of cyclophosphamide to patients with advanced cancer, *Cancer Res.* **44**:1275–1280.

Berenbaum, M. D., 1962, The effect of cytotoxic agents on the production of antibodies to THB vaccine in the mouse, *Biochem. Pharmacol.* **11**:29–44.

Berenbaum, M. S., 1967, Immunosuppressive agents on the cellular kinetics of the immune response, in: *Immunity, Cancer, and Chemotherapy: Basic Relationship in the Cellular Level* (E. Michich, ed.), Academic Press, New York, pp. 217–241.

Bevan, M. J., 1975, The major histocompatibility complex determines susceptibility to cytotoxic T cells directed against minor histocompatibility antigens, *J. Exp. Med.* **142**:1349–1364.

Bonavida, B., 1977, Antigen-induced cyclophosphamide-resistant suppressor T cells inhibit the *in vitro* generation of cytotoxic cells from one-way mixed leukocyte reactions, *J. Immunol.* **119**(4):1530–1533.

Boyer, C. M., Kreider, J. W., and Bartlett, G. L., 1982, Regulation of the expression of adoptive tumor rejection immunity by recipient cyclophosphamide-sensitive cells, *Cancer Res.* **42**:2211–2215.

Brock, N., and Hohorst, H. J., 1963, Activation of cyclophosphamide *in vivo* and *in vitro*, *Arzneim. Forsch. (Drug Res.)* **13**:1021–1026.

Broder, S., Uchiyama, T., Muul L., Goldman, C., Sharrow, S., Poplak, D., and Waldman, T., 1981, Activation of leukemic pro-suppressor cells to become suppressor effector cells: Influence of cooperating normal cells, *N. Engl. J. Med.* **304**:1382–1387.

Cantor, H., and Boyse, E. A., 1975, Functional subclasses of T lymphocytes bearing different Ly antigens I, *J. Exp. Med.* **143**:1376–1389.

Cantor, H., and Gershon, R. K., 1979, Immunological circuits: Cellular composition, *Fed. Proc.* **38**:2058.

Cantor, H., McVay-Boudreau, L., Hugenberger, J., Naridord, K., Shen, F. W., and Gershon, R. K., 1978, Immunoregulatory circuits among T-cell sets II, *J. Exp. Med.* **147**:1116–1125.

Connors, T. A., Grover, P. L., and McLoughlin, A. M., 1970, Microsomal activation of cyclophosphamide *in vivo*, *Biochem. Pharmacol.* **19**:1533–1535.

Connors, T. A., Cox, P. J., Farmer, P. B., Foster, A. B., and Jarman, M., 1974, Some studies of the active intermediates formed in the microsomal metabolism of cyclophosphamide and isophosphamide, *Biochem. Pharmacol.* **23**:115–129.

Cowens, J. W., Ozer, H., Ehrke, J., Colvin, M., and Mihich, E., 1981, Inhibition of the development of suppressor cells in culture by 4-hydroperoxycyclophosphamide, *Fed. Proc.* **40**:1096.

Cowens, J. W., Ozer, H., Ehrke, M. J., Greco, W. R., Colvin, M., and Mihich, E., 1984, Inhibition of the development of suppressor cells in culture by 4-hydroperoxycyclophosphamide, *J. Immunol.* **132**(1):95–100.

Cupps, T. R., Edgar, L. C., and Fauci, A. S., 1982, Suppression of human B lymphocyte function by cyclophosphamide, *J. Immunol.* **128**(6):2453–2457.

Debre, P., Waltenbaugh, C., Dorf, M. E., and Benacerraf, B., 1976, Genetic control of specific immune suppression. IV. Responsiveness to the random copolymer L-glutamic acid[50]-L-tryosine[50] induced in BALB/c mice by cyclophosphamide, *J. Exp. Med.* **144**:277–281.

DeWys, W. D., and Kight, N., 1969, Kinetics of cyclophosphamide damage: Sublethal damage repair and cell-cycle-related sensitivity, *J. Natl. Cancer Inst.* **42**:155–163.

Diamantstein, T., Willinger, E., and Reiman, J., 1979, T-suppressor cells sensitive to cyclophosphamide and to its *in vitro* active derivative 4-hydroperoxycyclophosphamide control the mitogenic response of murine splenic B cells to dextran sulfate, *J. Exp. Med.* **150**:1571–1576.

Diamantstein, T., Klos, M., Hahn, H., and Kaufmann, S. H. E., 1981, Direct *in vitro* evidence for different susceptibilities to 4-hydroperoxycyclophosphamide of antigen-primed T cells regulating humoral and cell-mediated immune responses to sheep erythrocytes: A possible explanation for the inverse action of cyclophosphamide on humor and cell-mediated immune responses, *J. Immunol.* **126**(5):1717–1719.

Dietrich, F. M., and Dukor, P., 1968, Characteristic features of immunosuppression by steroids and cytotoxic drugs, *Int. Arch. Allergy Appl. Immunol.* **34**:32–48.

Doherty, P. C., Blanden, R. V., and Zinkernagel, R. M., 1976, Specificity of virus-immune effector T cells for H-2K or H-2D compatible interactions: Implications for H-antigen diversity, *Transplant. Rev.* **29**:89–124.

Engleman, E., and McDevitt, H., 1978, A suppressor T cell of the MLR specific for the HLA-D region in man, *J. Clin. Invest.* **61**:828–838.

Fefer, A., Einstein, A. B., Cheever, M. A., and Berenson, J. R., 1976, Models for syngeneic adoptive chemoimmunotherapy of murine leukemias, *Ann. N.Y. Acad. Sci.* **276**:573–583.

Ferguson, R. M., and Simmons, R. L., 1978, Differential cyclophosphamide sensitivity of suppressor and cytotoxic cell precursors, *Transplantation (Baltimore)* **25**:36–38.

Fujimoto, S., Greene, M. I., and Sehon, A. H., 1976a, Regulation of the immune response to tumor antigens. I. Immunosuppressor cells in tumor-bearing hosts, *J. Immunol.* **116**:791–799.

Fujimoto, S., Greene, M. I., and Sehon, A. H., 1976b, Regulation of the immune response to tumor antigens. II. The nature of immunosuppressor cells in tumor-bearing hosts, *J. Immunol.* **116**:800–806.

Gill, H. K., and Liew, F. Y., 1978, Regulation of delayed-type hypersensitivity. III. Effect of cyclophosphamide on the suppressor cells for delayed-type hypersensitivity to sheep erythrocytes, *Eur. J. Immunol.* **8**(3):172–176.

Glaser, M., 1979a, Augmentation of specific immune response against a syngeneic SV40-induced sarcoma in mice by depletion of suppressor T cells with cyclophosphamide, *Cell. Immunol.* **48**:339–345.

Glaser, M., 1979b, Regulation of specific cell-mediated cytotoxic response against SV-40-induced tumor associated antigens by depletion of suppressor T cells with cyclophosphamide in mice, *J. Exp. Med.* **149**:774–779.

Gordon, J., Salch, W. S., and Maclean, L. D., 1970, A graft versus host reaction given by human immunocompetent cells: A test for anti-human lymphocyte serum, in: *Pharmacological Treatment in Organ and Tissue Transplantation* (A. Bertelli and A. P. Monaco, eds.), Excerpta Medica Foundation, Amsterdam.

Green, D. M., 1958, The effects of nitrogen mustard [methyl bis (β-chloro-ethyl) amine HCl] on the immunological response and the rabbit. I. The effects of nitrogen mustard on the primary response to a bacterial antigen, *Br. J. Exp. Pathol.* **39**:192–198.

Greenberg, P. D., Cheever, M. A., and Fefer, A., 1981, Eradication of disseminated murine leukemia by chemoimmunotherapy with cyclophosphamide and adoptively transferred immune syngeneic Lyt-1^{+}2^{-} lymphocytes, *J. Exp. Med.* **154**:952–963.

Greene, M., Perry, L. L., and Benacerraf, B., 1979, Regulation of the immune response to tumor antigen. V. Modulation of suppressor T-cell activity *in vivo*, *Am. J. Pathol.* **95**:159–170.

Hancock, E. J., and Kilburn, D. G., 1982, The effects of cyclophosphamide on *in vitro* cytotoxic responses to a syngeneic tumor, *Cancer Immunol. Immunother.* **14**(1):54–58.

Hathcock, K. S., and Hodes, R. J., 1982, Interaction of T cell subsets in the regulation of cytotoxic T lymphocyte responses, *Fed. Proc.* **41**:818.

Hellström, I., and Hellström, K. E., 1978, Cyclophosphamide delayed 3-methylcholanthrene sarcoma induction in mice, *Nature* **275**:129–130.

Hengst, J. C. D., Mokyr, M., and Dray, S., 1980, Importance of timing in cyclophosphamide therapy of MOPC-315 tumor bearing mice, *Cancer Res.* **40**:4135–2141.

Hengst, J. C., Mokyr, M. B., and Dray, S., 1981, Cooperation between cyclophosphamide tumoricidal activity and host anti-tumor immunity in the cure of mice bearing large MOPC-315 tumors, *Cancer Res.* **41**(6):2163–2167.

Howard, J. G., and Shand, F. L., 1979, The nature of drug-induced B cell tolerance, *Immunol. Rev.* **43**:43–68.

Huber, B., Devinsky, O., Gershon, R. K., and Cantor, H., 1976, Cell-mediated immunity: Delayed-type hypersensitivity and cytotoxic responses are mediated by different T-cell subclasses, *J. Exp. Med.* **143**:1534–1539.

Hurme, M., 1979, Differential cyclophosphamide sensitivity of precursor cells in allogeneic and H-2 restricted cytotoxic responses, *J. Exp. Med.* **149**:290–294.

Jandinski, J., Cantor, H., Tadakuma, T., Peauy, D. L., and Pierce, C. W., 1976, Separation of helper T cells from suppressor T cells expressing different Ly components, *J. Exp. Med.* **143**:1382–1390.

Jokipii, A. M. M., and Jokipii, L., 1973, Suppression of cell-mediated immunity by cyclophosphamide: Its independence of concomitant B cell response, *Cell. Immunol.* **9**:477–481.

Jones, J. W., Brody, G. L., Oneal, R. M., and Haines, R. F., 1963, Prolongation of skin homografts in rabbits, using cyclophosphamide, *J. Surg. Res.* **3**:189–198.

Katz, S. I., Parker, D., and Turk, J. L., 1974, B-cell suppression of delayed hypersensitivity reactions, *Nature* **251**:550–551.

Kaufmann, S. H., Hahn, H., and Diamantstein, T., 1980, Relative susceptibilities of T cell subsets involved in delayed-type hypersensitivity to sheep red blood cells to the *in vitro* action of 4-hydroperoxycyclophosphamide, *J. Immunol.* **125**(3):1104–1108.

Kawaguchi, S., 1970, Studies on the induction of immunological paralysis to bovine γ-globulin in adult mice. II. The effect of cyclophosphamide, *Immunology* **19**:291–299.

Kerckhaert, J. A., van den Berg, G. J., and Hofhuis, F. M., 1974a, Influence of cyclophosphamide on the delayed hypersensitivity in the mouse after immunization with histocompatibility antigen, *J. Immunol.* **113**(6):1801–1808.

Kerckhaert, J. A. M., van den Berg, G. J., and Willers, J. M. N., 1974b, Influence of cyclophosphamide on the delayed hyersensitivity of the mouse, *Ann. Immunol.* **125**:415–426.

Kettman, J., 1972, Delayed hypersensitivity: Is the same population of thymus-derived cells responsible for cellular immunity reactions and the carrier effect? *Immunol. Commun.* **1**:289–299.

L'Age-Stehr, J., and Diamantstein, T., 1978, Induction of autoreactive T lymphocytes and their suppressor cells by cyclophosphamide, *Nature* **271**:663–665.

Lagrange, P. H., Mackaness, G. B., and Miller, T. E., 1974a, Influence of dose and route of antigen injection on the immunological induction of T cells, *J. Exp. Med.* **139**:528–542.

Lagrange, P. H., Mackaness, G. B., and Miller, T. E., 1974b, Potentiation of T-cell-mediated immunity by selective suppression of antibody formation with cyclophosphamide, *J. Exp. Med.* **139**(6):1529–1539.

Lando, Z., Teitelbaum, D., and Arnon, R., 1979, Effect of cyclophosphamide on suppressor cell activity in mice unresponsive to EAE, *J. Immunol.* **123**(5):2156–2160.

Larson, F. S., and Sparck, J. V., 1983, Effect of cyclophosphamide on spleen cell suppressor activity and tumour growth in mice, *Acta Pathol. Microbiol. Immunol. Scand.* **91**(5):323–333.

Livingston, P. O., DeLeo, A. B., Jones, M., and Oettgen, H. F., 1983, Comparison of approaches for augmenting the serologic response to the individually specific methylcholanthrene-induced sarcoma—Meth A: Pretreatment with cyclophosphamide is most effective, *J. Immunol.* **131**(5):2601–2605.

Lubaroff, D. M., and Waksman, B. H., 1968, Bone marrow as a source of cells in reactions of cellular hypersensitivity. I. Passive transfer of tuberculin sensitivity in syngeneic systems, *J. Exp. Med.* **128**:1425–1435.

Lubet, R. A., and Carlson, D. E., 1978, Therapy of murine plasmacytoma MOPC 104E: Role of the immune response, *J. Natl. Cancer Inst.* **61**:897–903.

Mackaness, G. B., Lagrange, P. H., Miller, T. E., and Ishibashi, T., 1974, Feedback inhibition of specifically sensitized lymphocytes, *J. Exp. Med.* **139**:543–559.

McQuarrie, D. G., Condie, R. M., Meeker, W. R., Roller, F., and Varco, R. L., 1960, Effect of methyl bis (2-chlorethyl) amine upon survival of skin homografts in rats and rabbits, *Proc. Soc. Exp. Biol. Med.* **103**:278–282.

Maguire, H. C., and Ettore, V. L., 1967a, Enhancement of dinitrochlorobenzene (DNCB) contact sensitization by cyclophosphamide in guinea pigs, *J. Exp. Med.* **129**:103–121.

Maguire, H. C., Jr., and Ettore, V. L., 1967b, Enhancement of dinitrochlorobenzene (DNCB) contact sensitization by cyclophosphamide in the guinea pig, *J. Invest. Dermatol.* **48**:39–43.

Maguire, H. C., Jr., Mailbach, H. I., and Minisce, L. W., Jr., 1961, Inhibition of guinea pig anaphylactic sensitization with cyclophosphamide, *J. Invest. Dermatol.* **36**:235–236.

Mathe, G., Halle-Panneko, O., and Bourut, C., 1977, Effectiveness of murine leukemia chemotherapy according to the immune state: Reconsideration of correlations between chemotherapy, tumor cell killing, and survival time, *Recent Results Cancer Res.* **62**:9–12.

Merluzzi, V. J., Faanes, R. B., and Choi, Y. S., 1980, Recovery of the capacity for cytotoxic T cell generation in cyclophosphamide-treated mice by the addition of LYT-1/2-helper cells, *Int. J. Immunopharmacol.* **2**(4):341–344.

Milton, J. D., Carpenter, C. B., and Addison, I. E., 1976, Depressed T-cell reactivity and suppressor activity of lymphoid cells from cyclophosphamide-treated mice, *Cell. Immunol.* **24**:308–317.

Mitsuoka, A., Baba, M., and Morikawa S., 1976, Enhancement of delayed hypersensitivity by depletion of suppressor T cells with cyclophosphamide in mice, *Nature* **262**:77–78.

Mitsuoka, A., Morikawa, S., Baba, M., and Harada, T., 1979, Cyclophosphamide eliminates suppressor T cells in age-associated central regulation of delayed hypersensitivity in mice, *J. Exp. Med.* **149**:1018–1028.

Mokyr, M. B., and Dray S., 1983, Some advantages of curing mice bearing a large subcutaneous MOPC-315 tumor with a low dose rather than a high dose of cyclophosphamide, *Cancer Res.* **43**(7):3112–3119.

Mokyr, M. D., Hengst, J. C., and Dray, S., 1982, Role of antitumor immunity in cyclophospha-mide-induced rejection of subcutaneous nonpalpable MOPC-315 tumors, *Cancer Res.* **42**(3):974–979.

Moorehead, J. W., and Claman, H. N., 1974, Subpopulations of mouse T lymphocytes. I. "Thy-midine Suicide" of a major proliferating, PHA-responsive cell population present in spleen but not in lymph node, *J. Immunol.* **112**:333–338.

Morimoto, C., Distaso, J., Borel, Y., Schlossman, S., and Reinherz, E., 1982, Communicative interactions between subpopulations of human T lymphocytes required for generation of suppressor effector function in a primary antibody response, *J. Immunol.* **128**:1645–1650.

Ozer, H., Cowens, J. W., Nussbaum, A., Mihich, E., and Colvin, M., 1981, Human immunoreg-ulatory T subset function defined *in vitro* by cyclophosphamide metabolites, *Fed. Proc.* **40**:1075.

Ozer, H., Cowens, J. W., Colvin, M., Nussbaum-Blumenson, A., and Sheedy, D., 1982, In vitro effects of 4-hydroperoxycyclophosphamide on human immunoregulatory T subset function. I. Selective effects on lymphocyte function in T–B cell collaboration, *J. Exp. Med.* **155**:276–290.

Paul, R. D., Ghaffar, A., and Sigel, M. M., 1982, Selective action of alkylating agents against cells participating in suppression of antibody responses, *Int. J. Immunopharmacol.* **4**(3):159–166.

Pierce, C. W., and Kapp, J. A., 1976, Regulation of immune responses by suppressor T cells, *Contemp. Top. Immunobiol.* **5**:91–143.

Polak, L., and Turk, J. L., 1974, Reversal of immunological tolerance by cyclophosphamide through inhibition of suppressor cell activity, *Nature* **244**:654–656.

Poulter, L. W., and Turk, J. L., 1972, Proportional increase in the T lymphocytes in peripheral lymphoid tissue following treatment with cyclophosphamide, *Nature: New Biol.* **238**:17–18.

Ramshaw, I. A., Bretscher, P. A., and Parish, C. R., 1976, Regulation of the immune response: Suppression of delayed-type hypersensitivity by T cells from mice expressing humoral immunity, *Eur. J. Immunol.* **6**:674–679.

Ramshaw, I. A., Bretscher, P. A., and Parish, C. R., 1977, Regulation of the immune response. II. Repressor T cells in cyclophosphamide-induced tolerant mice, *Eur. J. Immunol.* **7**:180–185.

Reinherz, E., Kung, P., Breard, J., Goldstein, G., and Schlossman, S., 1980, T cell requirements for generation of helper functions in man: Analysis of the subsets involved, *J. Immunol.* **124**:1883–1887.

Rollinghoff, M., Starzinski-Powitz, A., Pfizenmaier, K., and Wagner, H., 1977, Cyclophospha-mide-sensitive T lymphocytes suppress the *in vivo* generation of antigen-specific cytotoxic T lymphocytes, *J. Exp. Med.* **145**:455–459.

Santos, G. W., 1967, Immunosuppressive drugs. I. *Fed. Proc.* **26**:910–913.

Santos, G. W., and Owens, A. H., 1965, A comparison of the effects of selected cytotoxic agents on allogeneic skin graft survival in rats, *Bull. Johns Hopkins Hosp.* **116**:327–340.

Santos, G. W., Owens, A. H., and Sensenbrenner, L. L., 1964, Effects of selected cytotoxic agents on antibody production in man: A preliminary report, *Ann. N.Y. Acad. Sci.* **114**:404–423.

Schwartz, A., Orbach-Arbouys, S., and Gershon, R. K., 1976, Participation of cyclophosphamide-sensitive T cells in graft-vs-host reactions, *J. Immunol.* **117**:871–875.

Schwartz, A., Askenase, P. W., and Gershon, R. K., 1978, Regulation of delayed-type hyper-sensitivity reactions by cyclophosphamide-sensitive T cells, *J. Immunol.* **121**(4):1573–1577.

Shand, F. L., 1978, The capacity of microsomally-activated cyclophosphamide to induce im-
munosuppression *in vitro*, *Immunology* **35**:1017–1025.
Shand, F. L., and Howard, J. G., 1978, Cyclophosphamide-inhibited B cell receptor regeneration
as a basis for drug-induced tolerance, *Nature* **271**:255–257.
Shand, F. L., and Howard, J. G., 1979, Induction *in vitro* of reversible immunosuppression and
inhibition of B cell receptor regeneration by defined metabolites of cyclophosphamide,
Eur. J. Immunol. **9**:17–21.
Shand, F. L., and Liew, F. Y., 1980, Differential sensitivity to cyclophosphamide of helper T
cells for humoral responses and suppressor T cells for delayed-type hypersensitivity, *Eur.
J. Immunol.* **10**:480–483.
Shearer, G. M., Rehn, T. G., and Schmitt-Verhulst, A. M., 1976, Role of the murine major
histocompatibility complex in the specificity of *in vitro* T cell mediated lympholysis against
chemically-modified autologous lymphocytes, *Transplant. Rev.* **29**:222–248.
Smith, J., Cowens, W., Nussbaum-Blumenson, A., Sheedy, D., Mihich, E., and Ozer, H., 1982,
Functional separation of human suppressor and cytotoxic T subsets defined *in vitro* by 4-
HC, *Fed. Proc.* **41**:797.
Smith, J., Mihich, E., and Ozer, H., 1985, In vitro effects of 4-hydroperoxycyclophosphamide
on human immunoregulatory T subset function. II. Selective effects on lymphocyte function
in T-T cell collaboration (submitted).
Spurr, C. L., 1947, Influence of nitrogen mustards on the antibody response, *Proc. Soc. Exp.
Biol. Med.* **64**:259–261.
Stender, H. S., Strauch, D., and Winter, H., 1961, Vergleichende Untersuchungen über die
Behinderung der Antikorpes Bildung durch Roentgenstrahlen und eines N-lost-Phospham-
idester, *Streihlentherapie* **115**:175–186.
Stevenson, H. C., Fauci, A. S., 1980, Differential effects of *in vitro* cyclophosphamide on human
lymphocyte subpopulations involved in B-cell activation, *Immunology* **39**(3):391–397.
Sy, M. S., Miller, S. D., and Claman, H. N., 1977, Immune suppression with supraoptimal doses
of antigen in contact sensitivity. I. Demonstration of suppressor cells and their sensitivity
to cyclophosphamide, *J. Immunol.* **119**(1):240–244.
Takamizawa, A., Matsumoto, S., Iwata, T., Tochino, Y., Katagiri, K., Yamaguchi, K., and Shir-
atori, O., 1975, Studies on cyclophosphamide metabolites and their related compounds. 2.
Preparation of an active species of cyclophosphamide and related compounds, *J. Med.
Chem.* **18**:376–383.
Taylor, R. B., and Basten, A., 1976, Suppressor cells in humoral immunity and tolerance, *Br.
Med. Bull.* **32**:152–157.
Thomas, Y., Susman, J., Irigoyen, O., Friedman, S., Kung, P. C., Goldstein, G., and Chess, L.,
1980, Functional analysis of human T cell subsets defined by monoclonal antibodies. I.
Collaborative T–T interactions in the immunoregulation of B cell differentiation, *J. Im-
munol.* **125**:2402–2408.
Thomas, Y., Susman J., Irigoyen, M., Friedman, S., Kung, P., Goldstein, G., and Chess, L., 1981,
Functional analysis of human T cell subsets defined by monoclonal antibodies. III. Regu-
lation of helper factor production by T cell subsets, *J. Immunol.* **126**:1948–1951.
Turk, J. L., and Parker, D., 1973, Further studies on B-lymphocyte suppression in delayed
hypersensitivity, indicating a possible mechanism for Jones-Mote hypersensitivity, *Im-
munology* **24**:751–758.
Turk, J. L., and Poulter, L. W., 1972, Selective depletion of lymphoid tissue by cyclophosphamide, *Clin. Exp. Immunol.* **10**(2):285–296.
Turk, J. L., Parker, D., and Poulter, L. W., 1972, Functional aspects of the selective depletion
of lymphoid tissue by cyclophosphamide, *Immunology* **23**:493–501.
Vadas, M. A., Miller, J. F. A. P., McKenzie, I. F. C., Chism, S. E., Shen, F. W., Boyse, E. A.,
Gamble, J. R., and Whitelaw, A. M., 1976, Ly and Ia antigen phenotypes of T cells involved
in delayed-type hypersensitivity and in suppression, *J. Exp. Med.* **144**:10–19.
van den Broek, A. A., 1971, Mechanism of immune suppression by nitrogen mustard and
cyclophosphamide, in: *Immune Suppression and Histophysiology of the Immune Response*
(thesis monograph), Drukkerij van Denderen, Groningen, pp. 47–82.

Varkila, K., and Hurme, M., 1983, The effect of cyclophosphamide on cytotoxic T-lymphocyte responses: Inhibition of helper T-cell induction *in vitro*, *Immunology* **48**(3):433–438.

Whisler, R. L., and Stobo, J. D., 1978, Suppression of humoral and delayed hypersensitivity responses by distinct T cell subpopulations, *J. Immunol.* **121**:539–542.

Whydehaag, F., Heijnen, C., Pot, K., and Ballieux, R., 1979, T–T interactions in the induction of antigen specific human suppressor T cells, *J. Immunol.* **123**:646–653.

Willers, J. M. N., and Sluis, E., 1975, The influence of cyclophosphamide on antibody formation in the mouse, *Ann. Immunol.* **126**(3):267–279.

Wood, M. L., and Monaco, A. P., 1979, Differential effect of cyclophosphamide on states of specific allograft unresponsiveness in immunosuppressed mice, *Transplantation* **27**(3):186–189.

Yachie, A., Miyawaki, T., Yokoi, T., Nagoki, T., and Taniguchi, N., 1982, Ia + cells generated by PWM stimulation within OKT4 + subset interact with OKT8 + cells for inducing active suppression on B cell differentiation, *J. Immunol.* **129**:103–106.

Yu, S., Lannin, D. R., Tsui-Collins, A. L., and McKhann, C. F., 1980, Effect of cyclophosphamide on mice bearing methylcholanthrene-induced fibrosarcomas, *Cancer Res.* **40**:2756–2761.

CHAPTER 5

THE IMMUNOMODULATORY ACTIVITY OF CERTAIN CANCER CHEMOTHERAPEUTIC AGENTS

FEDERICO SPREAFICO and ANNUNCIATA VECCHI

1. INTRODUCTION

The activity within the immune system of a composite series of cancer chemotherapeutic agents belonging to different chemical classes and believed to exert their antineoplastic effect through a variety of molecular mechanisms is briefly reviewed in this chapter. Thus only a fraction of all currently available anticancer drugs that are not discussed elsewhere in this volume shall be considered here. The basis for inclusion of compounds has essentially been threefold: (1) the large actual or potential clinical use of the agent; (2) availability of at least a minimum of information on its effect on the various components of the immune complex; and (3) the fact that their immunopharmacological activity appears to possess, for at least certain aspects, distinct features. With regard to the latter point, and as readily apparent from the following discussion, it should be emphasized, however, that also for the compounds considered here, existing knowledge on their immunological effects is in general quite limited, thus in most instances preventing conclusions based on a sufficiently detailed picture, both phenomenologically and mechanistically.

2. VINCRISTINE AND VINBLASTINE

The *Vinca rosea* alkaloids vincristine (VCR) and vinblastine (VLB) are widely employed cancer chemotherapeutic agents because of their effec-

FEDERICO SPREAFICO and ANNUNCIATA VECCHI ● Departments of Oncology and Immunology, Mario Negri Institute for Pharmacological Research, 20157 Milan, Italy.

tiveness in various types of human malignancies. The most generally accepted mechanism of action of these agents involves drug-induced microtubule dysfunction eventually leading to mitotic arrest, thus resembling the mechanisms of colchicine, another compound capable of disrupting microtubular assembly. It should be noted, however, that although VCR and VLB possess comparable *in vitro* capacity to bind to tubulin and block its polymerization these agents differ in their spectrum of anticancer activity as well as of clinical toxicity; neurotoxicity is the limiting side-effect of VCR, whereas that of VLB is leukopenia. It is thus possible that interference with other cellular structures, such as that repeatedly demonstrated with membranes (Rudolph *et al.*, 1977; Berlin and Fera, 1977), may be an important determinant of the *in vivo* activity of these compounds not only on cancer cells but also on immunocytes. These uncertainties on the mechanism of cellular action of *Vinca* alkaloids have their counterpart in the still substantial lack of knowledge on their effects on the various cells of the immune system: a number of important points of their immunomodulatory activity have not yet been systematically explored in man nor in experimental animals. Indeed, also in view of the fact that VCR and VLB are generally employed in combination with other antineoplastic agents, the clinical immunopharmacology of these drugs is practically nonexistent, and is restricted to studies performed more than two decades ago that considered only a very limited number of immune parameters (Santos *et al.*, 1964).

Various groups have reported that the administration to animals of VCR, VLB, and colchicine could inhibit primary antibody formation to T-dependent antigens such as sheep erythrocytes (Hersh, 1974). When single injections were used, inhibition could be observed only using relatively high and nearly toxic doses (i.e., with an effectiveness distinctly inferior to that of compounds such as cyclophosphamide), and was critically dependent on the timing of treatment relative to immunization. Depression of antibody response was only seen with drug administration after antigen. Drug injections concomitant with or prior to administration of antigen can on the other hand be associated with enhanced antibody response (Shek and Coons, 1977). The capacity of VCR and VLB to reduce antibody production has recently been confirmed also in *in vitro* systems (Ryoyama *et al.*, 1982), this study also showing that VCR was distinctly more effective than VLB in this regard. The exact mechanism(s) sustaining this reduced antibody production are still unclear. For instance, since the activity of VCR and VLB on the response to T-independent antigens does not appear to have been investigated, it is still unresolved whether this effect involves only T lymphocytes and/or macrophages or also direct effects on B cells. Since VCR and VLB are antimitotic agents, an effect on B-cell proliferation cannot be excluded in principle and thus could play a role in mediating the reduction of antibody levels, possibly together with inhibition of the secretory capacity of antibody-producing cells. A decreased immunoglobulin secretory capacity has been found in plasma cells after *in vitro* exposure to these agents, which is analogous to that seen for the secretion of other products by various other cell types (Antoine *et al.*, 1980). However, since this effect was seen at relatively high concentrations and contradictory data exist on this point after *in vivo* drug treatment (Teplitz *et al.*, 1975; Tartakoff *et al.*, 1977), the real importance of this mechanism still remains to be established.

If our understanding of VCR and VLB effects on B cells is still incomplete, existing knowledge on the activity of these compounds on T cells is also fragmentary. Available evidence suggests that the effects exerted may be complex, depending on the drug used, the dose employed, and the function examined. That VCR and VLB can inhibit cell-mediated reactivities was demonstrated by the finding reported two decades ago that animal treatment with these agents could prolong allograft survival and reduce delayed-type hypersensitivity reactions (Aisenberg and Wilkes, 1967). However, the effect observed was relatively modest despite the use of high doses. The response of human and animal lymphocytes to T mitogens such as concanavalin A (Con A) and phytohemagglutinin (PHA) can also be reduced by VLB or colchicine (Edelman *et al.*, 1973; Resch *et al.*, 1977; Steen and Lindmo, 1978). The main effect appears to be a prolongation of the lag phase and a reduction of the rate at which cells enter the S phase (Hall *et al.*, 1982), through biochemical mechanisms that are still under discussion but that do not involve early events of lymphocyte activation (Resch *et al.*, 1977; Steen and Lindmo, 1978). It is of interest, however, that treatment of lymphocytes with microtubule-disrupting agents does not necessarily decrease responsiveness to all stimulants. Under conditions reducing the response to Con A, colchicine increased lymphocyte blastogenesis by sodium periodate, a mitogen that requires cell–cell interaction to induce cellular proliferation (Stenzel *et al.*, 1978). In parallel, when colchicine was added to already ongoing mixed lymphocyte cultures, blastogenesis and generation of specific cytotoxic T effectors were inhibited, whereas early addition of the compound in low concentrations or brief pretreatment was associated with a significant increase in the response (Suthanthiran *et al.*, 1980). Although the mechanisms sustaining these effects are still speculative, it is noteworthy that similar dose-related opposite effects have been described to occur with VCR. It has been reported that the administration of a low VCR dose to mice was associated with an increase in the subsequent capacity of spleen cells to generate *in vitro* alloreactive T effectors, whereas higher doses (e.g., one half of the LD_{10}) were inhibitory (Bartocci *et al.*, 1980). Parallel findings were obtained when VCR was used *in vitro*, since low concentrations (0.01 μg/ml) were found to increase the generation of T effectors in contrast to the inhibition induced by higher (0.5–2 mg/ml) concentrations.

The inability of VCR treatment at relatively low doses to affect the proliferative capacity of the precursors of cytotoxic T effectors so that the generation of these elements, if not increased, was not reduced *vis-à-vis* controls, has been confirmed by other investigators who showed that VLB was significantly more inhibitory of these precursors than VCR. Conversely, VCR was more effective than VLB in inhibiting the development of antibody-producing cells *in vitro* (Ryoyama *et al.*, 1982).

Although no information is available for "mature" T suppressors, the generation of T suppressors is also sensitive to *Vinca* alkaloids, as first suggested by the finding that colchicine administration at the time of immunization was associated with marked augmentation of humoral responses (Shek *et al.*, 1977). This sensitivity has subsequently been confirmed in a study showing that VLB was again more effective in blocking the precursors of these elements than VCR, which was inhibitory only at relatively high, toxic doses *in vivo* or *in vitro* (Ryoyama *et al.*, 1982). Although no formal analysis of this question was performed, the data of this group would tend to suggest that the precursors of T suppressors are more sensitive than the precursors of T effectors to these drugs, which is analogous to sensitivities observed to other cancer chemotherapeutics such as cyclophosphamide.

With regard to the effect of VCR and VLB on effector T cells, a reduced capacity to express cytotoxicity has been described after *in vivo* and *in vitro* treatment (Borel, 1976); however, this decrease was relatively modest and observable only at high drug doses. On the other hand, it has also been shown that VLB and colchicine did not affect mitogen-induced release of lymphotoxin by human lymphocytes (Resch *et al.*, 1977). Lymphocyte-mediated antibody-dependent cytotoxicity against virus-infected target cells was reduced by *in vitro* exposure to VCR but only at concentrations of 1 μg/ml or higher (Bolivar *et al.*, 1980), whereas it has been reported that low concentrations (0.01–0.1 μg/ml) of VCR produced a marked increase in murine natural killer (NK) cells effector capacity (De Vecchis *et al.*, 1982). The mechanism of this effect, which does not appear to involve inactivation of NK suppressors, is unknown, nor is it known whether a similar activation occurs after *in vivo* administration of the drug. From all these data, it would appear therefore that, except at quite high doses, at which these drugs are frankly inhibitory, VLB and especially VCR can relatively spare and possibly increase, at least in selected circumstances, the effector capacity of cells of the T lineage and their generation from the appropriate precursors. In this context, it may be relevant to mention that in a murine lymphoma model, VCR was capable of effectively synergizing with host antitumor reactivity (Riccardi *et al.*, 1980). A low VLB dose administered at the time of immunization of mice with an otherwise nonprotective specific vaccine, was also capable of inducing a high degree of T-cell-mediated protection against *Pseudomonas aeruginosa* (Pier and Markham, 1982).

In comparison to effects on other cells of the immune system, the effects of VCR and VLB on macrophages have been the object of greater attention. These agents together with colchicine have in fact frequently been employed as tools for investigating the role of microtubules in phagocyte functions. In spite of this, various aspects of these drugs' activities on these elements remain unclear. Moreover, since most studies have been conducted with *in vitro* exposure to relatively high drug concentrations, the relevance of these results to more realistic *in vivo* conditions remains to be proven. When monocytes are exposed to colchicine or VLB, concomitant with changes from a gliding to a more ameboid and tortuous form of locomotion, a rounding of the cell occurs with an increased tendency for the nucleus to be eccentrically located and with alterations in the shape of pseudopods (Zakhireh and Malech, 1980). Spontaneous motility of human and animal macrophages [but apparently not that of polymorphonuclear neutrophils (PMN)] has, however, been reported to be increased after *in vitro* exposure to these compounds in concentrations of 10^{-6} M (Pick and Abrahamer, 1973), providing a further example of the biphasic dose–response curve shown by these agents on various immunocytes. On the other hand, the response of monocytes and PMN to chemoattractants is reduced in the presence of colchicine and VLB in concentrations equal to or higher than 10^{-6} M (Zakhireh and Malech, 1980), and macrophages also become unresponsive to the lymphokine migration inhibition factor (MIF) (Pick, 1979). In parallel, deuterium oxide, a compound stabilizing microtubules by preventing their depolymerization, reduces spontaneous macrophage migration and enhances their responsiveness to MIF (Pick, 1979), a finding that has been taken to support the view that MIF, possibly through prostaglandin-mediated changes in the activity of adenylcyclase and thus cyclic AMP, induces tubulin stabilization and thus a greater cellular rigidity and an increased strength of adhesion to substrates (Pick, 1979). Although colchicine and VLB were shown in early studies to inhibit phagocytosis and metabolic responses to particle ingestion in PMN (Bodel, 1976; Lehrer, 1973), the effect of these compounds on macrophage phagocytosis is less clear, and no study appears to have been performed after *in vivo* therapeutic treatment. Thus it has been reported that lysosomal fusion was inhibited at concentrations of colchicine as low as 10^{-6} M, that the drug was effective at high but not at low concentrations, or that it had no effect at any concentration through 10^{-3} M (Pesanti and Axline, 1975). It may be noted that even in studies reporting an inhibition of lysosomal enzyme induction by colchicine following pinocytic or phagocytic stimuli, no reduction in the intracellular digestion of bacteria by macrophages was observed (Pesanti and Axline, 1975). Colchicine and VLB *in vitro* have also been shown to stimulate macrophages (but not lymphocytes) to synthesize and release high amounts of prostaglandins of the E series (PGEs) possibly mobilizing arachidonic acid from phospholipids by stimulating phospholipases (Gemsa *et al.*, 1980). Although no *in vivo* data are available on this point, since PGEs are known to unspecifically modulate a wide variety of leukocyte activities, this effect may at least be a component of the antiinflammatory activity of these drugs. The effect of VCR and VLB on effector macrophage function is also uncertain. After exposure to VLB or colchicine, the cytotoxic activity of stimulated animal macrophages on cultured tumor cells has in fact been reported as being unaffected by some investigators (Keller, 1974) and reduced by others (Sharma and Piessens, 1978; Martin *et al.*, 1981). Of interest as an additional indication of the dose dependency of these drugs' effects is the recent finding that the capacity of macrophages to mediate antibody-dependent cytotoxicity (ADCC) is inhibited by high (10^{-4} M) concentrations of VLB or colchicine, but greatly augmented at lower, therapeutically more relevant ones (Ralph and Nakoinz,

1982). Since these drugs bind to microtubules within minutes whereas the stimulation of ADCC was only observable after several hours, it has been hypothesized that the mechanism involved could be an accumulation of toxic mediators within the cells secondary to drug-induced alteration in microtubules assembly. However, since VLB enhances macrophage capacity to form rosettes with antibody-coated erythrocytes (Medgyesi *et al.*, 1980), possibly through modulation of Fc membrane receptors (Ercolani and Schulte, 1983), it cannot be excluded that a greater capacity to bind target cells may also play a role. A paucity of information exists on the effects of VCR and VLB on the production of lymphomonocytic mediators. In addition to the previously mentioned lack of effects of VLB and colchicine on the production by lymphocytes of lymphotoxin, *in vitro* treatment with these compounds has been shown not to reduce the release by these cells of a lymphokine having osteoclast activity capacity (Resch *et al.*, 1977). Furthermore, the production of interleukin 1 (IL 1) in cultures of both previously stimulated and unstimulated macrophages was actually stimulated by prior exposure to low concentrations of VLB or colchicine in short pulses (Bodel, 1976; Stosic-Grujicic and Simic, 1982). Whether this augmented release of IL 1, a factor currently believed to be an obligatory signal for interleukin 2 production and thus T-cell proliferation, plays a role in the reported stimulatory effects of VCR and VLB on certain T-lymphocyte functions, is as yet unknown.

Semisynthetic *Vinca* alkaloids, such as vindesine, possessing clinical antineoplastic activity have recently become available. Treatment of melanoma patients with short courses of vindesine has been reported to induce no significant lymphopenia nor to affect T-lymphocyte responsiveness to antigens such as purified protein derivative, candidin, or allogeneic cells (Retsas *et al.*, 1981). Although these findings would suggest that vindesine is not a powerful immunodepressant, this information is too limited to permit reaching conclusions on the immunointerfering capacity of this compound.

In conclusion, it would appear that VCR and VLB possess a complex immunopharmacological activity with dose-dependent inhibitory or stimulatory effects on at least certain immune fractions. Although in principle the latter type of effects could have an interest in explaining the antineoplastic effectiveness of these drugs and may lead to a better manipulation of host anticancer reactivities, much more work is needed before this potential can be substantiated.

3. ADENOSINE DEAMINASE INHIBITORS

Several observations indicate that lymphocytes require physiological levels of adenosine deaminase (ADA) for maintenance of proper function, proliferation, and viability. Although present in almost all mammalian tissues, ADA levels are highest in lymphoid organs such as the thymus, spleen, and lymph nodes; the activity of this enzyme is increased in antigenically stimulated cells in addition to being markedly increased in blast cells from acute lymphocytic leukemia patients. More importantly, a congenital defect in this enzyme is present in a proportion of children with severe combined immunodeficiency disease (SCID). On this basis and in spite of the fact that the biochemical mechanism(s) responsible for lymphotoxicity in ADA deficiency are still controversial (Carson *et al.*, 1981), a good deal of interest has centered in the past decade on the search for ADA inhibitors as potential anticancer and immunomodulating agents and as selective lymphotoxic compounds not affecting other types of proliferating cells. This potential thus justifies discussion of ADA inhibitors in this chapter in spite of the still limited experience with such compounds not only in the clinic but also under experimental conditions. Although various ADA inhibitors have been synthesized, studies on their *in vivo* effects have so far been limited to only two such compounds, i.e., erythro-9-(2-hydroxy-3-nonyl)adenine (EHNA) and 2'-deoxycoformycin (DCF). The first is a synthetic aliphatic alcohol analog of adenine and is a relative weak and reversible ADA inhibitor, whereas DCF, an antibiotic of microbial origin, is a stoichiometric, tightly binding, irreversible, and thus more potent, inhibitor of this enzyme. Since, according to available evidence, the effect on immune cells of EHNA and DCF appear qualitatively similar, these substances will be discussed together.

Initial studies on the effect of ADA inhibitors on immune cells were conducted *in vitro* and were focused on responsiveness to mitogens. Using human lymphocytes, EHNA was found to inhibit the responsiveness to PHA and, to a lesser degree, Con A and pokeweed mitogen, but only at relatively high concentrations (i.e., in excess of those needed to inhibit ADA) and with long incubation of the lymphocytes with the drug prior to mitogen addition to cultures. Much lower drug concentrations, *per se* noninhibitory, on the other hand were effective if combined with adenosine. The depression was higher when [^{3}H]leucine rather than [^{3}H]thymidine incorporation was measured (Carson and Seegmiller, 1976; Hirschhorn and Sela, 1977). Essentially similar results have been reported with DCF, in the sense that the drug alone was poorly depressive and that inhibition was markedly potentiated by the simultaneous exposure of the cells to 2'-deoxyadenosine or adenosine, the former being clearly more effective than the latter (Uberti *et al.*, 1979; Glazer, 1980). Data available on the effect of ADA inhibitors on effector lymphocytes are contrasting. Under conditions in which lymphocyte responsiveness was inhibited, exposure to EHNA and 2'-deoxyadenosine was in fact reported not to affect the expression of nonspecific cytotoxicity induced in human lymphocytes by PHA (Simmonds *et al.*, 1978). In contrast, the lytic capacity of specifically sensitized murine lymphocytes could be decreased by EHNA, with 2–3 times lower drug concentrations needed if these effectors were also exposed to 2'-deoxyadenosine (Wolberg *et al.*, 1975). Whether this discrepancy is a reflection of the fact that different types of effector mechanisms and/or different subpopulations of cells from different species were tested remains unresolved. It is thus still impossible to conclude whether in addition to their demonstrated interference with lymphocyte activation, ADA inhibitors can also directly affect effector T-cell function.

Studies with EHNA *in vivo* have been limited. Repeated treatment with this compound was reported to delay the rejection of tumor, skin, and pancreatic islet allografts across non-H-2 histocompatibility barriers in mice (Lum *et al.*, 1979). However, the effects were modest even at high doses. Although various aspects of the actions of these agents on the immune system do not appear to have been investigated yet, comparatively more information is available for DCF which, as expected from the *in vitro* data, has proved to be a more potent immunodepressant than EHNA in animals. However, the effect observed is markedly influenced by the experimental conditions employed in regard not only to the animal species and strain used, but especially in regard to the treatment schedule employed. In fact, although lymphoid organ depletion can be induced with single injections of high DCF doses, repeated courses are generally associated with more consistent and important changes in lymphoid organ histopathology and immune function, with continuous infusion as the most lymphotoxic mode of treatment. Thus, the continuous infusion for 5 days of DCF doses in the 0.5 mg/kg range, which inhibited ADA by at least 80%, was associated with a decrease of circulating murine lymphocytes to 30%, marked atrophy of lymphoid organs, reduced antibody production, prolongation of allograft survival across strong histocompatibility barriers, impairment of delayed hypersensitivity, and a striking decrease in the response to the T-cell mitogens Con A and PHA as well as to the B-cell mitogen lipopolysaccharide (LPS). Although this treatment was associated with some general toxicity, it is of note that nonlymphoid organs were not histologically affected nor were bone marrow stem cells reduced in their number and differentiating capacity (Tedde *et al.*, 1979, 1980; Trotta *et al.*, 1981). Although differences exist between reports, it appears that qualitatively similar but less severe defects are seen when the same DCF dose administered by daily injections is used (Burridge *et al.*, 1977; Sordillo *et al.*, 1981), possibly because of the rapid clearance (2 hr) of the drug from the circulation allowing a recovery of ADA levels through synthesis of new protein or turnover of cells. A greater antileukemic activity was seen clinically when using constant DCF infusion than when using bolus injections (Benjamin *et al.*, 1980).

With regard to the question of the sensitivity to ADA inhibition of the different lymphocyte populations and subsets, various points remain unresolved. Available evidence supports the concept that although B cells are not intrinsically resistant to ADA inhibitors, these elements are less sensitive than T lymphocytes, as indicated by the finding that, when DCF treatments of medium severity are used, the decrease in T-cell numbers in lymphoid organs is more marked than for B cells, and the responsiveness to T mitogens more profoundly impaired than that to B-cell stimulants such as LPS (Sordillo *et al.*, 1981). Human T cells have been reported to have distinctly higher ADA levels than B cells (Sullivan *et al.*, 1977; Tung *et al.*, 1976). Also relevant in this context are the facts that a number of SCID patients demonstrate more T-cell than B-cell abnormalities (Cooper *et al.*, 1973; Carson *et al.*, 1981) and that normal T lymphocytes enable patients' B cells to produce immunoglobulins (Seeger *et al.*, 1976). Furthermore, another ADA inhibitor, coformycin, has been reported not to interfere with precursor maturation into mature immunoglobulin-secreting cells, while blocking the maturation of T precursors (Ballet *et al.*, 1976). In rats it has been found that ADA levels are three- to tenfold higher in thymocytes than in spleen or lymph node cells and that the highest enzyme levels are present in cortical thymocytes. On the other hand, thymocyte precursors and immature cortical thymocytes appear to possess low ADA levels (Barton *et al.*, 1979). However, it is not known whether different T-cell subpopulations in the periphery vary in their ADA levels and may thus be differentially affected by inhibitors of this enzyme. Although the finding that a repeated treatment with ADA inhibitors is required to observe immune impairment would be taken to suggest that mature T effectors may be less sensitive to these drugs than their proliferating precursors, direct information is not available on the possibility that different T-cell subpopulations (e.g., helper and suppressor) may vary in their susceptibility to drugs such as DCF. Although given the close functional connections between T lymphocytes and macrophages, ADA inhibitors would be expected to at least indirectly affect monocyte–macrophage functional capacity, this point does not appear to have yet been directly investigated. Similarly unresolved is whether ADA inhibitors modulate the function of other cells such as NK cells, believed to be related to T lymphocytes, and whether these drugs can affect the production and/or responsiveness to lymphokines. NK defects have recently been observed in a proportion of SCID patients with ADA defects. However, just as the clinical manifestations of SCID are heterogenous, so could be the biochemical abnormalities basic to the disease; accordingly, findings in these patients may not be totally representative of effects induced by ADA inhibitors.

4. CISPLATIN

Cis-diamine dichloroplatinum (II) (*cis*DDP) is now well established as a potent chemotherapeutic agent with proven activity against a widening list of human malignancies when employed singly or in combination with other antineoplastic agents. This compound has a direct cytotoxic activity on tumor cells in culture that is generally thought to derive from direct damage to the DNA template thus leading to inhibition of DNA synthesis. Although a paucity of data still exists on the immunological effects of *cis*DDP, inclusion of the compound in this chapter appears justified not only by its expanding use in the clinics but also by the fact that evidence, although mostly indirect, supports the possibility that the immunomodulatory capacity of this compound may play a role in its antineoplastic effectiveness. We shall therefore review first existing information on the effects of *cis*DDP on immune reactivity and then examine the possible interrelationship between these effects and tumor growth.

Administration of *cis*DDP to laboratory animals is associated with lymphopenia and cellular depletion in lymphoid organs, most evident in the thymus and spleen, whereas lymph nodes have been reported to be only marginally affected even at very high doses (Thompson and Gale, 1971). Single drug doses when administered to rodents either before or after sensitization, but in close proximity to it, can cause inhibition of primary antibody production to antigens such as sheep erythrocytes with a dose–response curve that is exponential, as would be expected from an alkylating agent (Khan and Hill, 1971; Berenbaum, 1971). However, it is important to note that marked depressions in this reactivity (i.e., over 90% decreases in the number of antibody-producing cells in the spleen) are only observed employing dose near the LD_{10} (Berenbaum, 1971). Also, in view of the fact that no data exist on the effect of *cis*DDP on the response to T-independent antigens, whether this reduction in antibody formation is mediated solely by effects on T cells or also on B lymphocytes is unresolved. Cell-mediated reactivities can also be inhibited by this drug, as indicated by its capacity to prolong allograft survival across non-H-2- and H-2-incompatible barriers (Brambilla *et al.*, 1974; Khan *et al.*, 1972). However, the prolongation of H-2-incompatible murine skin allografts was moderate even at very high doses, with repeated treatments being no more effective than single injections (Brambilla *et al.*, 1974). Graft-versus-host reactivity induced in F_1 mice by parental cells was also decreased by *cis*DDP at single doses above 5 mg/kg given at the time of sensitization or by postreatment with repeated lower doses (Khan and Hill, 1972). Administration of the compound to rodents has also been shown to be associated with a decreased lymphoid cell response to polyclonal activators such as Con A or PHA (Wierda and Pazdernik, 1979; Howle *et al.*, 1971). This effect was apparent already 24 hr after dosing with 6 mg/kg, i.e., before marked changes in spleen cellularity, with full recovery of both mitogen responses and organ cellularity on day 7 (Wierda and Pazdernik, 1979). Of interest, results from both single dose, time course analysis and dose–response studies indicated that the responsiveness to the T mitogen Con A was more sensitive than that to the B mitogen LPS, a finding that has been taken as indirect support for the possibility than platinum compounds may be more toxic for T than B lymphocyte function (Wierda and Pazdernik, 1979). Although *in vitro cis*DDP has been found to be more inhibitory of the proliferation of human leukemic T than of that of B cells (Ohnuma *et al.*, 1978), more direct information is needed before firm conclusions can be reached on this point. Interference by *cis*DDP on mitogen-induced blastogenesis has also been observed with human cells. PHA-stimulated lymphocytes exposed for 24 hr to drug concentration of 10^{-6}–10^{-5} M showed clearly reduced DNA synthesis (Howle *et al.*, 1971); however, exposure of already stimulated cells to these concentrations for only 1 hr was associated with only marginal or no effects. Similarly, no depression was observed after treatment of normal human lymphocytes with 10^{-5} M *cis*DDP for 1 hr prior to stimulation with mitogens or specific antigens (Kleinerman and Zwelling, 1982). It should be noted in this context that when standard doses are given to man by intravenous push, the resulting plasma concentration of active drug are in the range of $1–10 \times 10^{-6}$ M for less than 1 hr (De Conti *et al.*, 1973). In general analogy to these *in vitro* data, single injections of *cis*DDP to tumor patients by one push were associated with a decreased lymphocyte responsiveness to mitogens observable already within minutes after drug administration but with prompt recovery in 1–2 days after treatment discontinuation (Khan and Hill, 1973). Immunoglobulin and Con A receptor capping were inhibited in *cis*DDP-treated murine splenocytes (Tsokos and Choi, 1980). However, the significance of this finding is uncertain since this effect was seen after a number of hours of exposure at drug concentrations that clearly reduced cell survival.

Immunostimulatory effects of *cis*DDP have also been reported. *In vitro* treatment of human mononuclear cells with concentrations of this drug as low as 10^{-9} M for 15 min, i.e., at concentrations 1000-fold lower than those needed to induce detectable DNA damage or to produce cytotoxic effects in cultured malignant cells, has been shown to induce an accelerated and markedly enhanced (up to 300%) expression of monocyte-mediated spontaneous cytotoxicity (Kleinerman *et al.*, 1980b). This effect has been shown not be mediated by inactivation of suppressor cells but to be dependent on a direct stimulation by the drug of the effector cells, through mechanisms whose biochemical basis has not yet been investigated. The depressed spontaneous monocyte-mediated cytotoxicity versus erythrocytic targets present in advanced cancer patients was reported to be increased threefold during combination chemotherapy that contained *cis*DDP (Kleinerman *et al.*, 1980a; Kleinerman and Zwelling, 1982). Although the effector cell was not characterized, an increase in lymphoid cell-mediated cytotoxicity against tumor target cells upon *in vitro* addition of the drug has also been described by others (Mally *et al.*, 1980). More recently, in investigations of murine T-cell-mediated cytotoxicity generated in a mixed lymphocyte-tumor cell reaction, it has been reported that *in vitro* addition of *cis*DDP at the beginning of the culture resulted in augmentation of the response carried out in conditions of supraoptimal sensitization, i.e., in the conditions more likely to occur in a tumor-bearing host, whereas no effect or slight inhibition was seen when conditions for optimal *in vitro* sensitization were used (Schlaefli *et al.*, 1983). Interestingly, when the lymphocytes were obtained from animals treated with *cis*DDP or the analog *cis*-dichloro-*trans*-dihydroxy-*bis*-isopropylamine platinum (IV) (CHIP) at doses below their optimal therapeutic level also, an augmentation of T cytotoxicity generation was seen using both supraoptimal and suboptimal sensitization conditions. In the same study, evidence was also obtained that *cis*DDP and CHIP did not influence preformed T effector cells and that the latter compound at doses effective in causing an augmented generation of T-cell-mediated cytotoxicity also interfered with the development of nonspecific suppressor cells, whereas an LD_{50} dose was necessary to reduce the development of antigen-specific suppressor cell activity. Furthermore, responder cells from CHIP-treated donors exhibited a lower sensitivity to both antigen-specific and nonspecific suppressors than responder cells from untreated mice (Schlaefli *et al.*, 1983). In further confirmation of the possibility that, at therapeutic doses or concentrations, platinum compounds may induce stimulatory effects, another group has recently described that *in vitro* exposure to *cis*DDP to human leukocytes was associated with an increase in the number of autorosette-forming T cells and in NK-cell-mediated cytotoxicity (Cupissol *et al.*, 1983). Interestingly, the same group has observed that treatment of patients with solid tumors with 100 mg/m^2 *cis*DDP given intravenously did not alter delayed-type hypersensitivity skin tests to a battery of recall antigens, and was associated with significant increases in autorosetting T lymphocytes as well as in NK activity. Although the number of patients examined in this and other studies (Kleinerman *et al.*, 1980a) is still very limited, it may be worth mentioning that an increase in NK activity has also been observed in tumor-bearing rats treated with *cis*DDP (D. Cupissol, J. J. Akouala, and B. Serrou, personal communication).

Available evidence, still in large measure fragmentary, thus suggests that in addition to depressive effects generally of limited degree and duration and mostly seen at high, nearly, or frankly toxic drug doses, the immuno-modulatory activity of *cis*DDP may also comprise restoration or actual stimulation of at least certain immune reactivities both *in vivo* and at realistic drug concentrations *in vitro*. A number of indirect findings have also been described in the last decade supporting the possibility that the antineoplastic effectiveness of this compound may be not solely dependent on its direct action on tumor cell proliferation but may also involve immunomodulation. Among the first findings suggesting such a possibility was the observation that rats cured by *cis*DDP of a transplanted leukemia were protected against subsequent challenges with the same tumor (Kociba *et al.*, 1970). It has also been reported that murine tumor cells treated with *cis*DDP and other platinum-pyrimidine complexes at concentrations two orders of magnitude lower than those that are frankly cytotoxic and retaining viability *in vitro* were unable to grow *in vivo*, yet the hosts developed resistance versus reimplants of nontreated tumor cells (Rosenberg, 1975; Sarna and Sodhi, 1978). Similar findings have been obtained also in other murine systems (Page *et al.*, 1977). These results have been taken to suggest that *cis*DDP can modify tumor cell immunogenicity and/or antigenicity, and the hypothesis was advanced that this effect may be reconducible to its mutagenic activity or to its capacity to bind to membrane nucleic acids, thus leading to the unmasking of stronger antigens on the cell surface (Rosenberg, 1975). However, it should be emphasized that direct evidence supporting an altered immunogenicity of *cis*DDP-treated neoplastic cells has not yet been obtained. Indirectly in favor of the possibility that tumorous regression after *cis*DDP treatment may involve host participation are the findings that corticosteroids decrease the number of cures produced by *cis*DDP in animals, whereas coadministration of an immunostimulator augmented *cis*DDP effectiveness in poorly responsive tumor systems (Rosenberg, 1975). Murine tumors regressing after treatment with this compound have also been described as becoming heavily infiltrated with macrophages and lymphocytes (Sodhi and Aggarwal, 1974). In conclusion, a still limited but suggestive number of observations favor the view that *cis*DDP possesses a complex immunomodulatory activity and that this activity can be a determinant of its antitumor effectiveness. However, it is clear that a substantial amount of work still needs to be done before reaching firm conclusions on the relative roles of direct and indirect (i.e., modified immunogenicity of tumor cells and spared or inceased host reactivity) mechanisms in the anticancer capacity of this agent.

5. DACARBAZINE

Dacarbazine [5(3,3'-dimethyl-1-triazenyl)-1 H-imidazole-4-carboxamide (DTIC)] has been until recently the only cancer chemotherapeutic agent with demonstrable, although weak, clinical effectiveness when employed as a single agent in malignant melanoma. Inclusion of DTIC in this chapter is warranted not only on the basis of this relatively large clinical use, but also in consideration of the fact that this compound can be regarded as a prototype agent in exemplifying another aspect of the complex interaction of cancer chemotherapeutics with tumor cells and host reactivity, i.e., the capacity that at least some of these drugs have to modify the antigenicity of malignant cells. Although a capacity to induce tumor xenogenization (Kobayashi, 1978) has also been reported for a number of other antitumor agents following the initial data of Mihich and colleagues with methylglyoxal-*bis*(guanylhydrazone) (Mihich, 1969; Kitano *et al.*, 1971), DTIC has been the drug that has been most largely employed in studies of this phenomenon (Bonmassar *et al.*, 1979).

The direct activity of DTIC on the immune system has so far been the object of relatively limited investigations. In mice, this compound has been shown to be a very potent immunodepressant, with single injections of otherwise well-tolerated doses capable of producing profound and very long-lasting decreases in the number of antibody-producing cells after primary as well as secondary immunization (Vecchi *et al.*, 1976; Giampietri *et al.*, 1978). This inhibition is best seen with drug treatment before sensitization. Although the drug can undoubtedly affect T cells and accessory elements (see the following discussion), no direct information is available on the susceptibility of B lymphocytes to DTIC; the mechanisms at the basis of this humoral depression are therefore still uncertain. DTIC was also capable of markedly impairing the capacity of mice to reject H-2-incompatible allografts, single drug pretreatments reducing this reactivity for over 60 days, i.e., for a much longer duration than seen with equitoxic doses of other potent immunodepressants such as cyclophosphamide (Vecchi *et al.*, 1976; Giampietri *et al.*, 1978). In the same species, DTIC treatments were also incapable of synergizing with T-cell-mediated host reactivity in effecting the rejection of leukemia cells incompatible for multiple minor histocompatibility loci (Riccardi *et al.*, 1980). In addition, spleen cells obtained from drug-treated mice were incapable of mounting a graft-versus-host reaction (GVHR) when infused in allogeneic recipients and were incapable of generating cytotoxic T cells *in vitro*. On the other hand, DTIC treatment of an already ongoing GVHR was ineffective (Giampietri *et al.*, 1978). Although these findings may be taken to suggest that effector T cells may be relatively insensitive to the drug whereas the precursors of these elements would be susceptible, more direct information is needed before conclusions can be reached on the existence of a differential susceptibility to DTIC among the various T-cell subsets. When administered *in vivo* this drug has also been shown to depress the spontaneous or Bacillus-Calmette-Guerin-stimulated cytolytic capacity *vis-à-vis* tumor target cells of murine macrophages (Mantovani *et al.*, 1980). Conversely, at otherwise potently immunodepressive doses, DTIC did not significantly reduce on a unit cell number basis NK-mediated cytotoxicity (Mantovani *et al.*, 1978) and did not reduce the localized resistance expressed by certain lymphoid organs (e.g., spleen) against Hh-incompatible cells of hematopoietic origin, a reactivity believed not to be mediated by T cells but rather by elements having close functional resemblance with NK effectors (Bonmasser *et al.*, 1980).

Information on the immunopharmacological activity of DTIC in man is at present extremely limited, with contrasting findings between groups as well as with the animal data. In the first study, a depression of humoral antibody production was seen in cancer patients given DTIC doses as low as 150–450 mg/m^2 (Cheema *et al.*, 1970). Conversely, another group has reported that total doses of 750–1250 mg/m^2 depressed the responsiveness to typhoid vaccine and the expression of cutaneous hypersensitivity to primary sensitization in only a minority of melanoma patients, thus leading these investigators to conclude that DTIC was only moderately or not immunodepressive (Bruckner *et al.*, 1974). In support of this contention, the same group observed no decline in lymphocyte-mediated cytotoxicity against allogeneic or autologous melanoma target cells after 2–3 courses with DTIC at 150–250 mg/m^2 per day for 5 days at 3-week intervals, concomitant with no impairment in delayed cutaneous hypersensitivity to recall stimuli (Mitchell *et al.*, 1977). Although it cannot be excluded that, for reasons yet unknown, important species differences may exist in the immunosuppressive activity of DTIC, considering the demonstration of a marked and prolonged activity in rodents and the paucity of human data, it appears reasonable to withhold judgment on the nonimmunodepressive capacity of DTIC in men until further tests are conducted.

If thus many important aspects of the direct effects of DTIC on immune cells are still largely unknown, better documented is its capacity to modify tumor cell immunogenicity in experimental systems. Essentially, it has been found that poorly or nonimmunogenic, drug-resistant lymphoma cells recovered from DTIC-treated mice do not give rise to progressive tumors when retransplanted into normal immunocompetent syngeneic hosts in which a state of strong and long-lasting resistance is induced against the DTIC-treated cells as well as against the parental untreated tumor. On the other hand, lethal growths are seen when the same cells are transplanted in previously immunodepressed hosts, a finding that also indicates that the proliferative capacity of the drug-treated cells is not reduced (Bonmasser *et al.*, 1970; Bonmasser *et al.*, 1979; Nicolin *et al.*, 1976). Although relative long *in vivo* treatments with the drug are generally required to observe strong increases in immunogenicity (such that up to 10^7 DTIC-modified cells are rejected, whereas 1–10 cells of the nonexposed tumor will produce lethal growths, i.e., the immunogenic strength of these drug-modified elements is quantitatively comparable to that associated with products of the major histocompatibility complex), it is of note that detectable changes in tumor cell antigenicity can also be seen after single DTIC courses, and it has recently been reported that *in vitro* exposures to "activated" DTIC can also be effective in modifying tumor cell antigenic make up in such a way as to induce protective immunity into syngeneic hosts (Contessa *et al.*, 1979). Once induced, the increased immunogenicity detectable after DTIC exposure in leukemia and lymphoma cells (so far no data are available on the inducibility of such a modified immunogenicity in solid rodent neoplasms) is a stable and inheritable property of the tumor cells (i.e., maintained long after withdrawal of drug treatment), that thus become capable of evoking both *in vivo* and *in vitro* strong humoral and especially cell-mediated reactivities in which T lymphocytes, K cells, and macrophages appear to be the main effectors (Marelli *et al.*, 1982; Nicolin *et al.*, 1974; Riccardi *et al.*, 1978). On the other hand, DTIC-treated tumor cells have been shown to be less susceptible to NK lysis (Romani *et al.*, 1983), and effect not caused by a change in intrinsic susceptibility to NK- or T-cell-mediated damage but rather by lowered capacity of these cells to bind to NK effectors, presumably resulting from the alterations of cell surface components produced by the drug. Indirect and direct evidence has in fact been gathered consistent with the conclusion that this compound, while not affecting the expression of the normal histocompatibility antigens (Taramelli *et al.*, 1981), induces in tumor cells novel antigenic specificities not detectable in elements of the parental line, which are in general not cross-reactive between different sublines of the same tumor and whose nature is still unresolved. With regard to the mechanism sustaining this modified tumor antigenicity following DTIC exposure, several lines of evidence rule out the possibilities that the drug may act as a hapten, that it may activate a latent virus thus enabling the expression of virus-coded antigens, and that the strong immunodepressive activity of DTIC in mice (responsible for the fact that animals from which drug-resistant tumor cells possessing strong drug-induced neoantigens nevertheless die of progressive tumor growth) allows the emergence of immunogenic clones spontaneously present in the untreated neoplasm (Bonmasser *et al.*, 1979). Although direct evidence is still lacking, the most plausible mechanism is that the drug induces somatic mutations in cancer cells, with subsequent modifications in the structure of the cell membrane ultimately resulting in the expression of novel antigens. Also in support of such a mechanism are the findings that *in vitro* exposure of tumor cells to powerful mutagens can result in the appearance of highly immunogenic clonal sublines capable of growing in immunodepressed but not in intact syngeneic hosts (Boon and Kellerman,

1977), and that the capacity of DTIC to modify tumor antigenicity is reduced by quinacrine, a compound well known for its ability to reduce mutations in bacteria and mammalian cells (Giampietri *et al.*, 1980). No data are available at present on the capacity of DTIC to modify the antigenicity of human tumor cells.

6. NITROSOUREAS

Nitrosoureas (NUs) represent an important class of antitumor agents broadly employed clinically, especially in combination with other cancer chemotherapeutic agents, in the treatment of a variety of frequent human malignancies (Carter, 1981). In spite of this extended use, limited data are available on their immunological effects in both animals and man not only for the more recently developed analogs but also regarding compounds [i.e., 1,3-*bis*(2-chloroethyl)-1-nitrosourea (BCNU); 1-(2-chloroethyl)-3-cyclohexil-1-nitrosourea (CCNU); and 1-(2-chloroethyl)-3-(*trans*-4-methylcyclohexyl)-1-nitrosourea (MeCCNU)] that have been clinically employed for over a decade.

In mice, single BCNU doses were very active in decreasing humoral antibody formation to primary and secondary stimuli, whereas MeCCNU was somewhat less effective in this regard when employed at doses having comparable antineoplastic activity (Ghaffar *et al.*, 1978). At least in part this effect is sustained also by direct effects on B lymphocytes; results obtained using a T-independent antigen support the view that both resting and stimulated B cells are sensitive to these agents (Ghaffar *et al.*, 1981). Interestingly, it has been reported that B lymphocytes are more sensitive to BCNU than to MeCCNU (Ghaffar *et al.*, 1981). A decreased number of antibody-producing cells after primary sensitization with T-dependent antigens has also been observed in mice given single doses of other NUs, including CCNU, 2-[(chloro-2-ethyl)-3-nitrosureido]-D-glucopyranose (chlorozoticin), 1-(2-OH-ethyl)-3-(2-chloroethyl)-3-nitrosourea (HECNU), (chloro-2-ethyl)-1-(ribofuranosyl-iso-propylidene-2′,3′-*p*-nitrobenzoate-5′)-3-nitrosourea (RFCNU), and (chloro-2-ethyl)-1-(ribopyranosyl triacetate-2′,3′,4′)-3-nitrosourea (RFPCNU) (Spreafico *et al.*, 1981; Imbach *et al.*, 1975). Although on a mg/kg basis the degree of inhibition varied greatly between these compounds, at variance with the alleged differential potency of BCNU and MeCCNU, when the ED_{50} for antibody inhibition for these compounds was related to their optimal antileukemic dose, it was found that these agents were comparably effective in inducing this type of immune effect, whose severity did not correlate with the capacity of these drugs to reduce the number of bone marrow stem cells. NUs have also been found to reduce the capacity of mice to reject H-2-incompatible tumor grafts, with no substantial differences in potency being observable when classical NUs (e.g., BCNU and MeCCNU) and more recent derivatives such as HECNU and chlorozoticin are compared. (Spreafico *et al.*, 1981). However, the finding is noteworthy that, whereas the level of antineoplastic effectiveness of HECNU and chlorozoticin was comparable on sublines of murine leukemias of high and low immunogenicity, both BCNU and MeCCNU were clearly more effective in mice transplanted with the immunogenic sublines (Spreafico *et al.*, 1981), suggesting that at antitumor-effective doses in mice the immunological activity of these agents does not prevent the development of antitumor reactivity, which can thus synergize with their direct cytotoxic effect on malignant elements. Similar conclusions have been reached in other murine models (Riccardi *et al.*, 1980). BCNU and MeCCNU treatment of mice has also been shown to reduce lymphoid cell responsiveness to T and B mitogens (Ghaffar *et al.*, 1978) and a similar capacity has more recently been described for the newer sugar derivatives chlorozoticin, RPCNU, and RFCNU (Florentin *et al.*, 1983). Interestingly, maximal depression of responsiveness to PHA and Con A was seen in spleen cells 1 day after RFCNU injection, whereas it was on day 4 for chlorozoticin and on day 14 for RPCNU. Responsiveness to the B mitogen LPS was less impaired than that to T stimulants and the nadir was on day 14 for all compounds. In contrast to the inability of drug posttreatments to significantly modify delayed-type hypersensitivity, a definite increase in the expression of this reactivity was observed if mice were treated before sensitization with BCNU, MeCCNU, RPCNU, RFCNU, or chlorozoticin (Ghaffar *et al.*, 1978; Florentin *et al.*, 1983), with BCNU and MeCCNU being equally effective in this regard (Ghaffar *et al.*, 1978). Although the mechanism of this effect has not been investigated, it should be mentioned that BCNU has been found to affect T suppressor cells in the same species (Paul *et al.*, 1982). Although the data available are far from being conclusive on this point and it is possible that different analogs may quantitatively vary in this activity, it has been suggested that the progenitors of T suppressors may be sensitive to NUs whereas already developed effectors may be more resistant (Paul *et al.*, 1982).

Fragmentary information also exists with regard to NUs' effects on other immune cells in animals. The compound 1-(4-NH$_2$-2 methyl-5-pyrimidyl)-methyl-3-(2-chloroethyl)-3-NU (ACNU) has been reported (Saijo *et al.*, 1980) to reduce the number and the spontaneous cytotoxic activity of normal rat macrophages; however, the drug was without effects on the cytostatic capacity of BCG-stimulated macrophages obtained from normal or tumor-bearing hosts. The cytostatic activity of murine macrophages obtained after RPCNU, RFCNU, and chlorozoticin injection has also been found to be increased up to 14 days after treatment, and a similar increase was seen for macrophage phagocytosis. Chlorozoticin, but not RPCNU, RFCNU, BCNU, and MeCCNU, was additionally capable of enhancing 2- to 3-fold antibody-dependent cytotoxicity in mice at least when assessed against antibody-coated erythrocytes (Ghaffar *et al.*, 1978; Florentin *et al.*, 1983). At variance, single chlorozoticin injections reduced spleen NK activity (Florentin *et al.*, 1983), but no data on this activity exists for other NUs. These compounds have also been reported to affect target cell sensitivity to immune damage: the sensitivity of BCNU-pretreated tumor cells to macrophage-mediated cytotoxicity has in fact been shown to be increased (Nathan *et al.*, 1980) and a similar finding has been obtained for T-cell-mediated cytolysis (Hunyadi *et al.*, 1981). Although this effect has been ascribed to a drug-induced inhibition of the glutathione-redox cycle and tranglutaminase dependent on the carbamoylating activity of NUs, other mechanisms cannot be excluded as participating in this NU-increased immunosensitivity of tumor cells.

With regard to the immunological effects of NUs on human cells, RFCNU, RPCNU, and CCNU have been shown to variably affect lymphocyte responsiveness to PHA, Con A, and pokeweed mitogen when added *in vitro* at culture initiation (Levallois *et al.*, 1981). In general, an increase in blastogenesis was seen with pokeweed mitogen, whereas this facilitation was observed in only half of the subjects when PHA was used as mitogen, and inhibition was consistently obtained with Con A. These results led to the hypothesis of a selective toxicity for a suppressor cell population, but no data in support of this view are available. Decreases in PHA responsiveness have been seen up to 6 weeks after a single oral CCNU dose of 130 mg/m^2 in patients with multiple sclerosis (Shih *et al.*, 1983). This effect was seen in the absence of significant changes in the relative proportions of T and B cells and in NK activity, whereas this regimen was clearly capable of decreasing total white blood cell and lymphocyte counts in the periphery as well as immunoglobulin synthesis within the CNS.

7. CONCLUDING REMARKS

A number of points deserve brief comment because of their more general relevance that has emerged from the preceding discussion. In the first place, the compounds considered herein reinforce the conclusion (Spreafico *et al.*, 1982) that cancer chemotherapeutic agents are immunopharmacologically very heterogenous. Differences in immunological profiles can in fact be detected among chemically analogous compounds and also among drugs believed to exert their antiproliferative effect on transformed cells through similar if not identical biochemical mechanisms, although the mechanisms sustaining these complex differentials are at present in most cases unknown (Spreafico *et al.*, 1983). In this context, however, a growing body of evidence is in favor of the possibility that at least a number of the immune effects induced by these agents are not dependent on inhibition of immune cell proliferation but on more discrete functional effects. Second, although frequently fragmentary, the data discussed in the preceding section are in support of the contention that the immunological activity of anticancer chemicals should not be viewed solely under the optics of immunodepression, since at least a number of these compounds acting directly on immunocytes and/or on tumor cells (e.g., modifying their immunogenicity or immunosusceptibility) can modulate host reactivity toward neoplasms in complex ways. In view of the fact that the characteristics of their interaction with host immunity can be an important if not critical determinant of the antineoplastic effectiveness of a substantial number of clinically important antitumor agents (Spreafico and Mantovani, 1981), more extensive efforts in investigating both the phenomenological and mechanistic aspects of the immunopharmacology of cancer chemotherapeutic agents appear warranted toward the aim of gaining a better knowledge of their multifaceted mode of action, which in turn could lead to a better use of these drugs.

ACKNOWLEDGMENTS. This work was supported by Progetto Finalizzato Controllo della Crescita Neoplastica, CNR Contract No. 83.00973.96, and by a grant from Associazione Italiana Ricerche sul Cancro.

REFERENCES

Aisenberg, A. C., and Wilkes, B., 1967, Immunological tolerance induced by cyclophosphamide assayed by plaque spleen cell method, *Nature* **213**:498–499.

Antoine, J. C., Maurice, M., Feldmann, G., and Avrameas, S., 1980, *In vivo* and *in vitro* effects of colchicine and vinblastine on the secretory process of antibody-producing cells, *J. Immunol.* **125**:1939–1949.

Ballet, J. J., Insel, R., Merler, E., and Rosen, F. S., 1976, Inhibition of maturation of human precursor lymphocytes by coformycin, and inhibitor of the enzyme adenosine deaminase, *J. Exp. Med.* **143**:1271–1276.

Bartocci, A., Riccardi, C., and Bonmassar, E., 1980, *In vivo* or *in vitro* modulating effects of vincristine on the generation of allogeneic cytotoxic lymphocytes *in vitro, J. Immunopharmacol.* **2**:61–72.

Barton, R., Martiniuk, F., Hirschhorn, R., and Goldschneider, I., 1979, The distribution of adenosine deaminase among lymphocyte populations in the rat, *J. Immunol.* **122**:216–220.

Benjamin, R. S., Plunkett, W., Keating, M. J., Feun, L. C., Hug, V., Nelson, J. A., Boley, G. P., and Freireich, E. J., 1980, Phase 1 and biochemical pharmacological studies of deoxycoformycin, *Proc. Am. Assoc. Cancer Res.* **21**:337.

Berenbaum, M. C., 1971, Immunosuppression by platinum diamines, *Br. J. Cancer* **25**:208–211.

Berlin, R. D., and Fera, J. P., 1977, Changes in membrane microviscosity associated with phagocytosis: Effects of colchicine, *Proc. Natl. Acad. Sci. USA* **74**:1072–1076.

Bodel, P., 1976, Colchicine stimulation of pyrogen production by human blood leukocytes, *J. Exp. Med.* **143**:1015–1026.

Bolivar, R., Kohl, S., Pickering, L. K., and Walters, D. L., 1980, Effect of antineoplastic drugs on human leukocyte-mediated cytotoxicity against herpes simplex virus infected cells, *Cancer* **46**:1555–1561.

Bonmassar, E., Bonmassar, A., Vadlamudi, S., and Goldin, A., 1970, Immunologic alteration of leukemia cells in vivo after treatment with antitumor drugs, *Proc. Natl. Acad. Sci. USA* **66**:1089–1095.

Bonmassar, E., Fioretti, M. C., Nicolin, A., and Spreafico, F., 1979, Drug-induced modifications of tumor cell antigenicity, in: *Tumor-Associated Antigens and Their Specific Immune Response* (F. Spreafico and R. Arnon, eds.), Academic Press, New York, pp. 251–270.

Bonmassar, A., Riccardi, C., Rivosecchi-Merletti, P., Goldin, A., and Bonmassar, E., 1980, Transplantation resistance of drug-treated hybrid or allogeneic mice against murine lymphomas. I. Immunopharmacology studies, *Int. J. Cancer* **26**:819–829.

Boon, T., and Kellerman, O., 1977, Rejection by syngeneic mice of cell variants obtained by mutagenesis of a malignant teratocarcinoma cell line, *Proc. Natl. Acad. Sci. USA* **74**:272–275.

Borel, J.-F., 1976, Comparative study of *in vitro* and *in vivo* drug effects on cell mediated cytotoxicity, *Immunology* **31**:631–641.

Brambilla, G., Cavanna, M., and Maura, A., 1974, Effect of cis-diammine-dichloroplatinum (NSC-119875) on the allograft reaction in mice, *Cancer Chemother. Rep.* **58**:633–636.

Bruckner, H. W., Birnbaum Mokyr, M., and Mitchell, M. S., 1974, Effect of imidazole-4-carboxamide, 5-(3,3-dimethyl-1-triazeno) on immunity in patients with malignant melanoma, *Cancer Res.* **34**:181–183.

Burridge, P. W., Paetkau, V., and Henderson, J. F., 1977, Studies of the relationship between adenosine deaminase and immune function, *J. Immunol.* **119**:675–678.

Carson, D. A., and Seegmiller, J. E., 1976, Effect of adenosine deaminase inhibition upon human lymphocyte blastogenesis, *J. Clin. Invest* **57**:274–282.

Carson, D. A., Lakow, E., Wasson, D. B., and Kamatani, N., 1981, Lymphocyte dysfunction caused by deficiencies in purine metabolism, *Immunol. Today* **2**:234–238.

Carter, S. K., 1981, Design of clinical trials with nitrosourea, in: *Nitrosourea: Current Status and New Developments* (A. W. Prestayko, L. H. Baker, S. T. Crooke, S. K. Carter, and P. S. Schein, eds.), Academic Press, New York, pp. 411–416.

Cheema, A. R., Ohno, R., and Hersch, E. M., 1970, Immunosuppression studies in man and mice, *Abstracts X International Cancer Congress*, Houston, Texas, p. 189 (Abstract 304).

Contessa, A. R., Giampietri, A., Bonmassar, A., and Goldin, A., 1979, Increased immunogenicity of L1210 leukemia following short term exposure to DTIC in vivo or in vitro, *Cancer Immunol. Immunother.* **7**:71–76.

Cooper, M. D., Faulk, W. P., Fudemberg, H. H., Good, R. A., Hitzig, W., Kunkel, H., Rosen, F. S., Seligmann, M., Soothill, J., and Wedgwood, R. J., 1973, Classification of primary immunodeficiencies, *N. Engl. J. Med.* **288**:966–967.

De Conti, R. C., Toftn-ss, B. R., Lange, R. C., and Creasey, W. A., 1973, Clinical and pharmacological studies with cis-diamminedichloroplatinum (II), *Cancer Res.* **33**:1310–1315.

De Vecchis, L., Pastore, S., Migliorati, G., Giuliani, A., and Frati, L., 1982, Amplification of natural killer activity of mouse lymphocytes by vincristine, *Int. J. Tissue Reaction* **4**:283–289.

Edelman, G. M., Yahara, I., and Wang, J. L., 1973, Receptor mobility and receptor–cytoplasmic interactions in lymphocytes, *Proc. Natl. Acad. Sci. USA* **70**:1442–1446.

Ercolani, L., and Schulte, W. E., 1983, Metabolic and morphologic effects of colchicine on human T-lymphocyte expression of Fcu and Fc receptors, *Cell. Immunol.* **77**:222–232.

Florentin, I., Hayat, M., Kiger, N., Mathé, G., Maral, J., and Imbach, J. L., 1983, Comparative analysis of the immunopharmacological properties of three new nitrosourea analogues: RPCNU, RFCNU and chlorozotocin, *Int. J. Immunopharmacol.* **5**:201–210.

Gemsa, D., Kramer, W., Brenner, M., Till, G., and Resch, K., 1980, Induction of prostaglandin E release from macrophages by colchicine, *J. Immunol.* **124**:376–380.

Ghaffar, A., Lichter, W., Wellham, L. L., and Sigel, M. M., 1978, Effect of anticancer chemotherapeutic agents on immune reactions of mice. I. Comparison of two nitrosoureas: 1,3-bis(2-chloroethyl)-1-nitrosourea and 1-(2-chloroethyl)-3-(4-methylcyclohexyl)-1-nitrosourea, *J. Natl. Cancer Inst.* **60**:1483–1487.

Ghaffar, A., Paul, R. D., Lichter, W., Wellham, L. L., and Sigel, M. M., 1981, Selective action of alkylating agents on helper and suppressor functions, in: *Biological Relevance of Immune Suppression as Induced by Genetic, Therapeutic and Environmental Factors* (J. H. Dean and M. Paradathsingh, eds.), Van Nostrand Reinhold, New York, pp. 210–225.

Giampietri, A., Bonmassar, E., and Goldin, A., 1978, Drug induced modulation of immune responses in mice: Effects of 5-(3,3-dimethyl-1-triazeno)-imidazole-4-carboxamide (DTIC) and cyclophosphamide (CY), *J. Immunopharmacol.* **1**:61–86.

Giampietri, A., Fioretti, M. C., Goldin, A., and Bonmassar, E., 1980, Drug-mediated antigenic changes in murine leukemia cells: Antagonistic effects of quinacrine, an antimutagenic compound, *J. Natl. Cancer Inst.* **64**:297–301.

Glazer, R. I., 1980, Adenosine deaminase inhibitors: Their role in chemotherapy and immunosuppression, *Cancer Chemother. Pharmacol.* **4**:227–235.

Hall, D. J., O'Leary, J. J., and Rosenberg, A., 1982, Commitment and proliferation kinetics of human lymphocytes stimulated in vitro: Effects of colchicine on mitogen response, *J. Cell. Physiol.* **112**:157–161.

Hersh, E. M., 1974, Immunosuppressive agents, in: *Antineoplastic and Immunosuppressive Agents* (A. C. Sartorelli and D. G. Johns, eds.), Springer-Verlag, Berlin, pp. 577–617.

Hirschhorn, R., and Sela, E., 1977, Adenosine deaminase and immunodeficiency: An *in vitro* model, *Cell. Immunol.* **32**:350–360.

Howle, J. A., Thompson, H. S., Stone, A. E., and Gale, G. R., 1971, Cis-dichlorodiammineplatinum(II): Inhibition of nucleic acid synthesis in lymphocytes stimulated with phytohemagglutinin, *Proc. Soc. Exp. Biol. Med.* **137**:820–825.

Hunyadi, J., Szegedi, G., Szabo, T., Ahmed, A., and Laki, K., 1981, Increased cytotoxic sensitivity of YPC-1 tumor cells from mice treated with nitrosoureas, *Cancer Res.* **41**:1677–1681.

Imbach, J. L., Montero, J. L., Moruzzi, A., Serrou, B., Chenu, E., Hayat, M., and Mathé, G., 1975, The oncostatic and immunosuppressive action of new nitrosourea derivatives containing sugar radicals, *Biomedicine* **23**:410–413.

Keller, R., 1974, Mechanisms by which activated normal macrophages destroy syngeneic rat tumour cells "in vitro," *Immunology* **27**:285–298.

Khan, A., and Hill, J. M., 1971, Immunosuppression with cis-platinum (II) diamminodichloride: Effect on antibody plaque-forming spleen cells, *Infect. Immun.* **4**:320–321.

Khan, A., and Hill, J. M., 1972, Suppression of graft-versus-host reaction by cis-platinum (II) diaminodichloride, *Transplantation* **13**:55–57.

Khan, A., and Hill, J. M., 1973, Suppression of lymphocyte blastogenesis in man following cis-platinous diamminodichloride administration, *Proc. Soc. Exp. Biol. Med.* **142**:324–326.

Khan, A., Albayrak, A., and Hill, J. M., 1972, Effect of cis-platinous diamminodichloride on graft rejection: Prolonged survival of skin grafts against H_2-histocompatibility, *Proc. Soc. Exp. Biol. Med.* **141**:7–9.

Kitano, M., Mihich, E., and Pressman, D., 1971, Antigenic differences between L1210 and a subline resistant to methyl-glyoxal-bis-guanylhydrazone, *Proc. Am. Assoc. Cancer Res.* **12**:30.

Kleinerman, E. S., and Zwelling, L. A., 1982, The effect of cis-diammino-dichloroplatinum(II) on immune function *in vitro* and *in vivo*, *Cancer Immunol. Immunother.* **12**:191–196.

Kleinerman, E. S., Zwelling, L. A., Howser, D., Barlock, A., Young, R. C., Decker, J. M., Bull, J., and Muchmore, A. V., 1980a, Defective monocyte killing in patients with malignancies and restoration of function during chemotherapy, *Lancet* **2**:1102–1104.

Kleinerman, E. S., Zwelling, L. A., and Muchmore, A. V., 1980b, Enhancement of naturally occurring human spontaneous monocyte-mediated cytotoxicity by cis-diamminedichloroplatinum (II), *Cancer Res.* **40**:3099–3102.

Kobayashi, H., 1978, Xenogenization of tumor cells, *Gann Monogr. Cancer Res.* **21**:21–35.

Kociba, R. J., Sleight, S. D., and Rosenberg, B., 1970, Inhibition of Dunning ascitic leukemia and Walker 256 carcinoma with cis-diamminedichloroplatinum (II), *Cancer Chemother. Rep.* **54**:325–328.

Lehrer, R. I., 1973, Effects of colchicine and chloramphenicol on the oxidative metabolism and phagocytic activity on human neutrophils, *J. Infect. Dis.* **127**:40–48.

Levallois, C., Mani, J. C., Montero, J. L., Oiry, J., and Imbach, J. L., 1981, Action of three nitrosourea on human lymphocytes: Hypothesis of a specific effect on lymphocyte subpopulations, *Farmaco Ed. Sci.* **36**:947–956.

Lum, C. T., Sutherland, D. E. R., Eckhardt, J., Matas, A. J., and Najarian, J. S., 1979, Effect of an adenosine deaminase inhibitor on survival of mouse pancreatic islet allografts, *Transplantation* **27**:355–357.

Mally, M. B., Taylor, R. C., and Callewaert, D. M., 1980, Effects of platinum antitumor agents on *in vitro* assays of human antitumor immunity. II. Effects of cis-Pt$(NH_3)_2Cl_2$ on spontaneous cell-mediated cytotoxicity, *Chemotherapy* **26**:1–6.

Mantovani, A., Luini, W., Peri, G., Vecchi, A., and Spreafico, F., 1978, Effect of chemotherapeutic agents on natural cell-mediated cytotoxicity in mice, *J. Natl. Cancer Inst.* **61**:1255–1261.

Mantovani, A., Luini, W., Candiani, G. P., and Spreafico, F., 1980, Effect of chemotherapeutic agents on natural and BCG-stimulated macrophage cytotoxicity in mice, *Int. J. Immunopharmacol.* **2**:333–339.

Marelli, O., Mantovani, A., Franco, P., and Nicolin, A., 1982, Macrophage antitumor activity induced by the antigenic lymphoma L5178Y/DTIC subline, *Tumori* **68**:365–371.

Martin, F., Olsson, N. O., and Jeannin, J.-F., 1981, Effect of four agents that modify microtubules and microfilaments (vinblastine, colchicine, lidocaine, and cytochalasin B) on macrophage-mediated cytotoxicity to tumor cells, *Cancer Immunol. Immuother.* **10**:   –119.

Medgyesi, G. A., Foris, G., Deszö, B., Gergeby, J., and Bazin, H., 198   receptors of rat peritoneal macrophages immunoglobulin class specificity and sensitiv   y to drugs affecting the microfilament or microtubule system, *Immunology* **40**:317–323.

Mihich, E., 1969, Modification of tumor regression by immunological means, *Cancer Res.* **29**:2345–2350.

Mitchell, M. S., Birnbaum Mokyr, M., and Merrill Davis, J., 1977, Effect of chemotherapy and immunotherapy on tumor-specific immunity in melanoma, *J. Clin. Invest.* **59**:1017–1026.

Nathan, C. F., Arrick, B. A., Murray, H. W., De Santis, N. M., and Cohn, Z. A., 1980, Tumor cell anti-oxidant defences: Inhibition of the glutathione redox cycle enhances macrophage-mediated cytolysis, *J. Exp. Med.* **153**:766–782.

Nicolin, A., Bini, A., and Coronetti, E., 1974, Cellular immune response to a drug-treated L5178Y lymphoma subline, *Nature* **251**:654–655.

Nicolin, A., Spreafico, F., Bonmassar, A., and Goldin, A., 1976, Antigenic changes of L5178Y lymphoma after treatment with DTIC in vivo, *J. Natl. Cancer Inst.* **56**:89–93.

Ohnuma, T., Arkin, H., Minowada, J., and Holland, J. F., 1978, Differential chemotherapeutic susceptibility of human T-lymphocytes and B-lymphocytes in culture, *J. Natl. Cancer Inst.* **60**:749–752.

Page, R. H., Talley, R. M., and Livermore, D. H., 1977, The effect of cis-diamminodichloroplatinum and cyclophosphamide on immune response and tumor rejection in Balb/c and PL/JAX mice, *J. Clin. Hematol. Oncol.* **7**:105–113.

Paul, R. D., Ghaffar, A., and Sigel, M. M., 1982, Selective action of alkylating agents against cells participating in suppression of antibody responses, *Int. J. Immunopharmacol.* **4**:159–166.

Pesanti, E. L., and Axline, S. G., 1975, Colchicine effects on lysosomal enzyme induction and intracellular degradation in the cultivated macrophage, *J. Exp. Med.* **141**:1030–1046.

Pick, E., 1979, Mechanism of action of migration inhibitory lymphokines, in: *Biology of Lymphokines* (S. Cohen, E. Pick, and J. J. Oppenheim, eds.), Academic Press, New York, pp. 60–116.

Pick, E., and Abrahamer, H., 1973, Blocking of macrophage migration inhibitory factor action by microtubular disruptive drugs. *Int. Arch. Allergy Appl. Immunol.* **44**:215–220.

Pier, G. B., and Markham, R. B., 1982, Induction in mice of cell-mediated immunity to *Pseudomonas aeruginosa* by high molecular weight polysaccharide and vinblastine, *J. Immunol.* **128**:2121–2125.

Ralph, P., and Nakoinz, I., 1982, Augmentation of macrophage antibody-dependent killing of tumor targets by microtubule inhibitors, *Cell. Immunol.* **70**:321–329.

Resch, K., Bouillon, D., Gemsa, D., and Averdunk, R., 1977, Drugs which disrupt microtubules do not inhibit the initiation of lymphocyte activation, *Nature* **265**:349–351.

Retsas, S., Thomas, C., and Hobbs, J. R., 1981, The effect of Vindesine therapy on the *in vitro* immune response of patients with advanced malignant melanoma, *Clin. Oncol.* **7**:33–37.

Riccardi, C., Fioretti, M. C., Giampietri, A., Puccetti, P., and Goldin, A., 1978, Growth and rejection patterns of murine lymphoma cells antigenically altered following drug treatment in vivo, *Transplantation* **25**:63–68.

Riccardi, C., Bartocci, A., Puccetti, P., Spreafico, F., Bonmassar, E., and Goldin, A., 1980, Combined effects of antineoplastic agents and antilymphoma allograft reactions, *Eur. J. Cancer* **16**:23–33.

Romani, L., Migliorati, G., Bonmassar, E., Fioretti, M. C., 1983, Susceptibility of murine lymphoma cells treated with 5-(3,3-dimethyl-1-triazenyl)-1H-imidazole-4-carboxamide to NK-mediated cytotoxicity *in vitro*, *Int. J. Immunopharmacol.* **5**:299–306.

Rosenberg, B., 1975, Possible mechanisms for the antitumor activity of platinum coordination complexes, *Cancer Chemother. Rep.* **59**:589–598.

Rudolph, S. A., Greengard, P., and Malawista, S., 1977, Effects of colchicine on cyclic AMP levels in human leukocytes, *Proc. Natl. Acad. Sci.* **74**:3404–3408.

Ryoyama, K., Mace, K., Ehrke, M. J., and Mihich, E., 1982, The differential sensitivity of T cell immune functions to vincristine and vinblastine, *Int. J. Immunopharmacol.* **4**:187–194.

Saijo, N., Irimajiri, N., Ozaki, A., Shimizu, E., and Niitani, H., 1980, Effects of BCG and 1-(4-amino-2-methyl-5-pyrimidinyl)-methyl-3-(2-chloro-ethyl)-3-nitrosourea hydrochloride (ACNU) on cytostatic activity of macrophages in normal and tumour-bearing rats, *Br. J. Cancer* **42:**

Santos, G. W., Owens, A. H., Jr., and Sensenbrenner, L. L., 1964, Effects of selected cytotoxic agents on antibody production in man: A preliminary report, *Ann. N.Y. Acad. Sci.* **114:**404–423.

Sarna, S., and Sodhi, A., 1978, Chemoimmunotherapeutic studies on a fibrosarcoma with cis-diamminedichloroplatinum(II), *Ind. J. Exp. Biol.* **16:**1236–1239.

Schlaefli, E., Ehrke, M. J., and Mihich, E., 1983, The effects of dichloro-trans-dihydroxy-bis-isopropyl-amine-platinum IV on the primary cell-mediated cytotoxic response, *Immuno-pharmacology* **6:**107–122.

Seeger, R. C., Robins, R. A., Stevens, R. H., Klein, R. B., Waldman, D. J., Zelber, P. N., and Kessler, S. W., 1976, Severe combined immunodeficiency with B lymphocytes: In vitro correction of defective immunoglobulin production by addition of normal T lymphocytes, *Clin. Exp. Immunol.* **26:**1–10.

Sharma, S. D., and Piessens, W. F., 1978, Tumor cell killing by macrophages activated *in vitro* with lymphocyte mediators, *Cell. Immunol.* **38:**276–285.

Shek, P. N., and Coons, A. H., 1977, Effect of colchicine on the antibody response. I. Enhancement of antibody formation in mice, *J. Exp. Med.* **147:**1213–1227.

Shek, P. N., Waltenbaugh, C., and Coons, A. H., 1977, Effect of colchicine on the antibody response. II. Demonstration of the inactivation of suppressor cell activities by colchicine, *J. Exp. Med.* **147:**1228–1235.

Shih, W. W. H., Baumhefner, R. W., Tourtellotte, W. W., Haskell, C. M., Korn, E. L., and Fahey, J. L., 1983, Difference in effect of single immunosuppressive agents (cyclophosphamide, CCNU, 5-FU) on peripheral blood immune cell parameters and central nervous system immunoglobulin synthesis rate in patients with multiple sclerosis, *Clin. Exp. Immunol.* **53:**122–132.

Simmonds, H. A., Panayi, G. S., and Corrigall, V., 1978, A role for purine metabolism in the immune response: Adenosine-deaminase activity and deoxyadenosine catabolism, *Lancet* **1:**60–63.

Sodhi, A., and Aggarwal, S. K., 1974, Effects of cis-dichlorodiammine platinum (II) in the regression of sarcoma 1980: A fine structural study, *J. Natl. Cancer Inst.* **53:**85–101.

Sordillo, E. M., Ikehara, S., Good, R. A., and Trotta, P. P., 1981, Immunosuppression by 2'-deoxycoformycin: Studies on the mode of administration, *Cell. Immunol.* **63:**259–271.

Spreafico, F., and Mantovani, A., 1981, Immunomodulation by cancer chemotherapeutic agents and antineoplastic activity, in: *Pathobiology Annual* (H. L. Ioachim, ed.), Raven Press, New York, pp. 177–196.

Spreafico, F., Filippeschi, S., Falautano, P., Eisenbrand, G., Fiebig, H. H., Habs, M., Zeller, V., Berger, M., Schmähl, D., Van Putten, L. M., Smink, T., Csany, E., and Somfai-Relle, S., 1981, EORTC studies with novel nitrosoureas, in: *Nitrosoureas: Current Status and Developments* (A. W. Prestayko, L. H. Baker, S. T. Crooke, S. K. Carter, and P. S. Schein, eds.), Academic Press, New York, pp. 27–42.

Spreafico, F., Tagliabue, A., and Vecchi, A., 1982, Chemical immunodepressants, in: *Immunopharmacology* (P. Sirois, ed.), Elsevier, New York, pp. 315–347.

Spreafico, F., Alberti, S., Allegrucci, M., Canegrati, A., Colotta, F., Luini, W., Merendino, A., Pasqualetto, E., Romano, M., Sironi, M., and Vecchi, A., 1983, On the mode of action of immunodepressive agents, in: *Advances in Immunopharmacology 2* (J. W. Hadden, L. Chedid, P. DuKor, F. Spreafico, and D. Willoughby, eds.), Pergamon Press, New York, pp. 745–752.

Steen, H. B., and Lindmo, T., 1978, The effect of colchicine and colcemid on the mitogen induced blastogenesis of lymphocytes, *Eur. J. Immunol.* **8:**667–671.

Stenzil, K. H., Schwartz, R., Rubin, A. L., and Novogrodsky, A., 1978, Potentiation of lymphocyte activation by colchicine, *J. Immunol.* **121:**863–865.

Stosic-Grujicic, and Simic, M. M., 1982, Modulation of interleukin 1 production by activated macrophages: *In vitro* action of hydrocortisone, colchicine, and cytochalasin B, *Cell. Immunol.* **69**:235–247.

Sullivan, J. L., Osborn, W. R. A., and Wedgewood, R. J., 1977, Adenosine deaminase activity in lymphocytes, *Br. J. Haematol.* **37**:157–158.

Suthanthiran, M., Stenzel, K. H., Rubin, A. L., and Novogrodsky, A., 1980, Augmentation of proliferation and generation of specific cytotoxic cells in human mixed lymphocyte culture reactions by colchicine, *Cell. Immunol.* **50**:379–391.

Taramelli, D., Romani, L., Bonmassar, A., Goldin, A., and Fioretti, M. C., 1981, Expression of normal histocompatibility antigens in murine lymphomas treated with DTIC in vivo, *Eur. J. Cancer* **17**:411–420.

Tartakoff, A. M., Vassalli, P., and Detraz, M., 1977, Plasma cell immunoglobulin secretion: Arrest is accompanied by alterations of the Golgi complex, *J. Exp. Med.* **146**:1332–1345.

Tedde, A., Balis, M. E., Schonberg, R., and Trotta, P. P., 1979, Effects of 2'-deoxycoformycin infusion on mouse adenosine deaminase, *Cancer Res.* **39**:3044–3050.

Tedde, A., Balis, E. M., Ikehara, S., Pahwa, R., Good, R. A., and Trotta, P. P., 1980, Animal model for immune dysfunction associated with adenosine deaminase deficiency, *Proc. Natl. Acad. Sci. USA* **77**:4899–4903.

Teplitz, R. L., Mazie, J. C., Getson, I., and Barr, K. J., 1975, The effects of microtubular binding agents on secretion of IgM antibody, *Exp. Cell Res.* **90**:392–400.

Thompson, H. S., and Gale, G. R., 1971, *cis*-Dichlorodiammineplatinum(II): Hematopoietic effects in rats, *Toxicol. Appl. Pharmacol.* **19**:602–609.

Trotta, P. P., Tedde, A., Ikehara, S., Pahwa, R., Good, R. A., and Balis, M. E., 1981, Specific immunosuppressive effects of constant infusion of 2'-deoxycoformycin, *Cancer Res.* **41**:2189–2196.

Tsokos, G. C., and Choi, D. D., 1980, Inhibition of capping of immunoglobulin and Concanavalin A receptors by cis-diamminedichloroplatinum(II) in mouse spleen cells, *Cancer Lett.* **10**:261–267.

Tung, R., Silber, R., Quagliata, F., Conklin, M., Gottesman, J., and Hirschhorn, R., 1976, Adenosine deaminase activity in chronic lymphocytic leukemia, *J. Clin. Invest.* **57**:756–761.

Uberti, J., Lightbody, J. J., and Johnson, R. M., 1979, The effect of nucleosides and deoxycoformycin on adenosine and deoxyadenosine inhibition of human lymphocyte activation, *J. Immunol.* **123**:189–193.

Vecchi, A., Fioretti, M. C., Mantovani, A., Barzi, A., and Spreafico, F., 1976, The immunodepressive and hematotoxic activity of imidazole-4-carboxamide, 5-(3,3-dimethyl-1-triazeno) in mice, *Transplantation* **22**:619–624.

Wierda, D., and Pazdernik, T. L., 1979, Suppression of spleen lymphocyte mitogenesis in mice injected with platinum compounds, *Eur. J. Cancer* **15**:1013–1023.

Wolberg, G., Zimmerman, T. P., Hiemstra, K., Winston, M., and Chiu, L. C., 1975, Adenosine inhibition of lymphocyte-mediated cytolysis: Possible role of cyclic adenosine monophosphate, *Science* **187**:957–959.

Zakhireh, B., and Malech, H. L., 1980, The effect of colchicine and vinblastine on the chemotactic response of human monocytes. *J. Immunol.* **125**:2143–2153.

CHAPTER 6

EFFECT OF GLUCOCORTICOID HORMONES ON THE IMMUNE SYSTEM

ALBERTO MANTOVANI

1. INTRODUCTION

Glucocorticoids (GC) are used in the treatment of a wide range of diseases, particularly those with an inflammatory or immunological basis (Fauci *et al.*, 1976). Moreover, these agents are an important component of the chemotherapeutic armamentarium against neoplasia, having contributed to the therapeutic efficacy of regimens used in the treatment of such diseases as acute leukemias and lymphomas.

GC have profound effects on virtually every component of host defense mechanisms. The immunoregulatory activity of glucocorticoid hormones has fostered the use of these agents in immunologically based diseases. Moreover the interaction of GC with the immune system has proved an invaluable tool for dissection and analysis of basic aspects of the physiology of host defense mechanisms.

The immunoregulatory activity of glucocorticoid hormones is also relevant to their use in neoplastic diseases. A first aspect of the interaction of GC with immunocompetent cells relevant to the use of these compounds in neoplasia is their cytotoxicity for lymphoid cells, which can be demonstrated also in steroid-resistant species, such as man, at least on some cell subset or at some stages of cell activation (Galili *et al.*, 1980; Gailani *et al.*, 1973; Lippman *et al.*, 1974). It appears reasonable to assume that the mechanisms involved in cell killing are analogous for normal and malignant cells. Immunosuppressive activity is generally considered an important determi-

ALBERTO MANTOVANI ● Laboratory of Human Immunology, Mario Negri Institute for Pharmacological Research, 20157 Milan, Italy.

nant of infections occurring concomitantly with the use of chemotherapy. Finally, modulation of antineoplastic host defense mechanisms could also be relevant to the antitumor activity of GC. On the one hand it has been suggested that interference with immunity is an intrinsic limiting factor in the efficacy of anticancer agents: according to this view, chemotherapeutic drugs would be self defeating (Schwartz, 1968). On the other hand evidence has accumulated that several cancer chemotherapeutic agents, including GC (reviewed here), do not simply cause a nonspecific generalized inhibition of immune responsiveness but have selective effects on host defense mechanisms (see other chapters in this book). Therefore the relationship between antitumor efficacy and modulation of host resistance might be more complicated than expected on the somewhat simplistic assumption that chemotherapeutic agents act merely as depressants of immunity.

The effects of glucocorticoid hormones on host defense mechanisms have been repeatedly reviewed along with those of other immunosuppressive agents (Makinodan *et al.*, 1970; Bach, 1975; Mantovani, 1982; Mantovani and Tagliabue, 1983). Recently, Cupps and Fauci (1982) examined in depth the effects of GC on immunity in man. These reviews provide the framework for this chapter, which is intended to focus on the relationship between effects of GC on immunity and antitumor efficacy of these agents. In the first part of this article, the immunoregulatory effects of GC on various components of the immune system will be summarized. The main focus will be on those aspects of immunoregulation of immunity by GC that are deemed of relevance to neoplasia. Those aspects of the *in vivo* activity of GC on tumor growth and metastasis that may be related to the immunoregulatory activity of GC will then be considered. Finally, the relationship (if any) between the interaction with components of host defense mechanisms and antineoplastic efficacy of GC will be examined.

2. GENERAL CONCEPTS ON THE MODE OF ACTION OF GLUCOCORTICOIDS

The mechanism of action of glucocorticoid hormones has been the subject of a recent review (Chan and O'Malley, 1978) and will be only briefly summarized here with focus on cells involved in host defense mechanisms. GC bind to specific cytoplasmic receptors, and the steroid-hormone complex is translocated to the nucleus. Interaction with the genome eventually leads to synthesis of protein(s) in the cytoplasm and subsequent phenotypic alterations. In this series of events, the receptor step has been the one most extensively studied in cells of the immune system. All the cellular components of immunity have been shown to have high-affinity binding sites for glucocorticoid hormones. Thus, steroid receptors have been documented in lymphocytes (Lippman and Barr, 1977; Niefeld *et al.*, 1977; Smith *et al.*, 1977; Homo *et al.*, 1975), monocytes and macrophages (Werb *et al.*, 1978;

Ranelletti *et al.*, 1983a), and polymorphonuclear leukocytes (Peterson *et al.*, 1981; Murakami *et al.*, 1979) in humans and rodents.

Monocytes and polymorphs have been reported to have considerably higher numbers of high-affinity binding sites for GC than lymphoid cells (Lippman and Barr, 1977; Murakami *et al.*, 1979). The density of corticosteroid receptors in lymphocytes can also vary in different subpopulations and with cell cycle. Stimulation by mitogens or antigen increases glucocorticoid receptors (Niefeld *et al.*, 1977; Smith *et al.*, 1977), an effect probably dependent on increased expression (2- to 3-fold) of GC during the S and post-S phase of the cell cycle (Crabtree *et al.*, 1980). T and B lymphocytes have comparable numbers and density of glucocorticoid receptors (Klein *et al.*, 1980). Similarly human T cells with Fc receptors for IgG (Tγ) and for IgM (Tμ) do not differ significantly in number, affinity, and dissociation constant of intracytoplasmic receptors for GC (Fauci *et al.*, 1980). However, human peripheral blood T lymphocytes purified by E-rosette formation have more glucocorticoid receptors than cells obtained by passage through nylon wool (Distelhorst and Benutto, 1981). It may be important to note at this point that, since monocytes have higher numbers of binding sites for glucocorticoid hormones (Murakami *et al.*, 1979), minor variations in the contaminants of "purified" lymphocyte preparations can markedly affect results, and this methodological aspect should be taken into serious account in this type of studies.

Subpopulations of thymocytes differ markedly in glucocorticoid receptors. When human thymus cells were separated according to binding to peanut lectin, the more mature population (peanut negative) had approximately twice as many glucocorticoid receptors as the immature, peanut-positive population (Ranelletti *et al.*, 1981).

Neoplastic leukocytes of different lineage have high-affinity binding sites for glucocorticoid hormones (Gailani *et al.*, 1973; Lippman, 1973; Ranelletti *et al.*, 1983a; Shipman *et al.*, 1981; Werb *et al.*, 1978). It has been reported that there is a correlation between glucocorticoid receptors and response to therapeutic protocols that include GC (Bloomfield *et al.*, 1980; Lippman, 1973). However it must be emphasized that there are cell lines with high numbers of high-affinity binding sites for glucocorticoid hormones resistant to the cytotoxic action of these agents (Gailani *et al.*, 1973; Lippman *et al.*, 1974).

Although normal immunocyte populations are heterogeneous for the presence of glucocorticoid receptors, there seems to be little correlation between the presence of glucocorticoid-specific binding sites and susceptibility to the immunoregulatory activity of these compounds. T cells are generally more easily affected than B lymphocytes by glucocorticoid hormones (Cupps and Fauci, 1982), but there are no substantial differences in glucocorticoid receptors between the two cell populations (Klein *et al.*, 1980). Human T and B lymphocytes differ in their capacity to metabolize cortisol, and this difference could contribute to the different susceptibility of these populations (Klein *et al.*, 1980). Following *in vivo* administration in man, Tμ cells are preferentially depleted from the circulation compared to Tγ cells (Haynes and Fauci, 1978; Dupont *et al.*, 1983; Speigelberg *et al.*, 1979), a finding not expected on the basis of the above-mentioned data on glucocorticoid receptors in these cells (Fauci *et al.*, 1980). Immature peanut-positive thymus cells have more receptors but are less susceptible to the action of GC compared to mature peanut-negative thymocytes (Ranelletti *et al.*, 1981).

The expression of glucocorticoid receptors in cells of the immune system is a function of previous exposure to glucocorticoid hormones. *In vitro* culture of a human monocytic cell line with dexamethasone resulted in a decreased number of receptors, reversed upon further cultivation in the absence of the drug (Ranelletti *et al.*, 1983a). In two studies, *in vivo* administration of various GC resulted in a decrease in the number of GC binding sites in lymphocytes that in one case lasted up to 3 weeks (Schlechte *et al.*, 1982; Shipman *et al.*, 1983). In view of the expression of glucocorticoid receptors in lymphoid subsets (similar in T and B cells and in Tγ and Tμ cells) and of the changes in their relative proportions (relative increase in Tγ, see the following discussion), it is unlikely that these alterations in lymphocyte glucocorticoid receptors after administration of GC reflect changes in the percentages of lymphocytes.

Lymphoid cells from corticosteroid-sensitive species (e.g., mouse, rat, rabbit) are easily lysed by GC *in vitro*, whereas gross cytotoxicity of lymphocytes from steroid-resistant species (e.g., guinea pig and man) is usually not observed at physiologic or pharmacologic concentrations (Claman, 1972; Claman *et al.*, 1971). The marked heterogeneity among species in susceptibility to glucocorticoid hormones cautions against mechanical extrapolation of data obtained in corticoid-sensitive animals, such as mice, to man. Although unstimulated human lymphocytes (Claman *et al.*, 1971; Claman, 1972) are not appreciably killed by GC, activated T cells are susceptible to glucocorticoid cytotoxicity (Galili *et al.*, 1980). Susceptibility to cytotoxicity was restricted to certain types of activated T cells [e.g., from mixed lymphocyte reaction (MLR)]. Recently Cohen and Duke (1984) related killing of mouse thymocytes to activation of a calcium-dependent endonuclease that could cause a rapid DNA degradation, thus shedding new light into the mode of action of GC on immunocytes.

Among the various steps of the mode of action of GC at the subcellular level, only the presence and characteristics of cytoplasmic receptors have been studied extensively in cells of the immune system. Recently Hattori *et al.* (1983) studied the effect of lipomodulin on human natural killer (NK) cells. Lipomodulin is a protein induced by glucocorticoid hormones that inhibits phospholipase (Hirata *et al.*, 1980). Lipomodulin suppresses NK activity and antibody-dependent cellular cytotoxicity (ADCC) *in vitro* (Hattori *et al.*, 1983). Hence it can be speculated that glucocorticoid-induced inhibition of NK cytotoxicity (see the following discussion) is mediated, at last in part, by induction of this phospholipase-inhibitory protein.

3. IMMUNOREGULATORY ACTIVITY OF GLUCOCORTICOIDS

3.1. Macrophages

Macrophages are a major target of the immunoregulatory and antiin-flammatory effects of glucocorticoid hormones (summarized in Table I) as indicated, for instance, by peripheral blood counts of monocytes that are affected more than those of other leukocyte populations (Claman, 1983; Craddock, 1978; Fauci and Dale, 1974). As already mentioned, cells of the monocyte-macrophage lineage have high-affinity binding sites for GC. Glucocorticoid-binding macromolecules have been demonstrated in monocytes, macrophages, and macrophage cell lines (Ranelletti et al., 1983a; Werb et al., 1978). The dissociation constant of the receptors was within physiolog-

TABLE I

Some Effects of Glucocorticoids on Mononuclear Phagocytes

Function	Effect	References
Monocyte production	Slightly reduced	Thompson and Van Furth (1973)
Monocyte release from bone marrow	Reduced	Thompson and Van Furth (1973)
Monocyte extravasation	Reduced	Blussé van Oud Alblas et al. (1981a)
Monocyte differentiation	Blocked	Rinehart et al. (1982), Crawford et al. (1983), Ranelletti et al. (1983a)
Response to chemoattractants	Reduced	Rinehart et al. (1974)
Response to MIF	Reduced	Balow and Rosenthal (1973), Wahl et al. (1975)
Response to inducers of proliferation	Reduced	Duncan et al. (1982), Hamilton (1983)
Induction of Ia expression	Blocked	Snyder and Unanue (1982)
Production of IL 1	Reduced	Snyder and Unanue (1982)
Phagocytosis	Unaffected	Gadeberg et al. (1975)
Production of procoagulant	Reduced	Lyberg et al. (1982)
Production of plasminogen activator	Reduced	Vassalli et al. (1976)
Production of prostaglandins	Reduced	Bray and Gordon (1976)
Production of collagenase	Reduced	Crawford et al. (1983)
Induction of ADCC	Blocked	Ralph et al. (1978, 1982)
Tumor cytotoxicity	Blocked	Hibbs (1974), Keller (1974)

ical ranges and the specificity and affinity correlated with biological function (Werb *et al.*, 1978).

The effect of these drugs on the kinetics of promonocytes, monocytes, and macrophages was investigated by Van Furth and co-workers (Thompson and Van Furth 1970, 1973; Crofton *et al.*, 1978) in the mouse, a corticosteroid-sensitive species. GC have proved to be invaluable tools for investigation of the origin and kinetics of macrophages in normal and inflamed tissues (Thompson and Van Furth 1970, 1973; Crofton *et al.*, 1978, Blussé Van Oud Alblas *et al.*, 1981a,b). It was found that administration of GC induces a rapid decrease (within 3–6 hr) in the number of circulating monocytes. The duration of this effect was dependent on both the kind and the dose of the compound administered. In fact, after a single injection of 25 μg of water-soluble dexamethasone sodium phosphate, the monocytes reappeared in the circulation within 12 hr. Injection of 15 mg of insoluble hydrocortisone acetate, which formed a subcutaneous depot releasing the steroid, resulted in prolonged monocytopenia lasting at least 14 days. In the same study, hydrocortisone did not affect the number of macrophages already present in the peritoneal cavity, but the transit of mononuclear phagocytes from the circulation into the peritoneal cavity was arrested. When an inflammatory response in the peritoneal cavity of hydrocortisone-treated mice was induced by injection of newborn calf serum, the increase in the number of monocytes in the circulation and in the peritoneal cavity was suppressed. Since no lytic action of steroids on mononuclear phagocytes could be demonstrated, it was hypothesized that monocytopenia after hydrocortisone administration could result from diminished production of monocytes in the bone marrow, as a result of a cytostatic action on their direct precursor cells, or from inhibition of the release of monocytes from the bone marrow. Thompson and Van Furth (1973) showed that GC did not induce decreased mitotic activity of the promonocytes and caused only a moderate reduction of monocyte production.

Since the release of monocytes from the bone marrow was found to be influenced by hydrocortisone, it was concluded that this drug interferes with the release of newly formed monocytes from the bone marrow, resulting in an arrest of these cells in this compartment. Similarly to the above-mentioned results obtained in the mouse, a great fall in circulating monocytes (4–6 hr) after administration of GC was reported by Fauci and Dale (1974) who administered both 100 mg and 400 mg of hydrocortisone to normal volunteers. Based on the results obtained, these investigators also concluded that the dramatic depletion of circulating monocytes is probably caused by a redistribution of cells out of the circulation into other body compartments.

Blussé van Oud Alblas *et al.* (1981a,b) studied the effect of GC on the kinetics of pulmonary macrophages in mice. Hydrocortisone reduced the monocyte influx into lungs to 14% of normal and local production to 7%. The efflux of pulmonary macrophages was decreased to 12% of normal with an overall increase in turnover time. The accumulation of macrophages into inflamed pulmonary tissue was also inhibited by hydrocortisone.

As already mentioned, *in vivo* administration of GC has only marginal effects on mature resident macrophage counts while it causes profound monocytopenia (Thompson and Van Furth, 1970, 1973; Crofton *et al.*, 1978; Acero *et al.*, 1984). It was reported that GC are not grossly cytotoxic *in vitro* for mouse macrophages and do not appreciably affect the limited proliferative capacity *in vitro* of these cells (Thompson and Van Furth, 1970, 1973; Crofton *et al.*, 1978).

In contrast, the proliferation of myeloid precursors in colony-stimulating-factor (CSF) stimulated cultures of bone marrow is suppressed by GC *in vitro* (Ishii *et al.*, 1983; Mishell *et al.*, 1982). In this *in vitro* system, the myelosuppressive effect of GC is reportedly prevented by interleukin 1 (IL 1) (Mishell *et al.*, 1982). Using mouse mature peritoneal macrophages induced by thioglycollate, Norton and Munck (1980) reported that GC inhibit the proliferative capacity of macrophages. Growth factors or phorbol esters can induce DNA synthesis in murine macrophages: macrophage proliferation induced by both stimuli was blocked by GC (Hamilton, 1983). A similar inhibition of macrophage DNA synthesis by glucocorticoid hormones was reported by Neumann and Sorg (1983) with mouse-bone-marrow derived mononuclear phagocytes. Using a lymphocyte product that induces proliferation of macrophages, Hadden and co-workers (Duncan *et al.*, 1982) found that glucocorticoid modulation of macrophage proliferation was complex. At suboptimal concentrations of macrophage mitogenic factor (MMF), GC inhibited macrophage DNA synthesis, whereas at supraoptimal concentrations potentiation of the effect of MMF has been observed (Duncan *et al.*, 1982).

GC alter the differentiation of mononuclear phagocytes. Upon *in vitro* culture human blood monocytes undergo changes in morphology, biochemistry (increased protein, lysozomal enzymes, and 5′-nucleotidase), and function (enhanced tumoricidal activity). This transition from monocytes to macrophage like cells *in vitro* was inhibited by glucocorticoid hormones (Rinehart *et al.*, 1982). Similarly, differentiation of an established monocytic cell line was partially inhibited by dexamethasone (Ranelletti *et al.*, 1983a). *In vivo* or *in vitro* exposure to GC prevented the spontaneous fusion of rabbit alveolar macrophages to form multinucleated giant cells (Crawford *et al.*, 1983). Mononuclear phagocytes can express class II histocompatibility antigens (Ia) that play an important role in antigen presentation (reviewed by Unanue, 1981). The induction of Ia antigen expression in murine macrophages by lymphokines is prevented by *in vitro* exposure to GC (Snyder and Unanue, 1982). In this context it is of interest that topical or systemic administration of GC in guinea pigs (a corticoid-resistant species) resulted in diminished epidermal Langerhans cells identified on the basis of ATPase and Ia expression (Belsito *et al.*, 1982).

Since monocytes and macrophages are important for the development and expression of cellular immunity, the capability of corticosteroids to compromise the recruitment of these cells into inflammatory sites was further investigated in an attempt to better clarify the mechanisms at the basis of the depression of delayed-type reactivities caused by steroids (Claman, 1972; Jeter and Seebohm, 1952; Casey and McCall, 1971; Balow and Rosenthal, 1973; Weston *et al.*, 1973). Employing macrophage migration inhibition assays, Casey and McCall (1971) showed that methylprednisolone-treated rabbits previously immunized with Bacillus Calmette–Guérin had impaired development of delayed hypersensitivity to purified protein derivative (PPD). This observation was then confirmed and extended by Balow and Rosenthal (1973), who reported that hydrocortisone and dexamethasone, but not desoxycorticosterone, estrogens, testosterone, and progesterone, inhibit macrophage migration in guinea pigs. Interestingly, in this study it was reported that GC inhibited the responsiveness of macrophages to migration inhibitory factor (MIF) but did not affect the production of this lymphokine. Wahl *et al.* (1975) confirmed the inhibition of macrophage responsiveness to MIF, but they also found that steroids blocked the production of this mediator. Similarly, macrophage responsiveness to aggregation factor was completely inhibited by *in vitro* addition of cortisol at a concentration of 10^{-3} M, but the capability of producing this factor by lymphoid cells was not affected (Weston *et al.*, 1973). Rinehart *et al.* (1974) reported that hydrocortisone inhibits the responsiveness of human monocytes to lymphocyte-derived chemoattractants. At variance with data with human monocytes, guinea pig peritoneal macrophages were rendered unresponsive to MIF by steroids, but not to chemotactic lymphokine(s) (Wahl *et al.*, 1975). Masur *et al.* (1982) reported that hydrocortisone renders mouse macrophages unresponsive to lymphokines that activate the oxydative burst and killing of *Toxoplasma*. Thus it can be concluded that corticosteroids render macrophage refractory to certain lymphokines. Hydrocortisone is a known membrane-stabilizing agent (Weissman and Dingle, 1961), and functional membranes are thought to be important for normal lymphokine responsiveness (reviewed in Cohen *et al.*, 1979). The defective membrane functionality after corticosteroid could account for the lack of response to lymphokines of macrophages from steroid-treated animals (Casey and McCall, 1971; Balow and Rosenthal, 1973; Weston *et al.*, 1973).

In addition to causing monocytopenia, to inhibiting recruitment of mononuclear phagocytes at sites of inflammation, and to suppressing responsiveness to lymphokines, GC interfere with various macrophage functions such as production of plasminogen activator and of prostaglandins (Bray and Gordon, 1976; Vassalli *et al.*, 1976). Collagenase secretion by rabbit lung macrophages exposed *in vitro* or *in vivo* to GC was inhibited (Crawford *et al.*, 1983). Ralph and co-workers (1978, 1982) found that GC did not inhibit the baseline production of colony-stimulating activity, phagocytosis, and killing of antibody-coated targets by murine macrophage cell lines. In contrast, the same functions stimulated by bacterial lipopolysaccharides or PPD were suppressed by exposure to glucocorticoid hormones. In patients with autoimmune hemolytic anemia and in volunteers, glucocorticoid administration caused a dose-dependent reduction of monocyte Fc receptors (Fries *et al.*, 1983). The enhancement of procoagulant activity of monocytes exposed to mycobacteria was prevented by dexamethasone (Lyberg *et al.*, 1982). GC have also been shown to block the production of IL 1 by macrophages (Snyder and Unanue, 1982; Stŏsić-Grujičić and Simić, 1982; Bendtzen *et al.*, 1983), a subject that will be analyzed in more detail in a subsequent section of this chapter.

Mononuclear phagocytes are thought to play an important role in the defense mechanisms activated in the host by bacterial infections and tumors. Therefore several investigators have performed studies directed to elucidate the effect of corticosteroids on monocyte and macrophage functions in animals bearing infections (North, 1971) and tumors (Hibbs, 1974; Keller, 1974; Keller *et al.*, 1974; Schultz *et al.*, 1978; Cameron and Churchill, 1981). North (1971) reported that a single 2.5-mg dose of cortisone acetate given at the beginning of infection with *Listeria monocytogenes* in mice delays and suppresses blood monocyte accumulation at the infective foci in tissues. Since phagocytosis of macrophages does not seem to be affected by GC (Gadeberg *et al.*, 1975; Pruzanski *et al.*, 1983), the suppressed resistance to a wide range of bacterial infections (Germuth, 1956) in mice treated with corticosteroids can be more likely attributed to defective macrophage recruitment at the site of infection rather than to defective killing of the bacteria by mononuclear phagocytes.

However, the results obtained by investigating the *in vitro* effects of macrophages on tumor cells clearly indicate that GC can directly interfere with killing mechanisms. In fact, hydrocortisone and other steroids were observed to reduce the cytostatic and cytotoxic activity of *in-vivo-* (Hibbs, 1974) and *in-vitro-* (Keller, 1974; Schultz *et al.*, 1978) activated mouse and rat macrophages against several tumor cell lines. Furthermore, human-macrophage-mediated cytotoxicity against tumor cells was reported to be affected by hydrocortisone added to the *in vitro* cultures (Cameron and Churchill, 1981). Since it has been shown that macrophage–target-cell interaction is associated with the fusion of the two plasma membranes and transfer of lysosomes from the macrophage to the target cell (Hibbs, 1974; Chambers and Weiser, 1969), it was suggested that transfer of lysosomes may be a killing mechanism. Hydrocortisone could block the lysosome transfer (Hibbs, 1974; Keller, 1974; Schultz *et al.*, 1978; Cameron and Churchill, 1981) through the stabilization of cell membranes (Weissman and Dingle, 1961). It is of interest in this context that *in vivo* treatments with cortisone acetate abolish the nonspecific protection induced by *Corynebacterium parvum* in mice bearing the P815 mastocytoma (Scott, 1975). In addition to inhibiting the expression of macrophage cytotoxicity, GC can modulate the susceptibility of target cells to killing. Hydrocortisone prevented killing of actinomycin D sensitized to WEH1164 cells by human monocytes in a recently described assay system (Colotta *et al.*, 1984). GC at high concentrations have also been reported to protect tumor cells from lysis by antibody and complement or cytotoxic T lymphocytes (Schlager, 1982; Schlager and Ohanian, 1983).

3.2. T Cells

CG cause important changes in the relative and absolute number of leukocytes in the circulation, and T cells are markedly affected by these agents. Neutrophilic granulocytes are increased after administration of GC probably as a consequence of both stimulated release from the bone marrow and impaired migration out of the circulation (Dale *et al.*, 1974, 1975). In contrast glucocorticoid hormones decrease basophils (Dunsky *et al.*, 1979) and eosinophil counts (Kellgren and Janus, 1951). Circulating lymphocyte counts are markedly depressed soon after administration of GC and return to normal levels by 24 hr (Fauci and Dale, 1974). The mechanisms of corticosteroid-induced lymphopenia have been extensively studied and are probably different in corticosteroid-sensitive and -resistant species. In steroid-sensitive mice and rats GC cause massive lympholysis, whereas gross killing does not occur in steroid-resistant animals (man and guinea pig). In the latter species lymphopenia in peripheral blood results predominantly from a redistribution of the recirculating pool of peripheral blood lymphocytes (Fauci and Dale, 1975a). T cells identified by E-rosette formation or monoclonal antibodies are most markedly affected, whereas a less profound decline of B cells has been reported in some, but not all, studies (Fauci and Dale, 1974; Fauci, 1975a; Fan *et al.*, 1978; Slade and Hepburn, 1983). T-cell subsets are differentially affected by glucocorticoid hormones. T lymphocytes with an Fc receptor for IgM ($T\mu$) are preferentially depleted from the circulation, while the relative proportion of $T\gamma$ cells increases (Haynes and Fauci, 1978; Dupont *et al.*, 1983; Slade and Hepburn, 1983). In two studies helper and suppressor/cytotoxic subsets defined with monoclonal antibodies were studied in volunteers or kidney transplant recipients treated with GC (Dupont *et al.*, 1983; Slade and Hepburn, 1983). A disproportionate decrease of OKT4$^+$ (helper/inducer) cells was observed compared to OKT8$^+$ lymphocytes with a corresponding decrease of the T4 : T8 ratio (Dupont *et al.*, 1983; Slade and Hepburn, 1983). In agreement with the above-mentioned data, GC were not toxic *in vitro* to lymphocytes and did not alter the percentage of T4$^+$ or T8$^+$ cells (Slade and Hepburn, 1983).

The mechanisms responsible for glucocorticoid-induced alterations in T-cell subsets have not been completely elucidated. At least in humans and guinea pigs, gross cytotoxicity is not a critical determinant of these effects (Claman, 1972), and redistribution at extravascular sites appears to play a major role. The effect of GC on peripheral blood lymphocytes have been observed in splenectomized subjects, thus excluding a role for this organ in redistribution of lymphoid cells (Slade and Hepburn, 1983). After glucocorticoid administration in guinea pigs, lymphocytes enter the bone marrow (Fauci, 1975a). Migration to the bone marrow has also been described with human lymphocytes (Fauci, 1975b). Hence redistribution to the bone marrow could play a major role in glucocorticoid-induced lymphopenia, but the mechanisms of these effects remain unclear.

Low doses of prednisone *in vivo* have been reported to induce a reversible suppression of Ia antigen expression in human T cells stimulated with mitogens (Indiveri *et al.*, 1983). It is of interest that a similar inhibition of Ia expression has been reported also with macrophages as discussed in the previous section.

The results described so far were obtained in glucocorticoid-resistant species (human and guinea pig). Alterations in the relative proportions of lymphoid cell subpopulations have also been reported in the mouse, a steroid-sensitive species (Rogers and Matossian-Rogers, 1982). In this study, in addition to the peripheral blood compartment, lymphoid organs were also examined. An increase in the proportion of B cells analogous to that found in human blood was only observed in lymph nodes. In all organs, hydrocortisone caused a dose-dependent increase in Lyt 2^+ cells, which comprise both cytotoxic and suppressor T cells (Herzenberg *et al.*, 1976; Kimura and Wigzell, 1978).

In vitro or *in vivo* exposure to glucocorticoid hormones inhibits a number of T-cell-dependent functions in animals and humans. A number of reviews on the phenomenology of glucocorticoid suppression of T-cell functions are available, (Makinodan *et al.*, 1970; Bach, 1975; Cupps and Fauci, 1982) and these data are not reviewed in detail in this chapter.

GC, *in vitro* or *in vivo*, suppress the proliferative response to mitogens, soluble antigens, allogeneic cells, and the autologous mixed lymphocyte reaction (MLR). The latter response appears to be exquisitively sensitive to GC with suppression already in the physiological range of hormone concentrations (Ilfeld *et al.*, 1977; Katz and Fauci, 1979).

Suppressor cell function is modulated by GC and immunoregulation at this level has been suggested to play a role in the antitumor action *in vivo* of these agents (Schechter and Feldman, 1977). The generation of T suppressor cells for immunoglobulin production following exposure to concanavalin A (Con A) is blocked by glucocorticoid hormones in humans (Haynes and Fauci, 1979; Haynes *et al.*, 1979; Galanaud *et al.*, 1981). However the expression of suppressive activity by Con-A-induced cells is not affected by GC (Haynes and Fauci, 1979). Also naturally occurring human lymphocyte-mediated suppression has been reported to be blocked by GC (Haynes and Fauci, 1979). At variance with these observations, corticosteroids were reported to enhance the Con-A-generated suppressor cell function evaluated in MLR in man (Hirshberg *et al.*, 1980). The reason for these differences in the effects of GC on suppressor cell activity in different systems have not been elucidated. GC also interfere with suppressor cell function in mice. Bradley and Mischell demonstrated that suppressor T cells generated after immunization with heterologous erythrocytes were abolished by dexamethasone, whereas T helper cells were unaffected (Bradley and Mishell, 1982). This finding is of interest in view of the above-mentioned observation that GC result in an increased relative proportion of Lyt 2^+ cells, which mediate suppression (Rogers and Matossian-Rogers, 1982), and it stresses the importance of functional assays performed in parallel with phenotypic analysis.

3.3. B Cells

GC have been reported to have diverse effects on B-cell function. In corticoid-sensitive species humoral antibody production is inhibited by *in-vivo*-administered GC (reviewed by Bach, 1975). In contrast, in humans humoral antibody production in response to a number of soluble antigens has not been found affected by *in vivo* treatment with these agents (reviewed by Bach, 1975). However, decreases of various immunoglobulin classes, most notably IgG and IgA, have been reported (Butler and Rossen, 1973; Posey *et al.*, 1978). After *in vivo* treatment with GC, *in vitro* humoral antibody production in response to pokeweed mitogen has been reported diminished (Saxon *et al.*, 1978) or unaffected (Fauci *et al.*, 1977).

In vitro exposure to GC has been reported to have variable effects on humoral antibody production, from potentiation (Cooper *et al.*, 1979; Fauci *et al.*, 1977) to inhibition (Galanaud *et al.*, 1981). Methodological factors may in part contribute to this diversity of effects (Fauci *et al.*, 1976, 1980; Cupps and Fauci, 1982), which in any case stresses how this cell compartment is relatively resistant to suppression by these agents, in particular when proliferation and redistribution in extravascular compartments are considered.

3.4. Natural Killer Cells

In vivo administration of hydrocortisone or dexamethasone has been shown to inhibit NK activity in mice and humans (Hochman and Cudkowicz, 1977; Djeu *et al.*, 1979; Lotzova and Savary, 1981; Parrillo and Fauci, 1978; Oehler and Herberman, 1978). Suppressor cells for NK activity have been found in the spleen of glucocorticoid-treated mice, but their nature and actual *in vivo* relevance has not been completely defined (Hochman and Cudkowicz, 1979). Moreover GC suppress NK activity *in vitro* of lymphoid cells from both steroid-sensitive (mice) and -resistant (humans) animals (Parrillo and Fauci, 1978; Hoffman *et al.*, 1981; Bray *et al.*, 1983; Patek *et al.*, 1982; Cox *et al.*, 1983). NK cells and killer cells involved in ADCC are closely related cell populations, but GC seem to dissociate these two functions. In fact, unlike NK activity, human ADCC is reportedly less affected by GC (Parrillo and Fauci, 1978).

GC induce a phospholipase inhibitory protein lipomodulin (Hirata *et al.*, 1980). Phospholipase has been suggested to play a role in NK cytotoxicity (Hoffman *et al.*, 1981) that would fit a stimulus–secretion model (Quan *et al.*, 1982). Recently it has been directly shown that lipomodulin inhibits the expression of NK activity and ADCC (Hattori *et al.*, 1983). Thus it could be postulated that GC inhibit NK activity by inducing lipomodulin that, by blocking phospholipase, interferes with a critical step in the cascade of events leading to target cell lysis. Although this model is highly attractive, recent observations are not entirely compatible with it. The *in vitro* effect of dexamethasone on NK cells was reported to be immediate and transient, not reversed by arachidonate and independent of *de novo* protein synthesis (Bray *et al.*, 1983). Thus the mode of action of GC on NK cells remains to be fully elucidated.

3.5. Lymphokines

Analysis of the interaction of glucocorticoid hormones with the production and effect on target cells of soluble mediators of lymphocytes and macrophages has considerably improved our understanding of the mode of action of these agents. Snyder and Unanue (1982) reported that hydrocortisone inhibited the production of interleukin 1 (IL 1) by mouse macrophages exposed to bacterial lipopolysaccharides (LPS). In the same study they also showed that GC blocked the lymphokine-induced expression of Ia antigens by macrophages. Similar results were reported by Smith (1980), who studied mouse macrophages triggered by LPS under treatment with dexamethasone. Spontaneous or carrageenan-induced production of IL 1 by rat macrophages was suppressed by hydrocortisone *in vitro* (Stošić-Grujičić and Simić, 1982). In apparent contrast with these data in rodents, methylprednisolone did not affect the production of IL 1 by human monocytes exposed to a phorbol ester (Bendtzen and Peterson, 1982). However, subsequent studies (Bendtzen *et al.*, 1983; Lomnitzer *et al.*, 1983) revealed that methylprednisolone inhibited the production of lymphocyte-activating factor by monocytes cultured with PPD. It was not excluded that under those circumstances the glucocorticoid in fact acted upon contaminating T cells responsible for triggering the release of the monokine by mononuclear phagocytes.

Reconstitution experiments provided further evidence that block at the IL 1 level can be important in glucocorticoid-mediated immunosuppression at least *in vitro*. Exogenous IL 1 has been shown to prevent glucocorticoid inhibition of the murine primary humoral response *in vitro* and to protect helper but not suppressor T cells from these agents (Mishell *et al.* 1977, 1979, 1980; Bradley and Mishell, 1982). However, using human cells Bendtzen *et al.* (1983) failed to reconstitute the production of leukocyte migration inhibitory factor (LIF), inhibited by methylprednisolone, with exogenous IL 1. IL 1 has also been reported to counteract the myelosuppressive effect of dexamethasone *in vitro* in a system of granulocyte/macrophage colony formation in response to CSF (Mishell *et al.*, 1982). Ranelletti *et al.* (1983b) studied the role of accessory cells in suppression of mitogen responsiveness in blood lymphocytes and thymus cells. Monocytes or IL 1 reconstituted the dexamethasone-inhibited response to phytohemagglutinin of blood lymphocytes, but mononuclear phagocytes or IL 1 failed to reconstitute the response to thymocytes.

IL 1 triggers the release of interleukin 2 (IL 2) from T cells, and this event is blocked by GC in rodents and man (Smith *et al.*, 1980; Palacios and

Sugawara, 1982). Dexamethasone did not inhibit the acquisition of responsiveness to growth factors by T cells nor did it affect the mitogenic effect of exogenous IL 2 on T-cell blasts (Larsson, 1980; Palacios and Sugawara, 1982). These effects contrast with the site of action of the immunosuppressive antibiotic cyclosporin A, which blocked the acquisition of responsiveness to growth factors by resting T cells (Larsson, 1980). Thus, GC directly inhibit the production of IL 2 (Smith 1980, 1982; Palacios and Sugawara, 1982) and exogenous IL 2 reverted the glucocorticoid-induced inhibition of mitogen-triggered T-cell proliferation and of alloantigen-initiated clonal growth of cytotoxic T cells (Gillis *et al.*, 1979a,b; Smith *et al.*, 1980). GC have been reported to affect the production or effect on target cells of lymphokines other than IL 1 and IL 2. Inhibition of the production of LIF (Bendtzen *et al.*, 1983) and MIF (Wahl *et al.*, 1975) has been demonstrated. Moreover glucocorticoid hormones render macrophages unresponsive to various lymphokines. After treatment with GC, mononuclear phagocytes did not respond to MIF (Balow and Rosenthal, 1973; Wahl *et al.*, 1975), aggregation factor (Weston *et al.*, 1973), chemotactic lymphokine (Rinehart *et al.*, 1974) and mitogenic factors (Duncan *et al.*, 1982). Treatment with GC prevented the induction of Ia antigens in mouse macrophages by lymphokine supernatants (Snyder and Unanue, 1982). This lymphokine activity was subsequently shown to be mediated by interferon (IFN) (γ) (Steeg *et al.*, 1982). IFN secretion by macrophages was not modified by dexamethasone *in vitro* (Neumann and Sorg, 1983).

In conclusion, analysis of the effect of GC on the production and effect of lymphokines and monokines (summarized in Table II) has added a novel level of understanding of the mode of action of these agents. In particular, inhibition of secretion of IL 1 and IL 2 is likely to play a major role in the immunosuppressive activity by glucocorticoid hormones, and the block of responsiveness of macrophages to lymphocyte products may be critical for the inhibition of the effector phase of cell-mediated immunity. An important caveat concerning these studies on GC and on interleukins is that immunocytes have been exposed to drugs *in vitro*, and their effects *in vivo* at this level remain to be formally documented.

4. EFFECT ON TUMOR GROWTH AND METASTASIS

Glucocorticoid hormones are used in the treatment of a wide range of human neoplastic disorders. GC have antitumor activity *in vivo* in various murine experimental tumors of different histological origin (e.g., Agosin, 1952; Bhakoo *et al.*, 1981; Acero *et al.*, 1984). The *in vivo* antitumor activity of GC may reflect the antiproliferative effect of these agents on various cell lines (e.g., Grove *et al.*, 1977). Indirect evidence suggests that inhibition of tumor growth by glucocorticoid hormones may be related to interaction with specific receptors at last in some murine models (Braunschweiger *et al.*, 1982; Bhakoo *et al.*, 1981).

TABLE II

Modulation of the Production and Activity of Lymphokines and
Monokines by Glucocorticoids

Function	Effect	Selected references
IL 1 production	Inhibited	Smith (1980), Snyder and Unanue (1982)
IL 2 production	Inhibited	Smith (1980), Smith et al. (1980), Larsson (1980)
T-cell responsiveness to growth factors	Unaffected	Larsson (1980), Palacios and Sugawara (1982)
Production of LIF, MIF, macrophage mitogen factor	Inhibited	Wahl et al. (1975), Bendtzen et al. (1983), Duncan et al. (1982)
Macrophage production of IFN	Unaffected	Neumann and Sorg (1983)
Macrophage responsiveness to MIF, chemotactic and mitogenic factor	Inhibited	Balow and Rossenthal (1973), Masur et al. (1982), Rinehart et al. (1974), Duncan et al. (1982)
Lymphokine-induced Ia in macrophages	Inhibited	Snyder and Unanue (1982)

Although it is clear that GC can inhibit growth of primary tumor, metastatic dissemination can be augmented by these agents (Agosin 1952; Gasic and Gasic, 1957; Pomeroy, 1954; Moore and Kondo, 1958; Kondo and Tsuki, 1956; Nemeth et al., 1960; Stoker, 1968; Zeidman, 1962; Kallum and Saldeen, 1967; Sugarbaker et al., 1970; Fidler and Lieber, 1972; Bhakoo et al., 1981; Acero et al., 1984). For instance, in the first (to the best of the author's knowledge) of these observations in a syngeneic model, Agosin (1952) found that cortisone inhibited the growth of C3H spontaneous mammary adenocarcinoma but induced the appearance of metastasis. A more widespread distribution of metastases after treatment with glucocorticoid hormones has also been reported in humans with recurrent malignancy (Iversen and Hjort, 1958; Sherlock and Hartman, 1962). Enhanced metastasis is not caused by increased numbers of tumor cells leaving the primary site (Gasic and Gasic, 1957), although this point has not been extensively investigated. In fact enhanced metastasis is also observed when tumor cells are injected intravenously, thus excluding a contribution at the level of the primary tumor (Fidler and Lieber 1972; Acero et al., 1984). Tumors comprise subpopulations heterogenous in various biological properties and metastases can differ both among themselves and from primary tumors in several biological properties (see review by Poste and Fidler, 1980). Hence it could be argued that the different effects of GC on primary tumors and metastasis may be related to differences in the intrinsic properties of tumor cells that populate these two sites. To test this hypothesis, cells from metastases were transplanted intramuscularly, and the effects of hydrocortisone under these conditions were studied (Acero et al., 1984). As illustrated in Table III, hydrocortisone had similar effects on tumors originated by transplanting cells from the primary lesion and from metastases, with enhancement of secondaries and inhibition of intramuscular malignancy. Thus the divergent effects of GC on growth of primary tumors and metastasis are not related to differences in the intrinsic properties of tumor cell populations at these sites (Acero et al., 1984).

TABLE III
Divergent Effect of Hydrocortisone on Growth of Primary Madison 109 Carcinoma
and on Metastasis Formation

Mice transplanted intramuscularly with cells from:	Treatment[a]	Primary tumor weight (g)	Number of spontaneous lung metastases
Subcutaneous primary tumor	Saline	9.2 ± 0.3	11.5 ± 0.8
	Hydrocortisone	6.8 ± 0.3[b]	85.0 ± 6.4[b]
Lung secondaries	Saline	9.2 ± 0.6	22.7 ± 3.9
	Hydrocortisone	7.0 ± 0.3[b]	>100[b]

[a]Mice were treated with hydrocortisone (200 mg/kg administered subcutaneously) on days −1 and 10. On day 0 animals were inoculated with 10^5 tumor cells from either a subcutaneous lesion or lung secondaries (Acero et al., 1984).
[b]$p < 0.01$.

Metastasis is a multistep event (Poste and Fidler, 1980), and the augmentation by GC of secondary spread is not indiscriminate on all steps of the process. Release of neoplastic cells from the primary lesions does not seem to be affected (Gasic and Gasic, 1957; Acero et al., 1984). Moreover, once established, secondary deposits are not enhanced by hydrocortisone, but actually tumor growth at these sites is inhibited by GC as found at the primary lesion (Acero et al., 1984). Thus GC augment metastasis by affecting some early step of implantation and growth at secondary sites (Acero et al., 1984).

In addition to augmenting metastasis at sites already involved by the secondary spread under "normal" conditions, GC alter the pattern of metastasis. In fact, glucocorticoid hormones caused the appearance of extrapumonary metastases in tumors that otherwise colonize only in lungs (Pomeroy, 1954; Acero et al., 1984). It is noteworthy that similar observations have been reported in humans (Sherlock and Hartman, 1962; Iversen and Hjort, 1958).

5. ROLE OF HOST DEFENSE MECHANISMS IN REGULATION OF TUMOR GROWTH AND METASTASIS BY GLUCOCORTICOIDS

It has been suggested that host defense mechanisms play an important role in determining the ultimate antitumor efficacy of chemotherapy (Schwartz, 1968), but a relative paucity of systematic studies is available in this area (for review see Mantovani, 1982; Mantovani and Tagliabue, 1983; other chapters in this book). Evidence that, at least for some drugs, the therapeutic activity is the result of cooperation between host defense mechanisms and direct tumor cytotoxicity has been obtained through different approaches, by evaluating for instance the antineoplastic efficacy in specifically preimmunized or immunosuppressed hosts (Mihich, 1969; Moore and Williams,

1973; Radov et al., 1976; Stele and Pierce 1974; Heppner and Calabresi, 1972, 1976; Mantovani et al., 1979) or by utilizing sublines with different immunological properties (Giuliani et al., 1974; Mantovani et al., 1979) or by in vitro approaches (e.g., Colotta et al., 1984). Using these approaches it has been convincingly shown that immune resistance may contribute to the antitumor action of drugs such as arabinosylcitosine, cyclophosphamide, and Adriamycin®, at least in selected murine tumor models. The author is not aware of indications along this line for glucocorticoid hormones, except for a study suggesting that GC affected growth of the Lewis lung carcinoma by inhibiting T suppressor cells (Schechter and Feldman, 1977).

Host defense mechanisms have been suggested to promote tumor growth at least in some neoplasms and at certain phases of tumor progression (Prehn, 1977). In particular, evidence suggests that the macrophage infiltrate of neoplastic tissues can provide the conditions for optimal tumor growth, possibly by favoring angiogenesis and by providing growth factors for neoplastic cells (reviewed by Evans, 1982; Mantovani, 1984). In a series of murine tumors, hydrocortisone diminished the macrophage infiltrate of neoplastic tissues and concomitantly the growth of primary tumors (Acero et al., 1984). Since there was no correlation between in vivo macrophages suppression of tumor growth on the one hand and, on the other, glucocorticoid receptor content or in vitro susceptibility to glucocorticoid cytotoxicity of neoplastic cells, the possibility that interference with some host component was responsible for inhibition of neoplastic growth by hydrocortisone was explored. A role for NK cells or T lymphocytes was excluded on the basis of data obtained in mice with congenital or acquired defects of these reactivities. Hydrocortisone depleted the macrophage content of the neoplastic tissues, and admixture of macrophages to tumor cells reconstituted malignant growth in hydrocortisone-treated mice at least for the mFS6 sarcoma, but not for another sarcoma used in the same study (Table IV) (Acero et al., 1984). Thus these and other (Nelson et al., 1981) data strongly suggest that at least in some tumors glucocorticoid may inhibit neoplastic growth by reducing macrophage accumulation in neoplastic tissues, tumor-associated macrophages providing the optimal conditions for neoplastic proliferation by favoring angiogenesis and providing growth factors (Polverini et al., 1977; Mantovani, 1978). This mode of action of GC, formally demonstrated so far only in one tumor model (Acero et al., 1984), may be of interest in relation to the recently observed antitumor activity of combinations of these agents with heparin, which have been suggested to act by interference with angiogenesis (Folkman et al., 1983).

As discussed in the previous section, glucocorticoid hormones enhance metastasis in experimental animals and, possibly, in humans. The mechanisms of this effect of GC have not been elucidated. NK cells and macrophages have been suggested to act as a mechanism of restraint of the vascular phase of secondary spread of cancer cells and of the early steps of cell implantation and growth (for review see Mantovani, 1984; Introna and Mantovani, 1983). It is at this (these) level(s) that GC augment metastasis (Gasic and Gasic,

TABLE IV
Reconstitution of Tumor Growth by Macrophages in Monocytopenic
Hydrocortisone-Treated Mice[a]

Mice treated with:	Tumor cells	Tumor weight (g)	
		mFS6 sarcoma	MN/MCA sarcoma
Saline	Alone	2.8	2.7
	With thymocytes	2.7	2.8
	With macrophages	2.5	2.3
Hydrocortisone (200 mg,	Alone	1.4	1.5
subcutaneously,	With thymocytes	1.4	1.4
day +1 and 10)	With macrophages	2.3[b]	1.2

[a]Monocytopenic, hydrocortisone-treated mice were inoculated with 10^6 tumor cells alone, or mixed with the same number of peritoneal macrophages or of thymocytes, the latter used as a "filler" control (Acero et al., 1984). Tumor weight was determined on day 10 after tumor inoculation.
[b]$p < 0.01$ versus tumor cells alone or with thymocytes.

1957; Acero et al., 1984). Therefore one can speculate that inhibition of NK cells and mononuclear phagocytes contribute to enhancement of metastasis by GC (Acero et al., 1984). Effects on the vessel wall could also play a role in augmentation of secondaries by GC (Fidler and Lieber, 1972).

6. CONCLUDING REMARKS

GC have profound effect on virtually every component of host resistance, and in recent years studies on their immunoregulatory activity, in particular on lymphokine production and effect, have considerably improved the understanding of the mode of action of these agents. The relevance of immunoregulation to modulation of tumor growth and metastasis by glucocorticoid hormones remains to be firmly established. There is evidence that interference with components of the immune system that promote tumor growth may play a role in inhibition of primary tumor growth by GC. On the other hand, interference with macrophage and NK-mediated resistance could play an important role in the enhancement of metastasis by GC, a phenomenon for which there is evidence also in humans. A better understanding of the immunoregulatory activity of GC in relation to modulation of tumor growth and metastasis could contribute to a less empirical use of these agents in the treatment of neoplastic disorders.

ACKNOWLEDGMENT. Supported in part by C.N.R. (Oncology Project), Rome, Italy.

REFERENCES

Acero, R., Polentarutti, N., Bottazzi, B., Alberti, S., Ricci, M. R., Bizzi, A., and Mantovani, A., 1984, Effect of hydrocortisone on the macrophage content, growth, and metastasis of transplanted murine tumors, *Int. J. Cancer* **33**:95.

Agosin, M., Christen, R., Badinez, O., Gasic, G., Neghme, A., Pizzarro, O., and Jarpa, A., 1952, Cortisone-induced metastases of adenocarcinoma in mice, *Proc. Soc. Exp. Biol. Med.* **80**:128.

Bach, J. F., 1975, *The Mode of Action of Immunosuppressive Agents*, North Holland, Amsterdam.

Balow, J. E., and Rosenthal, A. S., 1973, Glucocorticoid suppression of macrophage migration inhibitory factor, *J. Exp. Med.* **137**:1031.

Belsito, D. V., Flotte, T. J., Lim, H. W., Baer, R. L., Thorbecke, G. J., and Gigli, I., 1982, Effect of glucocorticosteroids on epidermal Langerhans cells, *J. Exp. Med.* **155**:291.

Bendtzen, K., and Petersen, J., 1982, Effects of cyclosporin A (CyA) and methylprednisolone (MP) on the immune response. I. T-cell-activating factor abrogates CyA- but not MP-induced suppression of antigen-induced lymphokine production, *Immunol. Lett.* **5**:79.

Bendtzen, K., Petersen, J., and Søeberg, B., 1983, Effects of cyclosporin A (CyA) and methylprednisolone (MP) on the immune response. II. Further studies of the monocyte–T cell interactions leading to lymphokine production, *Acta Pathol. Microbiol. Immunol. Scand. Sect. C* **91**:159.

Bhakoo, H. S., Paolini, N. S., Milholland, R. J., Lopez, R. E., and Rosen, F., 1981, Glucocorticoid receptors and the effect of glucocorticoids on the growth of B16 melanoma, *Cancer Res.* **41**:1695.

Bloomfield, C. O., Smith, K. A., Peterson, B. A., Hildebrandt, L., Zaleskas, J., Gajl-Peczalska, K. J., Frizzera, G., and Munck, A., 1980, In vitro glucocorticoid studies for predicting response to glucocorticoid therapy in adults with malignant lymphoma, *Lancet* **1**:952.

Blussé van Oud Alblas, A., Van der Linde-Schriver, B., and Van Furth, R., 1981a, Origin and kinetics of pulmonary macrophages during an inflammatory reaction induced by intravenous administration of head-killed bacillus Calmette-Guérin, *J. Exp. Med.* **154**:235.

Blussé van Oud Alblas, A., Van der Linden-Schriver, B., and Van Furth, R., 1981b, The effect of glucocorticosteroids on the kinetics of pulmonary macrophages, *J. Reticuloendothel. Soc.* **30**:1.

Bradley, L. M., and Mishell, R. I., 1982, Differential effects of glucocorticosteroids on the functions of subpopulations of helper T lymphocytes, *Eur. J. Immunol.* **12**:91.

Braunschweiger, P. G., Ting, H. L., and Schiffer, L. M., 1982, Receptor-dependent antiproliferative effects of corticosteroids in radiation-induced fibrosarcomas and implications for sequential therapy, *Cancer Res.* **42**:1686.

Bray, M. A., and Gordon, D., 1976, Effects of antiinflammatory drugs on macrophage prostaglandin synthesis, *Br. J. Pharmacol.* **57**:461.

Bray, R., Abrams, S., and Brahmi, Z., 1983, Studies on the mechanism of human natural killer cell-mediated cytolysis. I. Modulation by dexamethasone and arachidonic acid, *Cell. Immunol.* **78**:100.

Butler, W. T., and Rossen, R. D., 1973, Effects of corticosteroids in immunity in man. I. Decreased serum IgG concentration caused by 3 or 5 days of high doses methylprednisolone, *J. Clin. Invest.* **52**:2629.

Cameron, D. J., and Churchill, W. H., 1981, Macrophage mediated cytotoxicity in man: Role of hydrocortisone, trypan blue, chloroquine, and prednisolone, *Int. J. Immunopharmacol.* **3**:77.

Casey, W. J., and McCall, C. E., 1971, Suppression of the cellular interactions of delayed hypersensitivity by corticosteroid, *Immunology* **21**:225.

Chambers, V. C., and Weiser, R. S., 1969, The ultrastructure of target cells and immune macrophages during their interaction "in vitro," *Cancer Res.* **29**:301.

Chan, L., and O'Malley, B. W., 1978, Steroid hormone action: Recent advances, *Ann. Intern. Med.* **89**:694.

Claman, H. N., 1972, Corticosteroids and lymphoid cells, *N. Engl. J. Med.* **287**:388.

Claman, H. N., 1983, Glucocorticosteroids. I. Anti-inflammatory mechanisms, *Hosp. Pract.* **18**:131.

Claman, H. N., Moorehead, J. W., and Benner, W. H., 1971, Corticosteroids and lymphoid cells in vitro. I. Hydrocortisone lysis of human, guinea pig, and mouse thymus cells, *J. Lab. Clin. Med.* **78**:499.

Cohen, J. J., and Duke, R. C., 1984, Glucocorticoid activation of a calcium-dependent endonuclease in thymocyte nuclei leads to cell death, *J. Immunol.* **132**:38.

Cohen, S., Pick, E., and Oppenheim, J. J. (eds.), 1979, *Biology of the Lymphokines*, Academic Press, New York.

Colotta, F., Introna, M., Peri, G., and Mantovani, A., 1984, Rapid killing of actinomycin D-treated tumor cells by human mononuclear cells. I. Effector cells belong to the monocyte-macrophage lineage, *J. Immunol.* **132**:936.

Cooper, D. A., Duckett, M., Petts, V., and Penny, R., 1979. Corticosteroid enhancement of immunoglobulin synthesis by pokeweed mitogen-stimulated human lymphocytes, *Clin. Exp. Immunol.* **37**:145.

Cox, W. I., Holbrook, N. J., and Friedman, H., 1983, Mechanism of glucocorticoid action on murine natural killer cell activity, *J. Natl. Cancer Inst.* **71**:973.

Crabtree, G. R., Muck, A., and Smith, K. A., 1980, Glucocorticoids and lymphocytes. II. Cell cycle-dependent changes in glucocorticoid receptor content, *J. Immunol.* **125**:13.

Craddock, C. G., 1978, Corticosteroid-induced lymphopenia, immunosuppression, and body defense, *Ann. Intern. Med.* **88**:564.

Crawford, S. W., Kang, A. H., and Mainardi, C. L., 1983, Interstitial collagenase secretion and giant cell formation from rabbit alveolar macrophages: Effects of dexamethasone, *Am. Rev. Respir. Dis.* **127**:46.

Crofton, R. W., Disselhoff-den Dulk, M. M. C., and Van Furth, R., 1978, The origin, kinetics, and characteristics of the kupffer cells in the normal steady state, *J. Exp. Med.* **148**:1.

Cupps, T. R., and Fauci, A. S., 1982, Corticosteroid-mediated immunoregulation in man, *Immunol. Rev.* **65**:133.

Dale, D. C., Fauci, A. S., and Wolff, S. M., 1974, Alternate-day prednisone: Leukocyte kinetics and susceptibility to infections, *N. Engl. J. Med.* **291**:1154.

Dale, D. C., Fauci, A. S., Guerry, D. I. V. and Wolff, S. M., 1975, Comparison of agents producing a neutrophilic leukocytosis in man: Hydrocortisone, prednisone endotoxin, and etiocholanolone, *J. Clin. Invest.* **56**:808.

Distelhorst, C. W., and Benutto, B. M., 1981, Glucocorticoid receptor content of T lymphocytes: Evidence for heterogeneity, *J. Immunol.* **126**:1630.

Djeu, J. Y., Heinbaugh, J. A., Vieira, W. D., Holden, H. T., and Herberman, R. B., 1979, The effect of immunopharmacological agents on mouse natural cell-mediated cytotoxicity and on its augmentation by Poly I:C, *Immunopharmacology* **1**:231.

Duncan, M. R., Sadlik, J. R., and Hadden, J. W., 1982, Glucocorticoid modulation of lymphokine-induced macrophage proliferation, *Cell. Immunol.* **67**:23.

Dunsky, E. H., Zweiman, B., Fischler, E., and Levy, D. A., 1979. Early effects of corticosteroids on basophils, leukocyte histamine, and tissue histamine, *J. Allergy Clin. Immunol.* **64**:426.

Dupont, E., Schandene, L., Devos, R., Lambermont, M., and Wybran, J., 1983, Depletion of lymphocytes with membrane markers of helper phenotype: A feature of acute and chronic drug-induced immunosuppression, *Clin. Exp. Immunol.* **51**:345.

Evans, R., 1982, Macrophages and neoplasms: New insights and their implication in tumor immunobiology, *Cancer Metast. Rev.* **1**:227.

Fan, P. T., Yu, D. T. Y., Clements, P. J., Fowlston, S., Eisman, J., and Bluestone, R., 1978, Effect of corticosteroids on the human immune response: Comparison of one and three daily 1 gm intravenous pulses of methylprednisolone, *J. Lab. Clin. Med.* **91**:625.

Fauci, A. S., 1975a, Mechanisms of corticosteroid action on lymphocyte subpopulations. I. Redistribution of the circulating T and B lymphocytes to the bone marrow, *Immunology* **28**:669.

Fauci, A. S., 1975b, Human bone marrow lymphocytes. I. Distribution of lymphocytes subpopulations in the bone marrow of normal individuals, *J. Clin. Invest.* **56**:98.

Fauci, A. S., and Dale, D. C., 1974, The effects of in vivo hydrocortisone on subpopulations of human lymphocytes, *J. Clin. Invest.* **53**:240.

Fauci, A. S., and Dale, D. C., 1975a, Alternate-day prednisone therapy and human lymphocyte subpopulations, *J. Clin. Invest.* **55**:22.

Fauci, A. S., and Dale, D. C., 1975b, The effect of hydrocortisone on the kinetics of normal human lymphocytes, *Blood* **46**:235.

Fauci, A. S., Dale, D. C., and Balow, J. E., 1976, Glucocorticosteorid therapy: Mechanisms of action and clinical considerations, *Ann. Intern. Med.* **84**:304.

Fauci, A. S., Pratt, K. R., and Whalen, G., 1977, Activation of human B lymphocytes. IV. Regulating effects of corticosteroids on the triggering signal in the plaque-forming response of human peripheral blood B lymphocytes to polyclonal activation, *J. Immunol.* **119**:598.

Fauci, A. S., Murakami, T., Brandon, D. D., Loriaux, D. L., and Lipsett, M. B., 1980, Mechanisms of corticosteroid action on lymphocyte subpopulations. VI. Lack of correlation between glucocorticosteroid receptors and the differential effects on glucocorticosteroids on T-cell subpopulations, *Cell. Immunol.* **49**:43.

Fidler, I. J., and Lieber, S., 1972, Quantitative analysis of the mechanism of glucocorticoid enhancement of experimental metastasis, *Res. Commun. Chem. Pathol. Pharmacol.* **4**:607.

Folkman, J., Langer, R., Linhardt, R. J., Haudenschild, C., and Taylor, S., 1983, Angiogenesis inhibition and tumor regression caused by heparin or a heparin fragment in the presence of cortisone, *Science* **221**:719.

Fries, L. F., Brickman, C. M., and Frank, M. M., 1983, Monocyte receptors for the Fc portion of IgG increase in number in autoimmune hemolytic anemia and other hemolytic states and are decreased by glucocorticoid therapy, *J. Immunol.* **131**:1240.

Gadeberg, O. V., Rhodes, J. M., and Larsen, S. O., 1975, The effect of various immunosuppressive agents on mouse peritoneal macrophages and on the "in vitro" phagocytosis of *Escherichia coli* O4:K3:H5 and degradation of ^{125}I-labeled BSA-antibody complexes by these cells, *Immunology* **28**:59.

Gailani, S., Minowada, J., Silvernail, P., Nassbaum, A., Kaiser, N., Rosen, F., and Shimaoka, K., 1973, Specific glucocorticoid binding in human hemopoietic cell lines and neoplastic tissue, *Cancer Res.* **33**:2653.

Galanaud, P., Crevon, M. C., Hillion, D., and Delfraissy, J. F., 1981, Hydrocortisone sensitivity of human in vitro antibody response: Different sensitivity of specific and nonspecific B-cell responses induced by the same agent, *Clin. Immunol. Immunopathol.* **18**:68.

Galili, N., Galili, U., Klein, E., Rosenthal, L., and Nordenskjöld, B., 1980, Human T lymphocytes become glucocorticoid-sensitive upon immune activation, *Cell. Immunol.* **50**:440.

Gasic, G., and Gasic, T., 1957, Study of vascular dissemination of tumor cells in cortisone-treated mice, *Br. J. Cancer* **11**:88.

Germuth, F. G., 1956, The role of adrenocortical steroids in infection, immunity, and hypersensitivity, *Pharmacol. Rev.* **8**:1.

Gillis, S., Crabtree, G. R., and Smith, K. A., 1979a, Glucocorticoid-induced inhibition of T cell growth factor production. I. The effect on mitogen-induced lymphocyte proliferation, *J. Immunol.* **123**:1624.

Gillis, S., Crabtree, G. R., and Smith, K. A., 1979b, Glucocorticoid-induced inhibition of T cell growth factor production. II. The effect on the in vitro generation of cytolytic T cells, *J. Immunol.* **123**:1632.

Giuliani, F., Casazza, A. M., and Di Marco, A., 1974, Virologic and immunologic properties and response to Daunomycin and Adriamycin of a nonregressing mouse tumor derived from a MSV-induced sarcoma, *Biomedicine* **21**:435.

Grove, G. L., Houghton, B. A., Cochran, J. W., Kress, E. D., and Cristofalo, V. J., 1977, Hydrocortisone effects on cell proliferation: Specificity of response among various cell types, *Cell Biol. Int. Rep.* **1**:147.

Hamilton, J. A., 1983, Glucocorticoids and prostaglandins inhibit the induction of macrophage DNA synthesis by macrophage growth factor and phorbol ester, *J. Cell. Physiol.* **115**:67.

Hattori, T., Hirata, F., Hoffman, T., Hizuta, A., and Herberman, R. B., 1983, Inhibition of human natural killer (NK) activity and antibody dependent cellular cytotoxicity (ADCC) by lipo-modulin, a phospholipase inhibitory protein, *J. Immunol.* **131**:662.

Haynes, B. F., and Fauci, A. S., 1978, The differential effect of in vivo hydrocortisone on kinetics of subpopulations of human peripheral blood thymus-derived lymphocytes, *J. Clin. Invest.* **61**:703.

Haynes, B. F., and Fauci, A. S., 1979, Mechanisms of corticosteroid action on lymphocyte subpopulations. IV. Effects of in vitro hydrocortisone on naturally occurring and mitogen-induced suppressor cells in man, *Cell. Immunol.* **44**:157.

Haynes, B. F., Katz, P., and Fauci, A. S., 1979, Mechanisms of corticosteroid action on lym-phocyte populations. V. Effect of in vivo hydrocortisone on the circulatory kinetics and function of naturally occurring and mitogen-induced suppressor cells, *Cell. Immunol.* **44**:169.

Heppner, G. H., and Calabresi, P., 1972, Suppression by cytosine arabinoside of serum-blocking factors of cell-mediated immunity to syngeneic transplants of mouse mammary tumors, *J. Natl. Cancer Inst.* **48**:1161.

Heppner, G. H., and Calabresi, P., 1976, Selective suppression of humoral immunity by anti-neoplastic drugs, *Annu. Rev. Pharmacol. Toxicol.* **16**:367.

Herzenberg, L. A., Okumura, K., Cantor, H., Sato, V. L., Shan, F., Boyse, E. A., and Herzenberg, L. A., 1976, T cell regulation of antibody responses: Demonstration of allotype-specific helper T cells, *J. Exp. Med.* **144**:330.

Hibbs, J. B., Jr., 1974, Heterocytolysis by macrophages activated by bacillus Calmette Guerin: Lysosome exocytosis into tumor cells, *Science* **184**:468.

Hirata, F., Schiffmann, E., Venkatasubramanian, K., Solomon, D., and Axelrod, J., 1980, A phospholipase A_2 inhibitory protein in rabbit neutrophils induced by glucocorticoids, *Proc. Natl. Acad. Sci. USA* **77**:2533.

Hirschberg, T., Brandazzo, B., and Hirschberg, H., 1980, Effects of methylprednisolone on the in vitro induction and function of suppressor cells in man, *Scand. J. Immunol.* **12**:33.

Hochman, P. S., and Cudkowicz, G., 1977, Different sensitivities to hydrocortisone of natural killer cell activity and hybrid resistance to parental marrow grafts, *J. Immunol.* **119**:2013.

Hochman, P. S., and Cudkowicz, G., 1979, Suppression of natural cytoxicity by spleen cells of hydrocortisone-treated mice, *J. Immunol.* **123**:968.

Hoffman, T., Hirata, F., Bougnoux, P., Fraser, B. A., Goldfarb, R. H., Herberman, R. B., and Axelrod, J., 1981, Phospholipid methylation and phospholipase A_2 activation in cytotox-icity by human natural killer cells, *Proc. Natl. Acad. Sci. USA* **78**:3839.

Homo, M., Duval, D., and Meyer, P., 1975, Étude de la liaison de la dexamethasone tritée dans les lymphocytes de sujets normaux et leucémiques, *C. R. Acad. Sci. (D) (Paris)* **280**:1923.

Ilfeld, D. N., Krakauer, R. S., and Blaese, M., 1977, Suppression of the human autologous mixed leukocyte reaction by physiologic concentrations of hydrocortisone, *J. Immunol.* **119**:428.

Indiveri, F., Scudeletti, M., Pende, D., Barabino, A., Russo, C., Pellegrino, M. A., and Ferrone, S., 1983, Inhibitory effect of a low dose of prednisone on PHA-induced Ia antigen expression by human T cells and on proliferation of T cells stimulated with autologous PHA-T cells, *Cell. Immunol.* **80**:320.

Introna, M., and Mantovani, A., 1983, Natural killer cells in human solid tumors, *Cancer Metast. Rev.* **2**:337.

Ishii, Y., Shinoda, M., and Shikita, M., 1983, Specificity of the suppressive action of glucocor-ticoids on the prliferation of monocyte/macrophages in the CSF-stimulated cultures of mouse bone marrow, *Exp. Hematol.* **11**:178.

Iversen, H. G., and Hjort, G. H., 1958, The influence of corticoid steroids on the frequency of spleen metastases in patients with breast cancer, *Acta Pathol. Microbiol. Scand.* **44**:205.

Jeter, W. S., and Seebohm, P. M., 1952, Effects of cortisone and acrenocorticotropic hormone on delayed hypersensitivity to 2,4-dinitrochlorobenzene in guinea pigs, *Proc. Soc. Exp. Biol. Med.* **80**:694.

Kallum, B., and Saldeen, T., 1967, Experimental investigation on influence of hydrocortisone on spread of transplanted rous rat sarcoma in syngeneic tumor-host system, *Acta. Pathol. Microbiol. Scand.* **70**:12.

Katz, P., and Fauci, A. S., 1979, Autologous and allogenic intercellular interactions: Modulation by adherent cells, irradiation, and in vitro and in vivo corticosteroids, *J. Immunol.* **123:**2270.

Keller, R., 1974, Mechanisms by which activated normal macrophages destroy syngeneic rat tumor cells in vitro, *Immunology* **27:**285.

Keller, R., Keist, R., and Ivatt, R. J., 1974, Functional and biochemical parameters of activation related to macrophage cytostatic effects on tumor cells, *Int. J. Cancer* **14:**675.

Kellgren, J. H., and Janus, O., 1951, The eosinopenic response to cortisone and A.C.T.H. in normal subjects, *Br. Med. J.* **2:**1183.

Kimura, A. K., and Wigzell, H., 1978, Cell surface glycoproteins of murine cytotoxic lymphocytes. I. T 145, a new cell surface glycoprotein selectively expressed on Lyt-1$^-$2$^+$ cytotoxic cells, *J. Exp. Med.* **147:**1418.

Klein A., Bessler, H., Hoogervorst-Spalter, H., Kaufman, H., Djaldetti, M., and Joshua, H., 1980, A difference between human B and T lymphocytes regarding their capacity to metabolize cortisol, *J. Steroid Biochem.* **13:**517.

Kondo, T., and Tsuki, K, 1956, On production of metastases from rat tumor by nitrogen mustard N-oxide, X-ray, and cortisone, *Gann* **47:**339.

Larsson, E.-L., 1980, Cyclosporin A and dexamethasone suppress T cell responses by selectively acting at distinct sites of the triggering process, *J. Immunol.* **124:**2828.

Lippman, M. E., 1973, Glucocorticoid-binding protein in human adult lymphoblastic leukemia, *J. Clin. Invest.* **52:**1715.

Lippman, M., and Barr, R., 1977, Glucocorticoid receptors in purified subpopulations of human peripheral blood lymphocytes, *J. Immunol.* **118:**1977.

Lippman, M. E., Perry, S., and Thompson, E. B., 1974, Cytoplasmic glucocorticoid-binding proteins in glucocorticoid-unresponsive human and mouse leukemic cell lines, *Cancer Res.* **34:**1572.

Lomnitzer, R., Phillips, R., and Rabson, A. R., 1983, The effect of hydrocortisone (HC) on sodium periodate and phytohemagglutinin-induced (^{3}H) thymidine incorporation and lymphokine production by human lymphocytes, *Clin. Immunol. Immunopathol.* **27:**378.

Lotzova, E., and Savary, C. A., 1981, Parallelism between the effect of cortisone acetate on hybrid resistance and natural killing, *Exp. Hematol.* **9:**766.

Lyberg, T., Closs, O., and Prydz, H., 1982, Effect of purified protein derivative and sonicates of *Mycobacterium leprae* and *Mycobacterium bovis* BCG on thromboplastin response in human monocytes in vitro, *Infect. Immun.* **38:**855.

Makinodan, T., Santos, G. W., and Quinn, R. P., 1970, Immunosuppressive drugs, *Pharmacol. Rev.* **22:**189.

Mantovani, A., 1978, Effects on in vitro tumor growth of murine macrophages isolated from sarcoma lines differing in immunogenicity and metastasizing capacity, *Int. J. Cancer* **22:**741.

Mantovani, A., 1982, The interaction of cancer chemotherapy agents with mononuclear phagocytes, *Adv. Pharmacol. Chemother.* **19:**35.

Mantovani, A., 1984, Origin and function of tumor-associated macrophages in human neoplasms, in: *Progress in Immunology V* (T. Tada, ed.), Academic Press, New York, pp. 1001–1008.

Mantovani, A., and Tagliabue, A., 1983, Modulation of mononuclear phagocytes by cancer chemotherapeutic agents, in: *The Reticuloendothelial System: A Comprehensive Treatise,* Volume 5: *Cancer* (R. B. Herberman and H. Friedman, eds.), Plenum Press, New York, pp. 253–278.

Mantovani, A., Polentarutti, N., Luini, W., Peri, G., and Spreafico, F., 1979, The role of host defense mechanisms in the antitumor activity of Adriamycin and Daunomycin in mice, *J. Natl. Cancer Inst.* **63:**61.

Masur, H., Murray, H. W., and Jones, T. C., 1982, Effect of hydrocortisone on macrophage response to lymphokine, *Infect. Immun.* **35:**709.

Mihich, E., 1969, Combined effects of chemotherapy and immunity against leukemia L1210 in DBA/2 mice, *Cancer Res.* **29:**848.

Mishell, R. I., Lucas, A., and Mishell, B. B., 1977, The role of activated accessory cells in preventing immunosuppression by hydrocortisone, *J. Immunol.* **119:**118.

Mishell, R. I., Bradley, L. M., Chen, Y. U., Grabstein, K. H., and Shiigi, S. M., 1979, Glucocorticosteroid response modifying factors derived from accessory cells, *Ann. N. Y. Acad. Sci.* **332**:433.

Mishell R. I., Shiigi, J. M., Mishell, B. B., Grabstein, K. H., and Shiigi, S. M., 1980, Prevention of the immunosuppressive effects of glucocorticosteroids by cell-free factors from adjuvant-activated accessory cells, *Immunopharmacology* **2**:233.

Mishell, R. I., Lee, D. A., Grabstein, K. H., and Lachman, L. B., 1982, Prevention of the in vitro myelosuppressive effects of glucocorticosteroids by interleukin 1 (IL 1), *J. Immunol.* **128**:1614.

Moore, G. E., and Kondo, T., 1958, Study of adjuvant cancer: Chemotherapy by model experiments, *Surgery* **44**:199.

Moore, M., and Williams, D. E., 1973, Contribution of host immuity to cyclophospamide therapy of a chemically-induced murine sarcoma, *Int. J. Cancer* **11**:358.

Murakami, T., Brandon, D., Rodbar, D., Loriaux, D. L., and Lipsett, M. B., 1979, Glucocorticoid receptor in polymorphonuclear leukocytes: A simple method for leukocyte glucocorticoid receptor characterization, *J. Steroid Biochem.* **10**:475.

Nelson, M., Nelson, D. S., and Hopper, K. E., 1981, Inflammation and tumor growth. I. Tumor growth in mice with depressed capacity to mount inflammatory responses: Possible role of macrophages, *Am. J. Pathol.* **104**:114.

Nemeth, L., Lapis, K., and Bihari, E., 1960, Irradiation or chemotherapy in Guerin rat carcinoma, *Acta Unio Int. Contra Cancrum* **16**:709.

Neumann, C., and Sorg., C., 1983, Regulation of plasminogen activator secretion, interferon induction, and proliferation in murine macrophages, *Eur. J. Immunol.* **13**:143.

Niefeld, J. P., Lippman, M. E., and Tormey, D. C., 1977, Steroid hormone receptors in normal human lymphocytes, *J. Biol. Chem.* **252**:2972.

North, R. J., 1971, The action of cortisone acetate on cell-mediated immunity to infection, *J. Exp. Med.* **134**:1485.

Norton, J. M., and Munk, A., 1980, In vitro actions of glucocorticoids on murine macrophages: Effects on glucose transport and metabolism, growth in culture, and protein synthesis, *J. Immunol.* **125**:259.

Oehler, J. R., and Herberman, R. B., 1978, Natural cell-mediated cytotoxicity in rats. III. Effects of immunopharmacologic treatments on natural reactivity and on reactivity augmented by polyinosinic-polycytidylic acid, *Int. J. Cancer* **21**:221.

Palacios, R., and Sugawara, I., 1982, Hydrocortisone abrogates proliferation of T cells in autologous mixed lymphocyte reaction by rendering the interleukin-2 producer T cells unresponsive to interleukin-1 and unable to synthesize the T cell growth factor, *Scand. J. Immunol.* **15**:25.

Parrillo, J. E., and Fauci, A. S., 1978, Comparison of the effector cells in human spontaneous cellular cytotoxicity and antibody-dependent cellular cytotoxicity: Differential sensitivity of effector cells to in vivo and in vitro corticosteroids, *Scand J. Immunol.* **8**:99.

Patek, P. Q., Collins, J. L., and Cohn, M., 1982, Activity and dexamethasone sensitivity of natural cytotoxic cell subpopulations, *Cell. Immunol.* **72**:113.

Peterson, A. P., Altman, L. C., Hill, J. S., Gosney, K., and Kadin, M. E., 1981, Glucocorticoid receptor in normal human eosinophils: Comparison with neutrophils, *J. Allergy Clin. Immunol.* **62**:212.

Polverini, P. J., Cotran, R. S., Gimbrone, M. A., Jr., and Unanue, E. R., 1977, Activated macrophages induce vascular proliferation, *Nature* **269**:804.

Pomeroy, T. C., 1954, Stduies on the mechanism of cortisone-induced metastases of transplanted mouse tumors, *Cancer Res.* **14**:201.

Posey, W. C., Nelson, H. S., Branch, B., and Pearlman, D. S., 1978, The effects of acute corticosteroid therapy for asthma on serum immunoglobulin levels, *J. Allergy Clin. Immunol.* **62**:340.

Poste, G., and Fidler, I. J., 1980, The pathogenesis of cancer metastasis, *Nature* **283**:139.

Prehn, R. T., 1977, Immunostimulation of the lymphodependent phase of neoplastic growth, *J. Natl. Cancer Inst.* **59**:1043.

Pruzanski, W., Saito, S., and DeBoer, G., 1983, Modulatory activity of chemotherapeutic agents on phagocytosis and intracellular bacterial activity of human polymorphonuclear and mononuclear phagocytes, *Cancer Res.* **43**:1420.

Quan, P. C., Ishizaka, T., and Bloom, B. R., 1982, Studies on the mechanism of NK cell lysis, *J. Immunol.* **128**:1786.

Radov, L. A., Haskill, J. S., and Korn, J. H., 1976, Host immune potentiation of drug responses to a murine mammary adenocarcinoma, *Int. J. Cancer* **17**:773.

Ralph, P., Ito, M., Broxmeyer, H. E., and Nakoinz, I., 1978, Corticosteroids block newly induced but not constitutive functions of macrophage cell lines: Myeloid colony-stimulating activity production, latex phagocytosis, and antibody-dependent lysis of RBC and tumor targets, *J. Immunol.* **121**:300.

Ralph, P., Williams, N., Nakoinz, I., Jackson, H., and Watson, J. D., 1982, Distinct signals for antibody-dependent and nonspecific killing of tumor targets mediated by macrophages, *J. Immunol.* **129**:427.

Ranelletti, F. O., Piantelli, M., Iacobelli, S., Musiani, P., Longo, P., Lauriola, L., and Marchetti, P., 1981, Glucocorticoid receptors and in vitro sensitivity of peanut-positive and peanut-negative thymocyte subpopulations, *J. Immunol.* **127**:849.

Ranelletti, F. O., Starace, G., Piantelli, M., Lambertenghi-Deliliers, G., and Revoltella, R. P., 1983a, Glucorticoid receptors and cortico-sensitivity in a human clonal monocytic cell line, CM-SM, *J. Cell. Physiol.* **116**:329.

Ranelletti, F. O., Musiani, P., Maggiano, N. Lauriola, L., and Piantelli, M., 1983b, Modulation of glucocorticoid inhibitory action on human lymphocyte mitogenesis: Dependence on mitogen concentration and T-cell maturity, *Cell. Immunol.* **76**:22.

Rinehart, J. J., Balcerzak, S. P., Sagone, A. L., and Lo Buglio, A. F., 1974, Effects of corticosteroids on human monocyte function, *J. Clin Invest.* **54**:1337.

Rinehart, J. J., Wuest, D., and Ackerman, G. A., 1982, Corticosteroid alteration of human monocyte to macrophage differentiation, *J. Immunol.* **129**:1436.

Rogers, P., and Matossian-Rogers, A., 1982, Differential sensitivity of lymphocyte subsets to corticosteroid treatment, *Immunology* **46**:841.

Saxon, A., Stevens, R. H., Ramer, S. J., Clements, P. J., and Yu, D. T. Y., 1978, Glucocorticoids administered in vivo inhibit human suppressor T lymphocyte function and diminish B lymphocyte responsiveness in in vitro immunoglobulin synthesis, *J. Clin. Invest.* **61**:922.

Schechter B., and Feldman, M., 1977, Hydrocortisone affects tumor growth by eliminating precursors of suppressor cells, *J. Immunol.* **119**:1563.

Schlager, S.I., 1982, Ability of tumor cells to resist humoral *vs.* cell-mediated immune attack is controlled by different membrane physical properties, *Biochem. Biophys. Res. Commun.* **106**:58.

Schlager, S. I., and Ohanian, S. H., 1983, Role of membrane lipids on the immunological killing of tumor cells. I. Target cell lipids, *Lipids* **18**:475.

Schlechte, J. A., Ginsberg B. H., and Sherman, B. M., 1982, Regulation of the glucocorticoid receptor in human lymphocytes, *J. Steroid Biochem.* **16**:69.

Schultz, R. M., Pavlidis, N. A., Stylos, W. A., and Chirigos, M. A., 1978, Cytotoxic activity of interferon-treated macrophages: Studies by various inhibitors, *Cancer Treat. Rep.* **62**:1889.

Schwartz, R. S., 1968, Are immunosuppressive anticancer drugs self-defeating? *Cancer Res.* **28**:1452.

Scott, M. T., 1975, In vivo cortisone sensitivity of non-specific antitumor activity of *Corynebacterium parvum*-activated mouse peritoneal macrophages, *J. Natl. Cancer Inst.* **54**:789.

Sherlock, P., and Hartman, W. H., 1962, Adrenal steroids and the pattern of metastases of breast cancer, *JAMA* **181**:313.

Shipman, G. F., Bloomfield, C. D., Smith, K.A., Peterson, B. A., and Munck, A., 1981, The effects of glucocorticoid therapy on glucocorticoid receptors in leukemia and lymphoma, *Blood* **58**:1198.

Shipman, G. F., Bloomfield, C. D., Gajl-Peczalska, K. J., Munck, A. U., and Smith, K. A., 1983, Glucocorticoids and lymphocytes. III. Effects of glucocorticoid administration on lymphocyte glucocorticoid receptors, *Blood* **61**:1086.

Slade, J. D., and Hepburn, B., 1983, Prednisone-induced alterations of circulationg human lymphocyte subsets, *J. Lab. Clin. Med.* **101**:479.

Smith, K. A., 1980, T-cell growth factor, *Immunol. Rev.* **51**:337.

Smith, K. A., 1982, T-cell growth factor and glucocorticoids: Opposing regulatory hormones in neoplastic T-cell growth, *Immunobiology* **161**:157.

Smith, K. A., Crabtree, G. R., Kennedy, S. J., and Munck, A., 1977, Glucocorticoid receptors and glucocorticoid sensitivity of mitogen stimulated and unstimulated human lymphocytes, *Nature* **267**:523.

Smith, K. A., Lachman, L. B., Oppenheim, J. J., and Favata, M. F., 1980, The functional relationship of the interleukins, *J. Exp. Med.* **151**:1551.

Snyder, D. S., and Unanue, E. R., 1982, Corticosteroids inhibit murine macrophage Ia expression and interleukin 1 production, *J. Immunol.* **129**:1803.

Spiegelberg, H. L., O'Connor, R. D., Simon, R. A., and Mathison, D. A., 1979, Lymphocytes with immunoglobulin E Fc receptors in patients with atopic disorders, *J. Clin. Invest.* **64**:714.

Steeg, P. S., Moore, R. N., Johnson, H. M., and Oppenheim, J. J., 1982, Regulation of murine macrophage Ia antigen expression by a lymphokine with immune interferon activity, *J. Exp. Med.* **156**:1780.

Steele, G., and Pierce, G. E., 1974, Effects of cyclophosphamide on immunity against chemically-induced syngeneic murine sarcomas, *Int. J. Cancer* **13**:572.

Stoker, T. A. M., 1968, The effect of cortisone therapy and limb exercise on the retention of V_2 tumour cells by the popliteal lymph node of the rabbit, *Br. J. Surgery* **55**:870.

Stošić-Grujičić, S., and Simić, M. M., 1982, Modulation of interleukin 1 production by activated macrophages: In vitro action of hydrocortisone, colchicine, and cytochalsin B, *Cell. Immunol.* **69**:235.

Sugarbaker, E. V., Cohen, A. M., and Ketcham, A. S., 1970, Facilitated metastatic distribution of the Walker 256 tumor in Sprague-Dawley rats with hydrocortisone and/or cyclophosphamide, *J. Surg. Oncol.* **2**:277.

Thompson, J., and Van Furth, R., 1970, The effect of glucocorticosteroids on the kinetics of mononuclear phagocytes, *J. Exp. Med.* **131**:429.

Thompson, J., and Van Furth, R., 1973, The effect of glucocorticosteroids on the proliferation and kinetics of promonocytes and monocytes of the bone marrow, *J. Exp. Med.* **137**:10.

Unanue, E. R., 1981, The regulatory role of macrophages in antigenic stimulation. II. Symbiotic relationship between lymphocytes and macrophages, *Adv. Immunol.* **31**:1.

Vassalli, J., Hamilton, J., and Reich, E., 1976, Macrophage plasminogen activator: Modulation of enzyme production by anti-inflammatory steroids, mitotic inhibitors, and cyclic neuclotides, *Cell* **8**:271.

Wahl, S. M., Altman, L. C., and Rosenstreich, D. L., 1975, Inhibition of in vitro lymphokine synthesis by glucocorticosteroids, *J. Immunol.* **115**:476.

Weissman, G., and Dingle, J., 1961, Release of lysosomal protease by ultraviolet irradiation and inhibition by hydrocortisone, *Exp. Cell Res.* **25**:207.

Werb, Z., Foley, R., and Munck, A., 1978, Interaction of glucocorticoids with macrophages: Identification of glucocorticoid receptors in monocytes and macrophages, *J. Exp. Med.* **147**:1684.

Weston, W. L., Claman, H. N., and Krueger, G. C., 1973, Site of action of cortisol in cellular immunity, *J. Immunol.* **110**:880.

Zeidman, I., 1962, The fate of circulating tumor cells. II. A mechanism of cortisone action in increasing metastases, *Cancer Res.* **22**:501.

CHAPTER 7

ANTICANCER AGENTS IN BONE MARROW TRANSPLANTATION

RAINER STORB

1. INTRODUCTION

The use of cancer therapy is limited by toxicity to the bone marrow owing to the sensitivity of marrow stem cells to the anticancer agents. Higher—and potentially curative—doses of anticancer therapy can be given when this is done together with replacement of the marrow by transplantation. Under those circumstances, anticancer drugs can be given in dosages limited only by nonmarrow toxicity. It follows that marrow transplantation would be most effective in the treatment of cancer originating from the hemopoietic tissues, while more limited benefit would be expected in the treatment of nonhemopoietic tumors. The high-dose anticancer therapy also serves to immunosuppress the patient.

Most patients with hematologic cancer have clonogenic tumor cells in their marrow. The use of their own marrow for transplantation requires the availability of effective and reproducible methods to purge the malignant cells from the marrow. Because of this limitation, most marrow grafts to date have been from healthy donors, monozygous twins, HLA-identical siblings, and also less well-matched family members (Thomas *et al.*, 1975; Storb and Thomas, 1983, 1984).

Initially considered experimental treatment applied only to end-stage patients with hematologic diseases, but experience has proved marrow transplantation to be more effective when used at an earlier stage of the patients' disease. The following discussion reviews donor–recipient selection, conditioning regimens, transplantation techniques, the origin and management

RAINER STORB • Fred Hutchinson Cancer Research Center, and Division of Oncology, Department of Medicine, University of Washington School of Medicine, Seattle, Washington 98104.

of opportunistic infections, the pathophysiology and management of graft-versus-host disease (GVHD), and clinical transplant results. The emphasis will be on the use of anticancer agents in marrow transplantation for malignant diseases.

2. GENERAL PRINCIPLES

2.1. The Source of Marrow

Most allogeneic transplants have been from siblings identical for HLA-A, -B, -DR, and -D as determined by serologic and mixed leukocyte culture techniques (Thomas et al., 1975; Storb and Thomas, 1983). Syngeneic grafts are from monozygous twins completely identical for all genetic loci and provide an ideal source of marrow. Since many patients have neither a twin nor an HLA-identical sibling, recent interest has focused at identifying acceptable alternative criteria for the selection of genotypically nonidentical donor–recipient combinations with similar HLA phenotypes (Clift et al., 1979; Hansen et al., 1983). Results with HLA-nonidentical parent–offspring or sibling pairs have been encouraging, with the longest patients now surviving for more than 7 years after transplantation. Equally interesting, successful grafts have been carried out with marrow from phenotypically HLA-identical unrelated donors (Hansen et al., 1980). The availability of marrow cryopreservation techniques has rekindled interest in the use of the patients' own marrow (autologous transplants).

2.2. Conditioning Treatment of the Recipient for Transplantation

The patient with severe combined immunologic deficiency disease usually requires no immunosuppressive conditioning because of the nature of the disease. All other recipients of marrow transplants require some form of immunosuppressive conditioning so that they will not reject the graft. The type of conditioning is influenced by the underlying disease.

A conditioning regimen commonly used in patients with aplastic anemia involves the administration of cyclophosphamide (CY), 50 mg/kg on each of 4 successive days, followed 36 hr later by marrow infusion (Storb et al., 1974a). Other regimens have included CY (120–200 mg/kg combined with either 3–10 greys (Gy) total body irradiation (TBI), with or without partial shielding of the lungs (Bortin et al., 1981; Elfenbein et al., 1983; Gale et al., 1981; Gluckman et al., 1981); thoracoabdominal irradiation (Devergie and Gluckman, 1982); or total lymphoid irradiation (Ramsay et al., 1980, 1983).

Patients with genetically determined nonmalignant disorders such as Wiskott–Aldrich syndrome (Kapoor et al., 1981; Ochs et al., 1982) or thalassemia major (Thomas et al., 1982a) who have normal or greater-than-normal marrow cellularity have been conditioned by CY (200 mg/kg) combined with either busulfan (2 mg/kg per day orally for 4 days) or dimethyl busulfan

(5 mg/kg intravenously) to not only provide immunosuppression but also eradicate the affected marrow. Another approach has involved procarbazine and antithymocyte globulin combined with TBI in patients with the Wiskott–Aldrich syndrome (Parkman *et al.*, 1978).

Patients with leukemia or other hematologic malignancies require not only immunosuppression but also high-dose chemoradiotherapy to kill the malignant cells. Thirteen years ago, patients with acute leukemia were conditioned by chemotherapy alone. The first regimens used CY in doses of at least 45 mg/kg per day for 4 days (Graw *et al.*, 1972; Santos *et al.*, 1972). Remissions were achieved; however, all patients relapsed. Another regimen known as BACT [bischloroethyl nitrosourea (BCNU), Adriamycin®, CY, 6-thioguanine] also resulted in successful engraftment and remissions (Graw *et al.*, 1974). Unfortunately, many patients died early from advanced illness, the toxicity of the regimen, the complications of the transplant. All but one patient who survived the early complications died of recurrent leukemia.

Santos *et al.* (1983) have recently described a conditioning regimen consisting of a combination of busulfan (4 mg/kg per day for 4 days) and CY (50 mg/kg per day for 4 days). It appears that long-term disease-free remission can be achieved. Zander *et al.* (1981) reported remissions in three of six patients with relapsed acute leukemia conditioned by a combination of CY, BCNU, and VP-16-25. Other drugs such as piperazinedione or acridinyl anisidide have been used in conditioning patients with acute leukemia for marrow transplantation, but definitive results are still lacking.

It is possible that some anticancer drugs alone or in combination with other drugs might be effective in eradicating leukemic cells. However, with the notable exception of the busulfan–CY combination (Santos *et al.*, 1983), the results to date have not been encouraging, and most transplant teams have involved TBI as the principal ingredient in the conditioning for marrow transplantation.

The early studies in rodents, dogs, and monkeys showing the feasibility of transplanting marrow from one animal to another were carried out after TBI. Because of the extensive laboratory experience with TBI, most conditioning regimens for marrow grafting in patients with leukemia have involved TBI. Irradiation is an excellent way of killing malignant cells, and it has the advantage of penetrating into those privileged sites where cancer cells might not be accessible to certain chemotherapeutic agents. In the early experience in Seattle with allogeneic grafts after 10 Gy TBI, six patients with acute lymphoblastic leukemia were transplanted while in relapse. Of these, five subsequently relapsed and only one patient is alive without leukemia 14 years later (Thomas *et al.*, 1977).

In an effort to kill more leukemic cells, the Seattle team began using a large dose of CY before the TBI (Thomas *et al.*, 1977). The basic regimen included CY, 60 mg/kg on each of 2 days, followed 3 days later by 10 Gy TBI given at dose rates of 5–8 cGy/min from two opposing ^{60}Co sources. Other transplant teams have used different dose rates (4–50 cGy/min) and single-source arrangements, usually linear accelerators. Over the past 7 years, in attempts to reduce radiation toxicity and perhaps increase the leukemic cell kill, TBI has been administered in several fractions, instead of a single dose. Radiation doses per fraction ranged from 1.25 to 6 Gy, and fractionation intervals from 3 to 24 hr with total doses ranging from 5 to 15.75 Gy (see the following discussion).

2.3. Bone Marrow Harvest and Infusion

After the conditioning treatment of the recipient is completed, multiple marrow aspirations are carried out under general or spinal anesthesia from the anterior and posterior iliac crests of the donor (Thomas and Storb, 1970). The marrow is then placed into heparinized tissue culture medium. After screening through wire mesh, the marrow is administered to the recipient by intravenous infusion, usually in an amount of $2-6 \times 10^8$ marrow cells per kg. The infused hemopoietic stem cells seed the marrow cavity and divide.

2.4. Supportive Care and Opportunistic Infections

The conditioning treatment with high doses of anticancer agents leads to severe pancytopenia that lasts for 2–4 weeks before marrow engraftment becomes evident (Thomas *et al.*, 1975; Storb and Thomas, 1983; Elfenbein *et al.*, 1983). Supportive care includes transfusion support, prophylactic hyperalimentation, antibiotics, and in some patients, protective environments. Severe impairment of immunologic parameters is seen during the first 4 months, as are serious bacterial, fungal, and viral infections (Witherspoon *et al.*, 1981, 1982; Clift *et al.*, 1974; Meyers *et al.*, 1982). Most troublesome are the interstitial pneumonias usually seen between days 30 and 100, with an incidence of 35–50% in allogeneic recipients (mortality effect 25–35%) compared to 17% (mortality effect 7%) in syngeneic recipients (Meyers *et al.*, 1982). Prophylaxis with trimethoprim–sulfamethoxazole has largely avoided the pneumonias caused by *Pneumocystis carinii*. Thirty to 40% of the pneumonias are idiopathic, perhaps the result of chemoradiation damage to the lungs. In approximately 60% of the cases, cytomegalovirus is found in the lung tissues and more than three-fourths of afflicted patients die. Treatment or prevention of cytomegalovirus pneumonias with adenine arabinoside, acyclovir, interferon, or combinations thereof have as yet not been successful.

Recently prophylactic treatment of patients with cytomegalovirus-hyperimmune globulin was reported to prevent cytomegalovirus infection after marrow grafting (O'Reilly *et al.*, 1983a; Meyers *et al.*, 1983).

Forty to fifty percent of all patients will show varicella-herpes zoster virus infections within 1 year after transplantation (Atkinson *et al.*, 1980). Treatment with acyclovir is advisable early after transplantation or when lesions spread beyond the originally involved dermatome.

2.5. Acute Graft-versus-Host Disease: Incidence, Pathophysiology, and Immunological Events

Theoretically, GVHD after allogeneic human marrow transplantation would be anticipated to occur in all cases owing to multiple differences for polymorphic minor histocompatability antigens even between HLA-identical donors and recipients. T lymphocytes in the marrow inoculum recognize these minor host antigens as foreign, become sensitized, proliferate, and attack host tissue cells, thereby producing the clinical picture of GVHD.

However, fortunately for the recipients, the practical experience has not entirely borne out these theoretical expectations (Storb, 1984). This was illustrated first by experiments in random-bred dogs. When dogs were given 9 Gy TBI, marrow grafts from DLA-identical littermates, and no postgrafting immunosuppression (Storb et al., 1973a), 55% of the animals died with acute GVHD within the first 150 days of transplantation. Surprisingly, however, 45% of the dogs failed to develop GVHD and went on to become healthy long-term survivors.

Similar findings were made in human patients who were treated by marrow grafts from HLA-identical siblings and given postgrafting immunosuppression with methotrexate for no more than 102 days (Storb et al., 1983a, 1984; Deeg et al., 1983). Only 35–45% of the patients developed significant acute GVHD, while the others either did not have clinically detectable GVHD (a majority) or showed only mild and transient GVHD (a minority).

However, although acute GVHD was seen less frequently in clinical practice than theoretically expected, its occurrence signified the advent of life-threatening complications. Almost 90% of patients with either no or only mild and transient acute GVHD can be expected to survive compared to only 45% of those with moderate to severe acute GVHD (Storb et al., 1983a).

The distinction between illness caused by the immunological attack by donor lymphoid cells against host organs and the consequences of this attack, disturbed organ function and infection, is subtle. For unclear reasons, the principal targets of acute GVHD in animals and man are skin, gastrointestinal tract, and liver (Thomas et al., 1975; van Bekkum and de Vries, 1967; Glucksberg et al., 1974; Grebe and Streilein, 1976). The clinical and histological criteria for and the grading system of acute GVHD have been described in detail previously (Thomas et al., 1975; Storb, 1984). GVHD manifests itself by skin rash, liver function abnormalities, abdominal pain, diarrhea, infections, and deficiencies of immunological function.

The severity of acute GVHD appears to increase with an increase in the degree of disparity for histocompatability antigens as illustrated by studies in canine littermates given 9 Gy of TBI, marrow grafts from either DLA-identical or haploidentical littermates, and postgrafting immunosuppression with methotrexate (Storb et al., 1973a, 1976). Survival was superior in recipients of DLA-identical grafts.

It is generally agreed that donor T cells cause acute GVHD (Grebe and

Streilein, 1976). One piece of evidence for this assumption is the observed benefit on GVHD from immunosuppressive agents (see the following discussion). Studies in mice using xenogeneic antilymphocyte serum and antitheta antibodies suggest that mature T cells transferred with the marrow cause acute GVHD (Muller-Ruchholtz *et al.*, 1976; Rodt *et al.*, 1974; Korngold and Sprent, 1983). In these experiments acute GVHD was prevented by *in vitro* incubation of marrow with antibody and complement, even when grafts were carried out across major histocompatibility barriers. So far, human studies using similar approaches have been less conclusive (Rodt *et al.*, 1981; Prentice *et al.*, 1982; Filipovich *et al.*, 1982; Martin *et al.*, 1983) and have not definitely ruled out the possibility that T cells recently matured from hemopoietic stem cells attain immunocompetence and attack the host.

Extensive *in vitro* experiments in animals and humans are in agreement with the assumption that T-cell proliferation in response to histocompatibility antigens of the host and the subsequent development of cytotoxic cells are the underlying cause of GVHD.

2.6. Relationship between Infections and Acute Graft-versus-Host Disease

The relationship between infection and acute GVHD is complex. The following generalizations can be made (see review in Storb, 1984; Storb *et al.*, 1983a; Deeg and Storb, 1984): (1) The lesions caused by many infections, e.g., cytomegalovirus and hepatitis, are difficult to distinguish from those caused by acute GVHD; (2) patients with acute GVHD are more often infected than those without GVHD; and (3) prevention of infection by a protective environment significantly reduces the incidence and delays the onset of acute GVHD, thereby increasing patient survival.

The first observation stresses the need for careful diagnostic procedures to distinguish between infections and GVHD, thereby enabling the physician to institute appropriate therapy.

The second observation can be explained in at least three different ways: (1) GVHD lesions in skin and intestinal tract open up portals of entry for bacteria and fungi; (2) GVHD may reactivate latent cytomegalovirus and herpes simplex virus (Dowling *et al.*, 1977); and (3) GVHD may produce an even more pronounced immunodeficiency than already exists early after grafting.

The third observation, the beneficial influence of laminar air flow room isolation on survival (Storb *et al.*, 1983a) is probably the result of two interrelated components: (1) All patients in a protective environment have a significantly lowered infection rate even if they do not have GVHD; and (2) the decreased incidence and delayed onset of acute GVHD further reduce the risk of fatal infection. The mechanisms by which the protective environment reduces GVHD remain conjectural. Mortality among lethally irradiated germ-free mice and also mice decontaminated with oral antibiotics and then given H-2-incompatible marrow grafts is significantly decreased as compared with mortality among conventionally treated mice (Heit *et al.*, 1973; Jones *et al.*, 1971; van Bekkum and Knaan, 1977). Perhaps enterobacteria invading the GVHD lesions of the gut share antigenic epitopes with mucosal epithelium, thereby activating additional lymphocyte clones to become cytotoxic to gut epithelium and to increase the mucosal damage (van Bekkum and Knaan, 1977). Similar mechanisms are thought to apply to skin GVHD.

2.7. Prevention of Acute Graft-versus-Host Disease

Many anticancer agents have immunosuppressive properties and, therefore, have been investigated for their effectiveness in preventing acute GVHD. To be effective, treatment with immunosuppressive agents must be started before GVHD becomes apparent. Methotrexate, cyclophosphamide, and cyclosporine have been found effective (see review in Storb, 1984; and Deeg and Storb, 1984). Methotrexate can prevent GVHD in mice, dogs, and monkeys. It appears to work best when continued for several months, and stable long-term survival can be achieved even in some DLA-nonidentical canine recipients. Cyclophosphamide can prevent acute GVHD in mice, rats, and monkeys but not in dogs. Cytosine arabinoside, procarbazine, and antilymphocyte serum immediately postgrafting were ineffective in dogs, whereas 6-mercaptopurine and azathioprine have shown some benefit. Cyclosporine is effective in mice, rats, and dogs. A combination of methotrexate given for 11 days and cyclosporine given for 100 days was found to be very effective in preventing acute GVHD in DLA-nonidentical unrelated dogs (35% long-term survival) and DLA-haploidentical littermates (75% long-term survival). This compares to 10% long-term survival with either drug alone. Treatment of rodents, dogs, and monkeys with antilymphocyte serum just before grafting resulted in some prolongation of survival.

An often used postgrafting regimen for human marrow grafting is based on canine studies and consists of methotrexate, 15 mg/m^2 24 hr after grafting and 10 mg/m^2 on days 3, 6, and 11 and weekly thereafter for the first 100 days (Thomas *et al.*, 1975; Storb *et al.*, 1973a). Another regimen is based on studies in rats and consists of cyclophosphamide, 7.5 mg/kg per day for five doses on alternate days beginning 24 hr after marrow grafting, followed by additional doses at irregular intervals (Santos and Kaizer, 1982). A third regimen involves cyclosporine given at a dose of 12.5 mg/kg per day orally (or 3 mg/kg per day intravenously) beginning 24 hr before marrow grafting and continued for a period of 6–12 months with gradually tapered doses (Deeg *et al.*, 1983; Storb *et al.*, 1984; Powles *et al.*, 1980a). Controlled clinical trials comparing these regimens of GVHD prevention to no immunosuppression have not been done in humans, and the rationale for the use of these drugs is based on controlled animal studies. A nonrandomized study in pediatric patients suggested that omission of methotrexate postgrafting did not lead to an increased incidence of acute GVHD.

The Seattle team has conducted two randomized trials in patients given HLA-identical marrow grafts for acute nonlymphoblastic leukemia in first remission and chronic myelogenous leukemia in chronic phase, comparing methotrexate to cyclosporine as single agents (Deeg *et al.*, 1983; Storb *et al.*, 1984). No significant difference in the incidence of acute GVHD was found in patients given cyclosporine nor was there an improvement in overall survival. Advantages of cyclosporine over methotrexate include faster marrow engraftment, less mucositis, a lessened need for platelet transfusions, and a significantly shorter hospital stay. Disadvantages of cyclosporine include (reversible) renal toxicity, hypertension, and neurotoxicity. A trial combining an 11-day course of methotrexate and a 6-month course of cyclosporine is underway.

Prophylactic antithymocyte globulin was evaluated in patients receiving standard methotrexate with the antithymocyte globulin begun either at day 7 or day 16 after transplantation (Weiden et al., 1979a; Doney et al., 1981a). Neither regimen changed the GVHD incidence, GVHD severity, or survival when compared to patients given methotrexate alone. Another study compared methotrexate to a combination of methotrexate, prednisone, and antithymocyte globulin (Ramsay et al., 1982). The combination produced a significant decrease in the incidence of acute GVHD without, however, improving overall survival or decreasing the incidence of subsequent chronic GVHD.

Other approaches at avoiding acute GVHD have centered on eliminating T lymphocytes from the marrow by in vitro treatment before infusion. In mice and rats grafted across major and minor histocompatibility barriers, acute GVHD can be prevented in most cases by treating the marrow with anti-T-cell antibodies with complete restoration of hemopoiesis in surviving animals (Muller-Ruchholtz et al., 1976; Rodt et al., 1974; Korngold and Sprent, 1983). Encouraging results have also been seen in some dogs given haploidentical littermate marrow grafts that were incubated in vitro with rabbit antithymocyte globulin (Kolb et al., 1979). This approach has now been applied to human marrow transplants using either antithymocyte globulin or monoclonal antibodies to human T cells (Rodt et al., 1981; Prentice et al., 1982; Filipovich et al., 1982; Martin et al., 1983). Initially, antibodies have been used without complement under the assumption that antibody-coated T cells would be removed by the recipient's reticuloendothelial system after infusion. However, acute GVHD continued to develop and survival of patients was not improved compared to that of patients treated with more conventional methods. Current trials are aiming at improving the results by the use of more appropriate antibodies, the addition of complement, or by coupling antibody with toxins such as ricin or ricin A chain, thus achieving more efficient cell kill. These studies are in progress at several centers and results are still very preliminary. The series of patients studied are small and the follow-up is short. However, engraftment does not appear to be a problem in HLA-identical donor–recipient combinations, while failure of engraftment or severe GVHD seem to be the rule in leukemia patients given HLA-nonidentical grafts. More effective conditioning regimens are needed to overcome the hurdle of "resistance" to HLA-nonidentical grafts before the value of marrow incubation techniques in this setting can be evaluated. Most disturbing has been the observation of a high rate of lymphoma in recipients of marrow incubated with the CT-2 antibody (Bozdech et al., 1983).

Removal of immunocompetent cells from the marrow has also been accomplished by treating the marrow with soybean agglutinin and sheep red blood cells (O'Reilly *et al.*, 1983b). Results with this approach in patients with severe combined immune deficiency given grafts of haploidentical parental marrow have been encouraging, while graft failure has also been a problem in patients with acute leukemia.

2.8. Treatment of Acute Graft-versus-Host Disease

A few studies in rodents have attempted treating established GVHD with either chemotherapeutic agents or antilymphocyte serum (see review in Storb *et al.*, 1974b). Owens and Santos (1971), using H-2-incompatible mice, suppressed clinically established GVHD with cyclophosphamide. Based in part on canine studies (Storb *et al.*, 1973b), treatment of acute GVHD has been tried in humans with prednisone, antithymocyte globulin, cyclosporine, and various monoclonal antibodies directed against T cells (Martin *et al.*, 1983; Doney *et al.*, 1981b). Variable responses to treatment have been seen with prednisone, antithymocyte globulin, and cyclosporine. As the repertoire of monoclonal anti-T-cell antibodies increases, reagents may be found that specifically interact with those T cells that are actively involved in acute GVHD.

Current therapy involves the use of methylprednisolone (2 mg/kg per day for 7–10 days). Antithymocyte globulin (10–15 mg IgG/kg given intravenously every other day for six or more doses) is employed in patients who do not respond to corticosteroids. Also, cyclosporine (3 mg/kg per day intravenously) may be used. Hyperalimentation, gut rest, and careful infection prophylaxis and therapy are important elements of supportive care.

2.9. Chronic Graft-versus-Host Disease

Chronic GVHD occurs with an incidence of 35–45% after transplantation of HLA-identical marrow. It may develop at any time between 3 and 15 months after grafting (Storb *et al.*, 1983b). Manifestations of chronic GVHD include skin lesions, severe buccal mucositis, keratoconjunctivitis, esophageal and vaginal strictures, large intestinal involvement, chronic liver disease, generalized wasting, and pulmonary insufficiency (Glucksberg *et al.*, 1974; Saurat *et al.*, 1975; Shulman *et al.*, 1980; Lawley *et al.*, 1977; Graze and Gale, 1979; Sullivan *et al.*, 1981, 1983). The clinical picture resembles that seen in systemic collagen vascular diseases, a similarity that is strengthened by the finding of circulating autoantibodies and immunoglobulin and complement depositions at the dermal–epidermal junction. Patients with chronic GVHD are severely immunologically deficient; in particular they are not able to form normal quantities of humoral antibodies in response to neoantigens and pneumococcal polysaccharides, do not convert from IgM to IgG antibody production upon antigenic challenge, and have B-cell and T-helper-cell defects in assays of *in vitro* immunoglobulin synthesis (Witherspoon *et al.*, 1981; Lum *et al.*, 1981). Not surprisingly, they suffer from recurrent and occasionally fatal bacterial infections (Atkinson *et al.*, 1982a).

Two independent factors appear to be associated with the development of chronic GVHD: acute GVHD and increasing patient age (Storb *et al.*, 1983b). Both the association between acute and chronic GVHD and the response of chronic GVHD to immunosuppressive therapy (see the following discussion) suggest that the disease is caused by a reaction of immunologically active cells to host antigens. This speculation is supported by *in vitro* findings showing the presence in patients with chronic GVHD of circulating lymphocytes with unidirectional reactivity in mixed leukocyte culture to host lymphocytes and also of lymphocytes cytotoxic to host skin fibroblasts (Tsoi *et al.*, 1980). These cells are not present among long-term survivors without GVHD.

The adverse effect of increasing patient age may be related to the inverse relationship between thymic epithelial function and age (Storb *et al.*, 1983b). Defective thymic function in older patients may result in defective maturation of lymphoid cells generated by the grafted marrow. Defective maturation may lead to impaired defenses against infection and lack of "specific" suppressor cells (Tsoi *et al.*, 1981) thought to be needed for the establishment and maintenance of graft–host tolerance. Attempts to test this speculation by transplantation of thymic tissue fragments from unrelated donors (Atkinson *et al.*, 1982b) and the injections of thymosine fraction V (Witherspoon *et al.*, 1983) in addition to the marrow graft have, however, not been successful. The late-onset chronic GVHD seen in older patients is generally less severe, less often fatal, and more responsive to immunosuppressive drug therapy than the chronic GVHD developing after acute GVHD.

Therapy of chronic GVHD with prednisone (1 mg/kg every other day) either alone or in combination with procarbazine, cyclophosphamide, or azathioprine (all at 1.5 mg/kg per day) given for periods of 9–12 months, has favorably affected and, in one-third of the cases, permanently arrested the adverse natural course of extensive chronic GVHD (Sullivan *et al.*, 1981, 1983). Early treatment is important to prevent disability and joint contractures. As a result of drug therapy, approximately one-half of the patients with extensive chronic GVHD are living with Karnofsky performance scores of 100% and an additional 25% with scores of 80–90%. However, it is important to realize that 25% of affected patients die with infections.

Prevention of chronic GVHD has been described by one transplant team that administered prednisone for 6–18 months after grafting (Forman *et al.*, 1982), while another team found no benefit from corticosteroid prophylaxis (Ringden *et al.*, 1982).

2.10. Immunological Reconstitution of the Marrow Grafting

Marrow transplant candidates either do not have a functional immune system before transplantation, such as is the case in patients with the severe combined deficiency disease, or their immune system is destroyed by the conditioning regimen used in preparation for transplantation. After transplantation, the patient's immune system is gradually repopulated by cells generated from infused hemopoietic stem cells. Many studies have described this second round of ontogeny of the immune system (see review by Witherspoon et al., 1984). The studies have shown that all marrow graft recipients; regardless of whether they received syngeneic or allogeneic grafts; regardless of the underlying disease; regardless of the conditioning regimen; regardless of whether they received postgrafting methotrexate, cyclosporine, cyclophosphamide, or other agents; and regardless of GVHD, had profound impairment of most immunological functions during the first 4–5 months after grafting. Subsequently, recipients of syngeneic and autologous grafts and those allogeneic recipients without chronic GVHD showed a return of immunological parameters to the normal or near normal range, suggesting that the main determinant for the speed of recovery was the time needed to produce sufficient numbers of functional lymphoid subsets, analogous to the situation in fetal life and early infancy. Those long-term survivors, however, who developed chronic GVHD, remained immunologically crippled. These patients failed to produce normal amounts of circulating antibody in response to a variety of antigens and were unable to convert from IgM to IgG antibody after antigenic challenge. A serious problem in patients with chronic GVHD was gram-positive bacterial infections. Poor antibody production seemed to be the result of a combination of factors including deficient B-cell function, lack of T-helper-cell activity, and in some cases the presence of T suppressor cells.

It was somewhat surprising that, despite poor immune reactivity during the first 4–5 months after grafting, most patients survived this period of greatest risk for infections. This may to some extent be the result of intensive care with broad spectrum antibiotics and antifungal agents, granulocyte transfusions, a "germ-free" laminar air flow room environment, and immunoglobulin infusions. To some extent it may be related to the transfer with the infused marrow of mature donor lymphoid cells already immune to certain pathogens but as yet unable to mount responses to new antigens. Finally, host immunity to certain pathogens may persist for some time after grafting, a speculation supported by the demonstration of persisting host produced isohemagglutinins for up to 7 months in patients given marrow from ABO-incompatible donors.

It would be attractive to develop means of accelerating the development of normal immunity after marrow transplantation. Attempts to do this by thymic tissue transplantation and the use of thymosin fraction V, however, have as yet been unsuccessful. Perhaps other more effective immune response modifiers will become available, enabling the clinician to shorten the period of highest risk for infection after marrow transplantation.

3. CLINICAL MARROW TRANSPLANT RESULTS

3.1. Acute Leukemia in Relapse

Many newly diagnosed patients with acute leukemia, in particular children with acute lymphoblastic leukemia, can be cured by treatment with chemotherapeutic agents. Once relapse has occurred, another remission can often be achieved, but the outlook is grim. Until the mid-1970s, marrow transplantation was employed only after failure of all other therapy in patients with acute nonlymphoblastic or lymphoblastic leukemia in advanced relapse. Between 1970 and 1975, 110 patients in relapse were given CY (60 mg/kg × 2) and 10 Gy TBI followed by allogeneic marrow grafts in Seattle, and 10% are alive and have been in unmaintained remission between 4 and 9 years (Thomas et al., 1977). Statistical analysis of the data showed that, if deaths from other causes were censored, 75% of all patients could be anticipated to have recurrent leukemia within 2 years of grafting. Marker studies indicated that recurrent leukemia usually originated from host cells that had survived high-dose chemoradiotherapy. These statistics improved when patients with acute nonlymphoblastic leukemia were transplanted early in first relapse (approximately 25% long-term survival) (Appelbaum et al., 1983).

3.2. Graft-versus-Leukemia Effect

Some of the cures of end-stage patients by marrow transplantations may have been achieved through leukemic cell kill through immune reactions of donor cells directed at non-HLA antigens on the surface of leukemic cells, the "graft-versus-leukemia effect." Retrospective analyses of clinical results were in agreement with this hypothesis (Weiden et al., 1979b, 1981; Gale, 1982). The chances of being in remission 2 years after grafting was higher among allogeneic transplant recipients with GVHD than in those without GVHD and in syngeneic recipients. When results in patients who had lived at least 150 days were studied, survival was 50% at 2 years for those who had grades II–IV acute GVHD compared to 25% for those with grades O–I acute GVHD. Eighty percent of patients with de novo chronic GVHD were alive at 2 years. Current clinical trials are aimed at manipulating GVHD and exploiting its apparent antileukemic effect in patients grafted in relapse.

3.3. Acute Leukemia in Remission

In early 1976 the Seattle team began to transplant patients with acute nonlymphoblastic leukemia in first or subsequent remission and those with acute lymphoblastic leukemia in second or subsequent remission after conditioning with the standard CY (60 mg/kg × 2) and 10 Gy of TBI. We expected to see improved disease-free survival since patients with acute nonlymphoblastic leukemia on chemotherapy show a median survival of less than 2 years and a 5-year survival usually no better than 20%, while patients with acute lymphoblastic leukemia who have relapsed at least once usually survive no more than 2 years.

3.4. Acute Nonlymphoblastic Leukemia

Results have borne out the expectations with respect to patients with acute nonlymphoblastic leukemia in first remission. Twelve of the first 22 patients have survived between 5¼ and 7¼ years after grafting (Thomas et *al.*, 1979a). These striking results continue to be seen with now more than 160 patients grafted in Seattle and many additional patients transplanted at several other transplant centers, not only in patients transplanted after TBI regimens but also in those conditioned with CY and busulfan (Thomas *et al.*, 1982b; Forman *et al.*, 1983; Powles *et al.*, 1980b; Kersey *et al.*, 1982; Thomas *et al.*, 1982c). The actuarial relapse rate has been on the order of 25%. Overall, 50% of patients with acute nonlymphoblastic leukemia in first remission appear to experience long-term cure of their disease. This figure is approximately 65% for patients less than age 30 and approximately 35% for patients aged 30–50 years.

A higher leukemic recurrence rate, on the order of 60%, is seen in patients with acute nonlymphoblastic leukemia grafted in second remission. Accordingly, their projected survival is only 25%, a result that is not better than when patients are grafted in first relapse (Buckner *et al.*, 1982a).

3.5. Acute Lymphoblastic Leukemia

Twenty-two patients with acute lymphoblastic leukemia in second or subsequent remission were given CY (60 mg/kg × 2) and a single dose of 10 Gy TBI followed by an HLA-identical sibling marrow graft between 1976 and 1978 in Seattle (Thomas *et al.*, 1979b). Their survival curve plateaus at 27% 5¾–7¼ years after grafting (Thomas *et al.*, 1979b). In a subsequent prospective study marrow transplantation proved to be superior to chemotherapy for patients who have relapsed at least once (Johnson *et al.*, 1981). The major problem was leukemic relapse in cells of host type with a projected incidence of 60%. Other conditioning regimens are now being explored with the aim of increasing the kill of malignant cells. The Sloan Kettering team described early results in 22 patients with acute lymphoblastic leukemia in second remission conditioned with 13.2 Gy of fractionated TBI combined with CY (Dinsmore *et al.*, 1983). Fourteen of the 22 are surviving in continuous complete remission for 12–34 (median 24) months. The team at Baltimore treated 28 patients with acute lymphoblastic leukemia in second or third remission with CY (50 mg/kg × 4) and TBI (3 Gy × 4 with shielding of the lung for the last TBI dose) (Santos, 1983). Fifteen of the 28 patients are remaining in remission between 2 and 41 months. The team at Cleveland used cytosine arabinoside (3000 mg/m² every 12 hr for 12 doses) followed by 12 Gy TBI in 6 fractions to treat 10 patients with acute lymphoblastic leukemia in second remission and have, as yet, not seen any leukemic recurrences with patients living between 4 and 27 months (Coccia *et al.*, 1983). These results, although still preliminary, are encouraging. The Seattle team grafted 12 patients in second to fourth remission following CY (60 mg/kg × 2) and 14 Gy TBI (Clift *et al.*, 1982a). Only 4 of the 12 patients are alive in unmaintained remission at 2–3 years, a result not better than that seen with CY and 10 Gy single-dose TBI. Further improvements in remission duration and survival may come from new preparative regimens, perhaps added therapy with antibodies directed against leukemic cells, the use of interferon, or consolidation chemotherapy before or after transplantation.

3.6. Chronic Granulocytic Leukemia

The results with marrow transplantation for the treatment of patients with chronic granulocytic leukemia in blast crisis have been similar to those in patients with acute leukemia in relapse. The estimated disease-free long-term survival for patients grafted in blast crisis is approximately 25% (Thomas *et al.*, 1984). The marrow cells in surviving patients do not show the Philadelphia chromosome, suggesting cure of the disease, a unique and impressive result.

Transplantation early in the course of chronic granulocytic leukemia promised to improve these results. The Seattle team began a clinical trial in 12 patients with the chronic form of the disease who had healthy monozygous twins to serve as marrow donors (Fefer *et al.*, 1982). Dimethly busulfan, 5 mg/kg intravenously, was given before CY (60 mg/kg × 2) and 10 Gy TBI given as a single dose. All 12 patients experienced complete remissions with disappearance of the Philadelphia chromosome. One died at 4 months in remission of interstitial pneumonia. Three relapsed cytogenetically 2–2½ years after transplantation. One of the three proceeded to blast crisis and died, while the other two have remained hematologically normal. Eight of the 12 are alive in apparent remission without the Philadelphia chromosome 3½–7¼ years after grafting.

Encouraged by these results, studies of transplantation were begun, using marrow from HLA-identical siblings for patients with chronic granulocytic leukemia in the accelerated or chronic phase. The Seattle team has treated 35 patients with the chronic form of disease with CY (60 mg/kg × 2) and 12 Gy TBI given in 6 fractions before the marrow graft and followed these patients for 8 months to 4½ years after grafting. The projected survival is on the order of 60% (Storb *et al.*, 1984; Clift *et al.*, 1982b). The Toronto Marrow Transplant Team reported 11 patients with chronic granulocytic leukemia in the accelerated phase (Messner *et al.*, 1981). The preparative regimen usually included cytosine arabinoside (100 mg/m² per day × 5), CY (60 mg/kg per day × 2), and 5 Gy TBI. Seven patients were alive 2–26 months after transplantation. The UCLA Marrow Transplant Team described eight patients with chronic granulocytic leukemia in chronic or accelerated phase prepared with CY and TBI (Champlin *et al.*, 1982). Six are alive 3–20 months posttransplant. Similar results have been reported by other transplant teams (Goldman *et al.*, 1982; McGlave *et al.*, 1982). Although a longer follow-up period is needed for full evaluation, it appears that more than one-half of the patients with chronic granulocytic leukemia can be cured of their disease when grafted during the chronic phase but that some patients will die early of complications of the transplant.

Results are less good when transplants are being carried out in the accelerated phase of chronic granulocytic leukemia. In Seattle, these patients are conditioned with the standard conditioning regimen of CY (60 mg/kg × 2) and 12 Gy TBI given in 6 fractions, and only 35% of the patients appear to become disease-free long-term survivors (Thomas *et al.*, 1984). The Minneapolis team has conditionied patients in the accelerated phase with cytosine arabinoside for 3 days, CY for 2 days and TBI (2.8 Gy on each of 3 days) and they reported that 7 of 16 patients so treated were alive between 10 and 24 months after grafting (McGlave et al., 1984).

3.7. Nature of Recurrent Leukemia

Blood genetic marker and cytogenetic and restriction enzyme techniques permit determination of the origin of both the normal and abnormal cells after marrow grafting. Most leukemic relapses after marrow grafting have been of the original leukemic type occurring in host cells that survived the conditioning regimens used. However, eight cases of leukemic relapse in donor-type cells have been reported (Schubach et al., 1982). Two of these have been immunoblastic lymphosarcomas, different from the patients' original diseases, while six have been in cells of the original leukemia type, including acute lymphoblastic, acute nonlymphoblastic, and chronic granulocytic leukemia. Analysis of the Seattle data suggests that approximately 5% of the recurrences may be anticipated to be in cells of the donor-type. The mechanism of these recurrences in donor-type cells is, of course, unknown. Perhaps transfection is involved.

3.8. Additional Conditioning Therapy to Prevent Recurrence of Leukemia

The reappearance of the original leukemic cell clone after high-dose chemoradiotherapy and marrow transplantation indicated a remarkably resistant population of cells. It seemed reasonable to attempt eradicating these cells by more vigorous chemotherapy before CY and TBI. Among the chemotherapeutic agents tried in Seattle are dimethyl busulfan, BCNU, and daunorubicin (Badger et al., 1982). These agents did not reduce the incidence of recurrent leukemia while increasing the toxicity of the conditioning regimen. At UCLA, a regimen known as SCARI which consisted of cytosine arabinoside, 6-thioguanine, and Adriamycin before CY and TBI was investigated (The UCLA Marrow Transplantation Group, 1977). Although the incidence of recurrent leukemia may have been reduced, the regimen was very toxic and consequently overall survival was not improved.

Current efforts to eradicate leukemic cells more effectively, thereby decreasing the leukemic recurrence rate and increasing survival in patients with leukemia grafted in relapse, have focused on the use of higher doses of TBI by means of fractionating the radiation. This has not as yet improved the results for patients with acute lymphoblastic leukemia grafted in relapse in Seattle with irradiation doses up to 15.75 Gy (Clift et al., 1982a), while survival of patients with acute nonlymphoblastic leukemia grafted in early relapse is 25% at 2–4 years (Appelbaum et al., 1983; Buckner et al., 1982b).

Additional modifications of conditioning regimens are discussed in Section 3.5.

3.9. Non-Hodgkin's Lymphoma

Eight patients with disseminated non-Hodgkin's lymphoma failed conventional chemotherapy, were conditioned with high-dose chemotherapy combined with TBI, and then given marrow transplants from healthy monozygous twins (Appelbaum *et al.*, 1981). One of the seven did not enter a remission and died. Seven had complete remissions. One of the seven died of pneumonia in remission, and a second relapsed and died of recurrent and progressive lymphoma. A third patient relapsed at 10 months, was successfully retreated with chemotherapy, and is alive in unmaintained remission 6¾ years after grafting. Four additional patients have now remained in remission for 2¾ to 12¾ years. These encouraging results have led to trials of treating non-Hodgkin's lymphoma with allogeneic, HLA-identical marrow grafts.

3.10. Other Malignancies

Marrow grafting following the standard conditioning regimen of CY and TBI has now also been successfully used for the treatment of patients with myelofibrosis, multiple myeloma, preleukemia, and hairy cell leukemia (Osserman, *et al.*, 1982; Storb *et al.*, 1983c; Cheever *et al.*, 1982).

Pilot studies are being undertaken with radiosensitive solid tumors such as neuroblastoma, ovarian, testicular, and small-cell lung cancer, usually after failure of other therapy, and with the exception of neuroblastoma, results have been poor. Perhaps treatment of solid tumor patients should be considered before their disease reaches the terminal stage.

3.11. Autologous Marrow Transplantation

The relative success of syngeneic and allogeneic marrow grafting and the availability of effective marrow cryopreservation techniques have reawakened interest in autologous transplantation. Autologous marrow grafts would get around the two major problems of syngeneic and allogeneic grafts, namely that only 25–40% of all patients have suitable donors, and the risk of GVHD encountered after allogeneic grafts.

The conditioning regimens used in autologous transplantation are generally those developed for allogeneic and syngeneic grafting. Of course, postgrafting immunosuppression therapy is not required. Early trials in patients with acute leukemia grafted in relapse using marrow collected in initial remission and stored without further *in vitro* treatment yielded no long-term disease-free survivors; the median duration of remission was 4–6 months (Dicke *et al.*, 1979; Santos *et al.*, 1981; Herzig *et al.*, 1980; Buckner *et al.*, 1983). This differed from results of syngeneic marrow transplants, where 20–30% long-term survival has been reported (Fefer *et al.*, 1981); it suggested that some of the leukemic recurrences were caused by the infusion of marrow contaminated by leukemic cells. As suggested by studies in dogs with spontaneous lymphoma (Weiden *et al.*, 1979c), however, prolonged disease-free survival has been seen after autologous transplantation for non-Hodgkin's lymphoma (Santos *et al.*, 1981; Herzig *et al.*, 1980; Appelbaum *et al.*, 1978), suggesting that tumor contamination of remission marrow is not an invariant feature of all hematologic cancers. Favorable results have also been reported in children with neuroblastoma (August *et al.*, 1983).

To obtain results with autologous marrow transplants comparable to those with syngeneic and allogeneic grafts, the marrow must be cleared of leukemic cells while retaining normal marrow stem cells. A number of researchers have reported that it is possible to completely remove malignant cells from tumor-marrow cell suspensions in rodents by pharmacologic (4-hydroperoxycyclophosphamide) and immunologic (antibodies) reagents (Economou *et al.*, 1978; Bast *et al.*, 1979; Trigg and Poplack, 1981, Thierfelder *et al.*, 1977; Sharkis *et al.*, 1980). Early results of phase I clinical trials applying 4-hydroperoxycyclophosphamide or antibody and complement to autologous human marrow grafts for acute leukemia or non-Hodgkin's lymphoma have been described (Kaizer *et al.*, 1981). A favorable feature of *in vitro* treatment of marrow is that absolute specificity of an antiserum or chemical reagent is not necessary as long as the tumor cells are eliminated and normal marrow cells spared. A potential serious limitation is that, in contrast to many animal tumors, spontaneous human leukemias may originate from precursors that closely resemble normal marrow stem cells and do not express those differentiation antigens that are characteristic of their progeny. Therefore, it is possible that despite complete removal of recognizable leukemic cells from a marrow inoculum, the disease might recur from infused leukemic progenitor cells. Clinical trials will help answer these questions (Kaizer *et al.*, 1981). The results of syngeneic and allogeneic transplantation will serve as the yardstick by which the results of autologous transplantation can be measured. Unfortunately, as discussed in previous sections, getting rid of the cancer cells in the patient is still a major problem.

4. CONCLUSIONS

"Rescue" by bone marrow transplantation has considerably augmented the usefulness of anticancer agents. Drugs and radiation can be administered without concern for marrow toxicity. For example, it was possible to raise the dose of TBI from approximately 3 Gy to close to 16 Gy. Similarly impressive increments have been observed with dimethyl busulfan while other chemotherapeutic drugs, when administered alone, are limited by nonmarrow toxicity, e.g., CY. Even so, CY conveys powerful immunosuppression necessary for the establishment of genetically foreign marrow grafts and also contributes considerable tumor cell kill when administered together with marrow-ablative agents such as TBI. Administration of otherwise lethal chemoradiotherapy combined with marrow rescue offers the only hope of cure for patients with acute leukemia once relapse has occurred and patients with chronic granulocytic leukemia in blast crises, accelerated and chronic phase. For patients with advanced hematologic malignancies, exploration of new, experimental chemotherapeutic agents given in conventional fashion is no longer acceptable since marrow transplantation can now cure many of these patients. For patients with chronic granulocytic leukemia in chronic phase, the risk of early death from complications of marrow grafting must be weighed against the benefit of long-term survival and cure. For patients less than 30 years of age with acute nonlymphoblastic leukemia in first remission, marrow grafting appears to be the therapy of choice, while for patients aged between 30 and 50 years, the choice between marrow grafting and chemotherapy is debatable.

Anticancer agents are not only useful in the conditioning regimen before transplantation, but they also have played a major role after transplantation, where they are used to modify immune reactions of donor T-cells against host tissues, thereby avoiding GVHD and establishing stable graft-host tolerance.

ACKNOWLEDGMENT. This investigation was supported by Grants CA 18029, CA 18221, CA 30924, CA 31787, and CA 15704, awarded by the National Cancer Institute, Department of Health and Human Services.

REFERENCES

Appelbaum, F. R., Herzig, G. P., Ziegler, J. L., Graw, R. G., Levine, A. S., and Deisseroth, A. B., 1978, Successful engraftment of cryopreserved autologous bone marrow in patients with malignant lymphoma, *Blood* **52**:85–95.

Appelbaum, F. R., Fefer, A., Cheever, M. A., Buckner, C. D., Greenberg, P. D., Kaplan, H. G., Storb, R., and Thomas, E. D., 1981, Treatment of non-Hodgkin's lymphoma with marrow transplantation in identical twins, *Blood* **58**:509–513.

Appelbaum, F. R., Clift, R. A., Buckner, C. D., Stewart, P., Storb, R., Sullivan, K. M., and Thomas E. D., 1983, Allogeneic marrow transplantation for acute nonlymphoblastic leukemia after first relapse, *Blood* **61**:949–953.

Atkinson, K., Meyers, J. D., Storb, R., Prentice, R. L., and Thomas, E. D., 1980, Varicella-zoster virus infection after marrow transplantation for aplastic anemia or leukemia, *Transplantation* **29**:47–50.

Atkinson, K., Farewell, V., Storb, R., Tsoi, M.-S., Sullivan, K. M., Witherspoon, R. P., Fefer, A., Clift, R., Goodell, B., and Thomas, E. D., 1982a, Analysis of late infections after human bone marrow transplantation: Role of genotypic nonidentity between marrow donor and recipient and of nonspecific suppressor cells in patients with chronic graft-versus-host disease, *Blood* **60**:714–720.

Atkinson, K., Storb, R., Ochs, H. D., Goehle, S., Sullivan, K. M., Witherspoon, R. P., Lum, L. G., Tsoi, M.-S., Sanders, J. E., Parr, M., Stewart, P., and Thomas E. D., 1982b, Thymus transplantation after allogeneic bone marrow graft to prevent chronic graft-versus-host disease in humans, *Transplantation* **33**:168–173.

August, C. S., Serota, F. T., Koch, P. A., Burkey, E., Schlesinger, H., Evans, A. E., and D'Angio, G. J., 1983, Bone marrow transplantation for relapsed stage IV neuroblastoma, in: *Recent Advances in Bone Marrow Transplantation* (R. P. Gale, ed.), Liss, New York, pp. 703–716.

Badger, C., Buckner, C. D., Thomas, E. D., Clift, R. A., Sanders, J. E., Stewart, P. S., Storb, R., Sullivan, K. M., Shulman, H., and Flournoy, N., 1982, Allogeneic marrow transplantation for acute leukemia in relapse, *Leuk. Res.* **6**:383–387.

Bast, R. C., Jr., Feeny, M., Greenberger, J. S., and Knapp, R. C., 1979, Elimination of leukemic cells from rat bone marrow using antibody and complement (C'), *Proc. Am. Assoc. Cancer Res. Am. Soc. Clin. Oncol.* **20:**239 (abstract).

Bortin, M. M., Gale, R. P., and Rimm, A. A. [for the Advisory Committee of the International Bone Marrow Transplant Registry], 1981, Allogeneic bone marrow transplantation for 144 patients with severe aplastic anemia, *JAMA* **245:**1132–1139.

Bozdech, M. J., Finlay, J. L. Trigg, M. E., Billing, R., Hong, R., Sugden, W., and Sondel, P. M., 1983, Monoclonal B-cell lymphoproliferative disorder following monoclonal antibody (CT2) T cell-depleted allogeneic bone marrow transplantation, *Blood* **62:**218a (abstract).

Buckner, C. D., Clift, R. A., Thomas, E. D., Sanders, J. E., Hackman, R., Stewart, P. S., Storb, R., and Sullivan, K. M., 1982a, Allogeneic marrow transplantation for patients with acute non-lymphoblastic leukemia in second remission, *Leuk. Res.* **6:**395–399.

Buckner, C. D., Clift, R. A., Thomas, E. D., Sanders, J. E., Stewart, P. S., Storb, R., Sullivan, K. M and Hackman, R., 1982b, Allogeneic marrow transplantation for acute non-lymphoblastic leukemia in relapse using fractionated total body irradiation, *Leuk. Res.* **6:**389–394.

Buckner, C. D., Stewart, P. S., Bensinger, W., Clift, R., Appelbaum, F., Martin, P., Sanders, J., Fefer, A., Lum, L., Storb, R., Hill, R., and Thomas, E. D., 1983, Critical issues in autologous marrow transplantation for hematologic malignancies, in: *Recent Advances in Bone Marrow Transplantation* (R. P. Gale, ed.), Liss, New York, pp. 599–613.

Champlin, R., Ho, W., Arenson, E., and Gale, R. P., 1982, Allogeneic bone marrow transplantation for chronic myelogenous leukemia in chronic or accelerated phase, *Blood* **60:**1038–1041.

Cheever, M. A., Fefer, A., Greenberg, P. D., Appelbaum, F., Armitage, J. O., Buckner, C. D., Sale, G. E., Storb, R., Witherspoon, R. P., and Thomas E. D., 1982, Treatment of hairy-cell leukemia with chemoradiotherapy and identical-twin bone-marrow transplantation, *N. Engl. J. Med.* **307:**479–481.

Clift, R. A., Buckner, C. D., Fefer, A., Lerner, K. G., Neiman, P. E., Storb, R., Murphy, M., and Thomas, E. D., 1974, Infectious complications of marrow transplantation, *Transplant. Proc.* **6:**389–393.

Clift, R. A., Hansen, J. A., Thomas, E. D., Buckner, C. D., Sanders, J. E., Mickelson, E. M., Storb, R., Johnson, F. L., Singer, J. W., and Goodell, B. W., 1979, Marrow transplantation from donors other than HLA-identical siblings, *Transplantation* **28:**235–242.

Clift, R. A., Buckner, C. D., Thomas, E. D., Sanders, J. E., Stewart, P. S., Sullivan, K. M., McGuffin, R., Hersman, J., Sale, G. E., and Storb, R., 1982a, Allogeneic marrow transplantation using fractionated total body irradiation in patients with acute lymphoblastic leukemia in relapse, *Leuk. Res.* **6:**401–407.

Clift, R. A., Buckner, C. D., Thomas, E. D., Doney, K., Fefer, A., Neiman, P. E., Singer, J., Sanders, J., Stewart, P., Sullivan, K. M., Deeg, J., and Storb, R., 1982b, The treatment of chronic granulocytic leukaemia in chronic phase by allogeneic marrow transplantation, *Lancet* **2:**621–623.

Coccia, P. F., Strandjord, S. E., Gordon, E. M., Novak, L. J., Shina, D. C., Lazarus, H. M., and Herzig, R. H., 1983, High dose cytosine arabinoside (Ara-C) and fractionated total body irradiation (F-TBI) as preparation for bone marrow transplantation (BMT) for childhood acute leukemia in remission: A preliminary report, *Proc. Am. Soc. Clin. Oncol.* **2:**175 (Abstract C680).

Deeg, H. J., and Storb, R., 1984, Graft-versus-host disease: Pathophysiological and clinical aspects, in: *Annual Review of Medicine,* Volume 35 (W. P. Creger, ed.), Annual Reviews, Palo Alto, California, pp. 11–24.

Deeg, H. J., Storb, R., Thomas, E. D., Kennedy, M. S., Flournoy, N., Buckner, C. D., Clift, R., Doney, K., Sale, G., Sanders, J., and Witherspoon, R., 1983, Marrow transplantation for acute nonlymphoblastic leukemia in first remission: Preliminary results of a randomized trial comparing cyclosporine and methotrexate for the prophylaxis of graft-versus-host disease, *Transplant. Proc.* **15:**1385–1388.

Devergie, A., and Gluckman, E., 1982, Bone marrow transplantation in severe aplastic anemia following Cytoxan and thoraco-abdominal irradiation, *Exp. Hematol.* **10** (Suppl. 10): 17–18.

Dicke, K. A., Zander, A., Spitzer, G., Verma, D. S., Peters, L. J., Vellekoop, L., Thomson, S.,

Stewart, D., Hester, J. P., and McCredie, K. B., 1979, Autologous bone marrow transplantation in relapsed adult acute leukemia, *Exp. Hemat.* **7**(Suppl. 5):170–187.

Dinsmore, R., Kirkpatrick, D., Flomenberg, N., Gulati, S., Kapoor, N., Shank, B., Reid, A., Groshen, S., and O'Reilly, R. J., 1983, Allogeneic bone marrow transplantation for patients with acute lymphocytic leukemia, *Blood* **62**:381–388.

Doney, K. C., Weiden, P. L., Storb, R., and Thomas, E. D., 1981a, Failure of early administration of antithymocyte globulin to lessen graft-versus-host disease in human allogeneic marrow transplant recipients, *Transplantation* **31**:141–143.

Doney, K. C., Weiden, P. L, Storb, R., and Thomas, E. D., 1981b, Treatment of graft-versus-host disease in human allogeneic marrow graft recipients: A randomized trial comparing antithymocyte globulin and corticosteroids, *Am. J. Hematol.* **11**:1–8.

Dowling, J. N., Wu, B. C., Armstrong, H. A., and Ho, M., 1977, Enhancement of murine cytomegalovirus infection during graft-versus-host reaction, *J. Infect. Dis.* **135**:990–994.

Economou, J. S., Shin, H. S., Kaizer, H., Santos, G. W., and Schron, D. S., 1978, Bone marrow transplantation in cancer therapy: Inactivation by antibody and complement of tumor cells in mouse syngeneic marrow transplants, *Proc. Soc. Exp. Biol. Med.* **158**:449–453.

Elfenbein, G. J., Mellits, E. D., and Santos, G. W. [for the Johns Hopkins Bone Marrow Transplant Program], 1983, Engraftment and survival after allogeneic bone marrow transplantation for severe aplastic anemia, *Transplant. Proc.* **15**:1412–1416.

Fefer, A., Cheever, M. A., Thomas, E. D., Appelbaum, F. R., Buckner, C. D., Clift, R. A., Glucksberg, H., Greenberg, P. D., Johnson, F. L., Kaplan, H. G., Sanders, J. E., Storb, R., and Weiden, P. L., 1981, Bone marrow transplantation for refractory acute leukemia in 34 patients with identical twins, *Blood* **57**:421–430.

Fefer, A., Cheever, M. A., Greenberg, P. D., Appelbaum, F. R., Boyd, C. N., Buckner, C. D., Kaplan, H. G., Ramberg, R., Sanders, J. E., Storb, R., and Thomas, E. D., 1982, Treatment of chronic granulocytic leukemia with chemoradiotherapy and transplantation of marrow from identical twins, *N. Engl. J. Med.* **306**:63–68.

Filipovich, A. H., Ramsay, N. K. C., Warkentin, P. I., McGlave, P. B., Goldstein, G., and Kersey, H. J., 1982, Pre-treatment of donor bone-marrow with monoclonal antibody OKT3 for prevention of acute graft-versus-host disease in allogeneic, histocompatible, bone-marrow transplantation, *Lancet* **1**:1266–1269.

Forman, S. J., Farbstein, M. J., Scott, E. P., Wolf, J. L., Spruce, W. E., Fahey, J. L., Nademanee, A., and Blume, K. G., 1982, Prevention and therapy of graft-versus-host disease, *N. Engl. J. Med.* **307**:376.

Forman, S. J., Spruce, W. E., Farbstein, M. J., Wolf, J. L., Scott, E. P., Nademanee, A. P., Fahey, J. L., Hecht, T., Zaia, J. A., Krance, R. A., Findley, D. O., and Blume, K. G., 1983, Bone marrow ablation followed by allogeneic marrow grafting during first complete remission of acute nonlymphocytic leukemia, *Blood* **61**:439–442.

Gale, R. P., 1982, Bone marrow transplantation in acute myelogenous leukemia in first remission: Evidence for an antileukemic effect of graft-versus-host disease, *Exp. Hematol.* **10**:20 (abstract).

Gale, R. P., Ho, W., Feig, S., Champlin, R., Teser, A., Arenson, E., Ladish, S., Young, L., Winston, D., Sparkes, R., Fitchen, J., Territo, M., Sarna, G., Wong, L., Paik, Y., Bryson, Y., Golde, D., Fahey, J., and Cline, M., 1981, Prevention of graft rejection following bone marrow transplantation, *Blood* **57**:9–12.

Gluckman, E., Barrett, A. J., Arcese, W., Devergie, A., and Degoulet, P., 1981, Bone marrow transplantation in severe aplastic anaemia: A survey of the European Group for Bone Marrow Transplantation (E.G.B.M.T.), *Br. J. Haematol.* **49**:165–173.

Glucksberg, H., Storb, R., Fefer, A., Buckner, C. D., Neiman, P. E., Clift, R. A., Lerner, K. G., and Thomas, E. D., 1974, Clinical manifestations of graft-versus-host disease in human recipients of marrow from HL-A-matched sibling donors, *Transplantation* **18**:295–304.

Goldman, J. M., McCarthy, D. M., Hows, J. M., Catovsky, D., Goolden, A. W., Baughan, A. S., Worsley, A. M., Gordon-Smith, E. C., Batchelor, J. R., and Galton, D. A. G., 1982, Marrow transplantation for patients in the chronic phase of chronic granulocytic leukaemia, *Lancet* **2**:623–625.

Graw, R. G., Jr., Yankee, R. A., Leventhal, B. G., Rogentine, G. N., Herzig, G. P., Halterman, R. H., Merritt, C. B., Carolla, R. L., Alvegard, T. A., Bull, J. M., McGinniss, M. H., Kreuger, G. R. D., Gullion, D. S., Lippman, M. F., Bleyer, W. A., Berad, C. W., Whang-Peng, J., Trapani, R. J., Terasaki, P. I., Steinberg, A. S., Gralnik, H. R., and Henderson, E. S., 1972, Bone marrow transplantation in acute leukemia employing cyclophosphamide, *Exp. Hematol.* **22:**118–125.

Graw, R. G., Jr., Lohrmann, H.-P., Bull, M. I., Decter, J., Herzig, G. P., Bull, J. M., Leventhal, B.. G., Yankee, R. A., Herzig, R. H., Krueger, G. R. F., Bleyer, W. A., Buja, M. L., McGinniss, M. H., Alter, H. J., Whang-Peng, J., Gralnick, H. R., Kirkpatrick, C. H., and Henderson, E. S., 1974, Bone-marrow transplantation following combination chemotherapy immuno-suppression (B.A.C.T.) in patients with acute leukemia, *Transplant. Proc.* **6:**349–354.

Graze, P. R., and Gale, R. P., 1979, Chronic graft versus host disease: A syndrome of disordered immunity, *Am. J. Med.* **66:**611–620.

Grobo, S. C., and Streilein, J. W., 1976, Graft-versus-host reactions: A review, *Adv. Immunol.* **22:**119–221.

Hansen, J. A., Clift, R. A., Thomas, E. D., Buckner, C. D., Storb, R., and Giblett, E. R., 1980, Transplantation of marrow from an unrelated donor to a patient with acute leukemia, *N. Engl. J. Med.* **303:**565–567.

Hansen, J. A., Beatty, P. G., Clift, R. A., Mickelson, E. M., Nisperos, B., and Thomas, E. D., 1983, The HLA system in clinical bone marrow transplantation, in: *Recent Advances in Bone Marrow Transplantation* (R. P. Gale, ed.), Liss, New York, pp. 739–756.

Heit, H., Wilson, R., Fliedner, T. M., and Kohne, E., 1973, Mortality of secondary disease in antibiotic-treated radiation chimeras, in: *Germfree Research: Biological Effects and Gnotobiotic Environment* (J. B. Heneghan, ed.), Academic Press, New York, pp. 477–485.

Herzig, G. P., Phillips, G. L., Fay, J., NaPombejara, C., and Wolff, S., 1980, Autologous bone marrow transplantation for treatment of hematologic malignancy, *J. Supramol. Struct. Suppl.* **4:**36 (Abstract 088).

Johnson, F. L., Thomas, E. D., Clark, B. S., Chard, R. L., Hartmann, J. R., and Storb, R., 1981, A comparison of marrow transplantation to chemotherapy for children with acute lymphoblastic leukemia in second or subsequent remission, *N. Engl. J. Med.* **305:**846–851.

Jones, J. M., Wilson, R., and Bealmear, P. M., 1971, Mortality and gross pathology of secondary disease in germfree mouse radiation chimeras. *Radiat. Res.* **45:**577–588.

Kaizer, H., Stuart, R. K., Colvin, M., Korbling, M., Wharam, M. D., and Santos, G. W., 1981, Autologous bone marrow transplantation in acute leukemia: A pilot study utilizing *in vitro* incubation of autologous marrow with 4-hydroperoxycyclophosphamide (4HC) prior to cryopreservation. *Proc. Am. Assoc. Cancer Res. Am. Soc. Clin. Oncol.* **22:**483 (Abstract C-587).

Kapoor, N., Kirkpatrick, D., Blaese, R. M., Oleske, J., Hilgartner, M. H., Chagante, R. S., Good, R. A., and O'Reilly, R. J., 1981, Reconstitution of normal megakaryocytopoiesis and immunologic functions in Wiskott–Aldrich syndrome by marrow transplantation following myeloablation and immunosuppression with busulfan and cyclophosphamide, *Blood* **57:**692–696.

Kersey, J. H., Ramsay, N. K. C., Kim, T., McGlave, P., Krivit, W., Levitt, S., Filipovich, A., Woods, W., O'Leary, M., Coccia, P., and Nesbit, M. E., 1982, Allogeneic bone marrow transplantation in acute nonlymphocytic leukemia: A pilot study, *Blood* **60:**400–403.

Kolb, H. J., Reider, I., Rodt, B., Netzel, B., Grosse-Wilde, H., Scholz, S., Schaffer, E., Kolb, H., and Thierfelder, S., 1979, Anti-lymphocytic antibodies and marrow transplantation. VI. Graft-versus-host tolerance in DLA-incompatible dogs after *in vitro* treatment of bone-marrow with absorbed antithymocyte globulin, *Transplantation* **27:**242–245.

Korngold, R., and Sprent, J., 1983, Lethal GVHD across minor histocompatibility barriers: Nature of the effector cells and role of the H-2 complex, *Immunol. Rev.* **71:**5–29.

Lawley, T. J., Peck, G. L., Moutsopoulous, H. M., Gratwohl, A. A., and Deisseroth, A. B,, 1977, Scleroderma, Sjögren-like syndrome, and chronic graft-versus-host disease, *Ann. Intern. Med.* **87:**707–709.

Lum, L. G., Seigneuret, M. C., Storb, R. F., Witherspoon, R. P., and Thomas, E. D., 1981, In vitro regulation of immunoglobulin synthesis after marrow transplantation. I. T-cell and B-cell deficiencies in patients with and without chronic graft-versus-host disease, *Blood* **58**:431–439.

Martin, P. J., Hansen, J. A., Remlinger, K., Torok-Storb, B., Storb, R., and Thomas, E. D., 1983, Murine monoclonal anti-human T cell antibodies for the prevention and treatment of graft-versus-host disease, in: *Recent Advances in Bone Marrow Transplantation* (R. P. Gale, ed.), Liss, New York, pp. 313–329.

McGlave, P. B., Kim, T. H., Hurd, D. D., Arther, D. C., Ramsay, N. K., and Kersey, J., 1982, Successful allogeneic bone-marrow transplantation for patients in the accelerated phase of chronic granulocytic leukaemia, *Lancet* **2**:625–627.

McGlave, P. B., Arthur, D. C., Weisdorf, D., Kim, T., Goldman, A., Hurd, D. D., Ramsay, N. K. C., and Kersey, J. H., 1984, Allogeneic bone marrow transplantation as treatment for accelerating chronic myelogenous leukemia, *Blood* **63**:219–222.

Messner, H. A., Curtis, J. E., and Norman, C., 1981, Allogeneic bone marrow transplantation in patients with CML prior to blastic crisis, *Blood* **58**(Suppl. 1):175a (abstract).

Meyers, J. D., Flournoy, N., and Thomas, E. D., 1982, Nonbacterial pneumonia after allogeneic marrow transplantation: A review of ten years' experience, *Rev. Infect. Dis.* **4**:1119–1132.

Meyers, J. D., Leszczynski, J., Zaia, J. A., Flournoy, N., Newton, B., Snydman, D. R. Wright, G. G., Levin, M. J., and Thomas, E. D., 1983, Prevention of cytomegalovirus infection by cytomegalovirus immune globulin after marrow transplantation, *Ann. Intern. Med.* **98**:442–446.

Muller-Ruchholtz, W., Wottge, H.-U., and Muller-Hermelink, H. K., 1976, Bone-marrow transplantation in rats across strong histocompatibility barriers by selective elimination of lymphoid cells in donor marrow, *Transplant. Proc.* **8**:537–541.

Ochs, H. D., Lum, L. G., Johnson, F. L., Schiffman, G., Wedgwood, R. J., and Storb, R., 1982, Bone marrow transplantation in the Wiskott–Aldrich syndrome: Complete hematological and immunological reconstitution, *Transplantation* **34**:284–288.

O'Reilly, R. J., Reich, L., Gold, J., Kirkpatrick, D., Dinsmore, R., Kapoor, N., and Condie, R., 1983a, A randomized trial of intravenous hyperimmune globulin for the prevention of cytomegalovirus (CMV) infections following marrow transplantation: Preliminary results, *Transplant. Proc.* **15**:1405–1411.

O'Reilly, R. J., Kapoor, N., Kirkpatrick, D., Cunningham-Rundles, S., Pollack, M. S., Dupont, B., Hodes, M. Z., Good, R. A., and Reisner, Y., 1983b, Transplantation for severe combined immunodeficiency using histoincompatibile parental marrow fractionated by soybean agglutinin and sheep red blood cells: Experience in six consecutive cases, *Transplant. Proc.* **15**:1431–1435.

Osserman, E. F., Dire, L. B., Dire, J., Sherman, W. H., Hersman, J. A., and Storb, R., 1982, Identical twin marrow transplantation in multiple myeloma, *Acta Haematol.* **68**:215–223.

Owens, A. H., Jr., and Santos, G. W., 1971, The effect of cytotoxic drugs on graft-versus-host disease in mice, *Transplantation* **11**:378–382.

Parkman, R., Rappeport, J., Geha, R., Belli, J., Cassady, R., Levey, R., Nathan, D. G., and Rosen, F. S., 1978, Complete correction of the Wiskott–Aldrich syndrome by allogeneic bone marrow transplantation, *N. Engl. J. Med.* **298**:921–927.

Powles, R. L., Clink, H. M., Spence, D., Morgenstern, G., Watson, J. G., Selby, P. J., Woods, M., Barrett, A., Jameson, B., Sloane, J., Lawler, S. D., Kay, H. E. M., Lawson, D., McElwain, T. J., and Alexander, P., 1980a, Cyclosporin A to prevent graft-versus-host in man after allogeneic bone-marrow transplantation, *Lancet* **1**:327–329.

Powles, R. L., Morgenstern, G., Clink, H. M., Hedley, D., Bandini, G., Lumley, H., Watson, J. G., Lawson, D. Spence, D., Barrett, A., Jameson, B., Lawler, S., Kay, H. E. M., and McElwain, T. J., 1980b, The place of bone-marrow transplantation in acute myelogenous leukemia, *Lancet* **1**:1047–1050.

Prentice, H. G., Janossy, G., Skeggs, D., Blacklock, H. A., Bradstock, K. F., Goldstein, G., and Hoffbrand, A. V., 1982, Use of anti-T-cell monoclonal antibody OKT3 to prevent acute graft-versus-host disease in allogeneic bone-marrow transplantation for acute leukaemia, *Lancet* **1**:700–703.

Ramsay, N. K. C., Kim, T., Nesbit, M. E., Krivit, W., Coccia, P. F., Levitt, S. H., Woods, W. G., and Kersey, J. H., 1980, Total lymphoid irradiation and cyclophosphamide as preparation for bone marrow transplantation in severe aplastic anemia, *Blood* **55:**344–346.

Ramsay, N. K. C., Kersey, J. H., Robison, L. L., McGlave, P. B., Woods, W. G., Krivit, W., Kim, T. H., Goldman, A. I., and Nesbit, M. E., Jr., 1982, A randomized study of the prevention of acute graft-versus-host disease, *N. Engl. J. Med.* **306:**392–397.

Ramsay, N. K. C., Kim, T. H., McGlave, P., Goldman, A., Nesbit, M. E., Jr., Krivit, W., Woods, W. G., Kersey, J. H., 1983, Total lymphoid irradiation and cyclophosphamide prior to bone marrow transplantation for patients with severe aplastic anemia, *Blood* **62:**622–626.

Ringden, O., Lonnqvist, B., Lundgren, G., Gahrton, G., Groth, C. G., Moller, E., Baryd, I., Johansson, B., Pihlstedt, P., and Gullbring, B., 1982, Experience with a cooperative bone marrow transplantation program in Stockholm, *Transplantation* **33:**500–504.

Rodt, H., Thierfelder, S., and Eulitz, M., 1974, Anti-lymphocyte antibodies and marrow transplantation. III. Effect of heterologous anti-brain antibodies on acute, secondary disease in mice, *Eur. J. Immunol.* **4:**25–29.

Rodt, H., Kolb, H. J., Netzel, B., Haas, R. J., Wilms, K., Gotze, Ch. B., Link, H., and Thierfelder, S., and the Munich Cooperative Group of Bone Marrow Transplantation, 1981, Effect of anti-T-cell globulin on GVHD in leukemic patients treated with BMT, *Transplant. Proc.* **13:**257–261.

Santos, G. W. [for the Johns Hopkins Marrow Transplantation Program], 1983, Allogeneic and syngeneic marrow transplantation for acute lymphocytic leukemia (ALL) in remission, *Blood* **62:**229a (abstract).

Santos, G. W., and Kaizer, H. [for the Johns Hopkins University Bone Marrow Transplantation Team], 1981, Current status of autologous marrow transplantation, in: *Cancer: Achievements, Challenges, and Prospects for the 1980s* (J. H. Burchenal and H. F. Oettgen, eds.), Grune and Stratton, New York, pp. 673–682.

Santos, G. W., and Kaizer, H., 1982, Bone marrow transplantation in acute leukemia, *Semin. Hematol.* **19:**227–239.

Santos, G. W., Sensenbrenner, L. L., Burke, P. J., Mullins, G. M., Bias, W. B., Tutschka, P. J., and Slavin, R. E., 1972, The use of cyclophosphamide for clinical marrow transplantation, *Transplant Proc.* **4:**559–564.

Santos, G. W., Tutschka, P.J., Brookmeyer, R., Saral, R., Beschorner, W. E., Bias, W. B., Braine, H. G., Burns, W. H., Elfenbein, G. J., Kaizer, H., Mellits, D., Sensenbrenner, L. L., Stuart, R. K., and Yeager, A. M., 1983, Marrow transplantation for acute nonlymphocytic leukemia following busulfan and cyclophosphamide, *N. Engl. J. Med.* **309:**1347–1353.

Saurat, J. H., Didier-Jean, L., Gluckman, E., and Bussel, A., 1975, Graft-versus-host reaction and lichen planus-like eruption in man, *Br. J. Dermatol.* **92:**591–592.

Schubach, W. H., Hackman, R., Neiman, P. E., Miller, G., and Thomas, E. D., 1982, A monoclonal immunoblastic sarcoma in donor cells bearing Epstein–Barr virus genomes following allogeneic grafting for acute lymphoblastic leukemia, *Blood* **60:**180–187.

Sharkis, S. J., Santos, G. W., and Colvin, M., 1980, Elimination of acute myelogenous leukemic cells from marrow and tumor suspensions in the rat with 4-hydroperoxycyclophosphamide, *Blood* **55:**521–523.

Shulman, H. M., Sullivan, K. M., Weiden, P. L., McDonald, G. B., Striker, G. E., Sale, G. E., Hackman, R., Tsoi, M. S., Storb, R., and Thomas, E. D., 1980, Chronic graft-versus-host syndrome in man: A long-term clinicopathological study of 20 Seattle patients, *Am. J. Med.* **69:**204–217.

Storb, R., 1984, Pathophysiology and prevention of graft-versus-host disease, in: *Advances in Immunobiology* (J. McCullough, ed.), Liss, New York, pp. 337–366.

Storb, R., and Thomas, E. D., 1983, Allogeneic bone-marrow transplantation, *Immunol. Rev.* **71:**77–102.

Storb, R., and Thomas, E. D., 1984, Current state of marrow transplantation, in: *Contemporary Hematology/Oncology*, Volume 3, (R. Silber, A. S. Gordon, and J. Lobue, eds.), Plenum, New York, pp. 235–266.

Storb, R., Rudolph, R. H., Kolb, H. J., Graham, T. C., Mickelson, E., Erickson, V., Lerner, K. G.,

Kolb, H., and Thomas, E. D., 1973a, Marrow grafts between DL-A-matched canine littermates, *Transplantation* **15**:92–100.

Storb, R., Kolb, H. J., Graham, T. C., Kolb, H., Weiden, P. L., and Thomas, E. D., 1973b, Treatment of established graft-versus-host disease in dogs by antithymocyte serum or prednisone, *Blood* **42**:601–609.

Storb, R., Thomas, E. D., Buckner, C. D., Clift, R. A., Johnson, F. L., Fefer, A., Glucksberg, H., Giblett, E. R., Lerner, K. G., and Neiman, P., 1974a, Allogeneic marrow grafting for treatment of aplastic anemia, *Blood* **43**:157–180.

Storb, R., Gluckman, E., Thomas, E. D., Buckner, C. D., Clift, R. A., Fefer, A., Glucksberg, H., Graham, T. C., Johnson, F. L., Lerner, K. G., Neiman, P. E., and Ochs, H., 1974b, Treatment of established human graft-versus-host disease by antithymocyte globulin, *Blood* **44**:57–75.

Storb, R., Weiden, P. L., Schroeder, M.-L., Graham, T. C., Lerner, K. G., and Thomas E. D., 1976, Marrow grafts between canine littermates homozygous or heterozygous for lymphocyte-defined histocompatibility antigens, *Transplantation* **21**:299–306.

Storb, R., Prentice, R. L., Buckner, C. D., Clift, R. A., Appelbaum, F., Deeg, H. J., Doney, K., Hansen, J. A., Mason, M., Sanders, J. E., Singer, J., Sullivan, K. M., Witherspoon, R. P., and Thomas, E. D., 1983a, Graft-versus-host disease and survival in patients with aplastic anemia treated by marrow grafts from HLA-identical siblings: Beneficial effect of a protective environment, *N. Engl. J. Med.* **308**:302–307.

Storb, R., Prentice, R. L., Sullivan, K. M., Shulman, H. M., Deeg, H. J., Doney, K. C., Buckner, C. D., Clift, R. A., Witherspoon, R. P., Appelbaum, F. R., Sanders, J. E., Stewart, P. S., and Thomas, E. D., 1983b, Predictive factors in chronic graft-versus-host disease in patients with aplastic anemia treated by marrow transplantation from HLA-identical siblings, *Ann. Intern. Med.* **98**:461–466.

Storb, R., Sanders, J. E., Ramberg, R., Witherspoon, R. P., Sullivan, K. M., Stewart, P., Sale, G. E., Doney, K., Deeg, H. J., Clift, R. A., Buckner, C. D., Appelbaum, F. R., and Thomas, E. D., 1983c, Marrow transplantation for treatment of preleukemia, *Exp. Hematol.* **11** (Suppl. 14):133 (Abstract 242).

Storb, R., Deeg, H. J., Thomas, E. D., Buckner, C. D., Clift, R. A., Flournoy, N., Kennedy, M. S., Doney, K., Appelbaum, F. R., Sanders, J. E., Stewart, P., Shulman, H., Sullivan, K. M., and Witherspoon, R. P., 1984, Preliminary results of prospective randomized trials comparing methotrexate and cyclosporine for prophylaxis of graft-versus-host disease after HLA-identical marrow transplantation, *Transplant. Proc.* **15**:2620–2623.

Sullivan, K. M., Shulman, H. M., Storb, R., Weiden, P. L., Witherspoon, R. P., McDonald, G. B., Schubert, M M., Atkinson, K., and Thomas, E. D., 1981, Chronic graft-versus-host disease in 52 patients: Adverse natural course and successful treatment with combination immunosuppression, *Blood* **57**:267–276.

Sullivan, K. M., Storb, R., Witherspoon, R., Shulman, H., Deeg, H. J., Schubert, M., Doney, K., Appelbaum, F., Tsoi, M.-S., Sale, G., Sanders, J., McDonald, G., and Thomas, E. D., 1983, Biology and treatment of chronic graft-versus-host disease, in: *Recent Advances in Bone Marrow Transplantation* (R. P. Gale, ed.), Liss, New York, pp. 331–342.

Thierfelder, S., Rodt, H., and Netzel, B., 1977, Transplantation of syngeneic bone marrow incubated with leukocyte antibodies. I. Suppression of lymphatic leukemia of syngeneic donor mice, *Transplantation* **23**:459–463.

Thomas, E. D., and Storb, R., 1970, Technique for human marrow grafting, *Blood* **36**:507–515.

Thomas, E. D., Storb, R., Clift, R. A., Fefer, A., Johnson, F. L., Neiman, P. E., Lerner, K. G., Glucksberg, H., and Buckner, C. D., 1975, Bone-marrow transplantation, *N. Engl. J. Med.* **292**:832–843, 895–902.

Thomas, E. D., Buckner, C. D., Banaji, M., Clift, R. A., Fefer, A., Flournoy, N., Goodell, B. W., Hickman, R. O., Lerner, K. G., Neiman, P. E., Sale, G. E. Sanders, J. E., Singer, J., Stevens, M., Storb, R., and Weiden, P. L., 1977, One hundred patients with acute leukemia treated by chemotherapy, total body irradiation, and allogeneic marrow transplantation, *Blood* **49**:511–533.

Thomas, E. D., Buckner, C. D., Clift, R. A., Fefer, A., Johnson, F. L., Neiman, P. E., Sale, G. E., Sanders, J. E., Singer, J. W., Shulman, H., Storb, R., and Weiden, P. L., 1979a, Marrow transplantation for acute nonlymphoblastic leukemia in first remission, *N. Engl. J. Med.* **301**:597–599.

Thomas, E. D., Sanders, J. E., Flournoy, N., Johnson, F. L., Buckner, C. D., Clift, R. A., Fefer, A., Goodell, B. W., Storb, R., and Weiden, P. L., 1979b, Marrow transplantation for patients with acute lymphoblastic leukemia in remission, *Blood* **54**:468–476.

Thomas, E. D., Buckner, C. D., Sanders, J., Papayannopoulou, T., Borgna-Pignatti, C., De Stefano, P., Sullivan, K. M., Clift, R. A., and Storb, R., 1982a, Marrow transplantation for thalassemia, *Lancet* **2**:227–228.

Thomas, E. D., Clift, R. A., and Buckner, C. D. [for the Seattle Marrow Transplant Team], 1982b, Marrow transplantation for patients with acute nonlymphoblastic leukemia who achieve a first remission, *Cancer Treat. Rep.* **66**:1463–1466.

Thomas, E. D., Clift, R. A., Hersman, J., Sanders, J. E., Stewart, P., Buckner, C. D., Fefer, A., McGuffin, R., Smith, J. W., and Storb, R., 1982c, Marrow transplantation for acute nonlymphoblastic leukemia in first remission using fractionated or single-dose irradiation, *Int. J. Radiat. Oncol. Biol. Phys.* **8**:817–821.

Thomas, E. D., Clift, R. A., and Storb, R., 1984, Indications for marrow transplantation, in: *Annual Review of Medicine*, Volume 35 (W. P. Creger, ed.), Annual Reviews, Palo Alto, California, pp. 1–10.

Trigg, M. E., and Poplack, D. G., 1981, Successful transplantation in mice of leukemic bone marrow incubated with cytotoxic anti-leukemic antibodies, *Exp. Hematol.* **9** (Suppl. 9):96 (Abstract 161).

Tsoi, M. S., Storb, R., Dobbs, S., Medill, L., and Thomas, E. D., 1980, Cell-mediated immunity to non-HLA antigens of the host by donor lymphocytes in patients with chronic graft-*vs*-host disease, *J. Immunol.* **125**:2258–2262.

Tsoi, M. S., Storb, R., Dobbs, S., and Thomas, E. D., 1981, Specific suppressor cells in graft-host tolerance of HLA-identical marrow transplantation, *Nature* **292**:355–357.

The UCLA Bone Marrow Transplantation Group, 1977, Bone marrow transplantation with intensive combination chemotherapy/radiation therapy (SCARI) in acute leukemia, *Ann. Intern. Med.* **86**:155–161.

van Bekkum, D. W., and de Vries, M. J., 1967, *Radiation Chimeras*, Logos Press, London.

van Bekkum, D. W., and Knaan, S., 1977, Role of bacterial microflora in development of intestinal lesions from graft-versus-host disease, *J. Natl. Cancer Inst.* **58**:787–790.

Weiden, P. L, Doney, K., Storb, R., and Thomas, E. D., 1979a, Antihuman thymocyte globulin for prophylaxis of graft-versus-host disease: A randomized trial in patients with leukemia treated with HLA-identical sibling marrow grafts, *Transplantation* **27**:227–230.

Weiden, P. L., Flourney, N., Thomas, E. D., Prentice, R., Fefer, A., Buckner, C. D., and Storb, R., 1979b, Antileukemic effect of graft-versus-host disease in human recipients of allogeneic-marrow grafts, *N. Engl. J. Med.* **300**:1068–1073.

Weiden, P. L, Storb, R., Deeg, H. J., Graham, T. C., and Thomas E. D., 1979c, Prolonged disease-free survival in dogs with lymphoma after total-body irradiation and autologous marrow transplantation consolidation of combination-chemotherapy-induced remissions, *Blood* **54**:1039–1049.

Weiden, P. L., Sullivan, K. M., Flournoy, N., Storb, R., Thomas, E. D., and the Seattle Marrow Transplant Team, 1981, Antileukemic effect of chronic graft-versus-host disease: Contribution to improved survival after allogeneic marrow transplantation, *N. Eng. J. Med.* **304**:1529–1533.

Witherspoon, R. P., Storb, R., Ochs, H. D., Flournoy, N., Kopecky, K. J., Sullivan, K. M., Deeg, H. J., Sosa, R., Noel, D. R., Atkinson, K., and Thomas, E. D., 1981, Recovery of antibody production in human allogeneic marrow graft recipients: Influence of time posttransplantation, the presence or absence of chronic graft-versus-host disease, and antithymocyte globulin treatment, *Blood* **58**:360–368.

Witherspoon, R. P., Kopecky, K., Storb, R. F., Flournoy, N., Sullivan K. M., Sosa, R., Deeg, H. J., Ochs, H. D., Cheever, M. A., Fefer, A., and Thomas, E. D., 1982, Immunological recovery in 48 patients following syngeneic marrow transplantation for hematological malignancy, *Transplantation* **33**:143–149.

Witherspoon, R. P., Hersman, J., Storb, R., Ochs, H., Goldstein, A. L., McClure, J., Noel, D., Weiden, P. L., and Thomas, E. D., 1983, Thymosin fraction 5 does not accelerate reconstitution of immunologic reactivity after human marrow grafting, *Br. J. Haematol.* **55:**595–608.
Witherspoon, R. P., Lum, L. G., and Storb, R., 1984, Immunologic reconstitution after human marrow grafting, *Semin. Hematol.* **21:**2–10.
Zander, A. R., Spitzer, G. Vellekoop, L., Verma, D., Minnhaar, G., and Dicke, K. A., 1981, New developments in bone marrow transplantation, *Cancer Bull.* **33:**286–295.

INDEX